English-Spanish Medical Dictionary and Phrase Book

Spanish-English

first edition 2013

ISBN is 1481830244
EAN-13 is 978-1481830249

by A.H. Zemback

Contents

	english	spanish
Introduction	How are you?	¿Cómo está?
	Good morning, good afternoon, good evening.	Buenos días, buenas tardes, buenas noches.
	My name is ...	Me llamo...
demographics	What is your name?	¿Cómo se llama usted?
	Pleased to meet you.	Mucho gusto.
	Do you speak English?	¿Habla usted inglés?
	Speak more slowly, please.	Hable más despacio, por favor.
	Repeat, please.	Favor de repetir.
	Come in, please.	Adelante, por favor.
	Sit down, please.	Siéntese, por favor.
	What province do you live in ?	¿En que provincia vive?
	What is your address?	¿Cuál es su dirección?
	What is your telephone number?	¿Su número de teléfono?
	Are you married?	¿Está casado (male)? ¿Está casada (female)?
	What is your age?	¿Cuántos años tiene?
Chief complaint	What is your health concern? (What can we do for you today?)	¿Cual es su problema médico? (¿Qué podemos hacer para usted hoy?)
	When did this problem start?	¿Cuándo comenzó este problema?
	Are you in pain now?	¿Tiene dolor ahora?
	Is the pain severe?	¿Está muy fuerte el dolor?
	Sharp or dull?	¿Agudo o débil?
	Touch the spot with one finger.	Muestrame el lugar donde tiene dolor con un dedo.
	What makes it better?	¿Qué alivia el dolor?
	What makes it worse?	¿Qué empeora el dolor?
	When do you get the pain...	¿Cuándo le da el dolor...
	At night? Before meals? After meals?	En la noche? Antes de comer? Después de comer?
	Have you been in the hospital before?	¿Ha estado hospitalizado alguna vez?
	What were you treated for?	¿De que lo antendieron?
Common complaints	My lower back hurts.	Me duele la parte inferior de la espalda.
	The pain goes down this leg.	El dolor baja por esta pierna.
	My neck is stiff.	Mi cuello está tieso.
	I have pain in my shoulder.	Yo tengo dolor en el hombro.
	This arm hurts.	Este brazo me duele.
	This wrist hurts.	Me duele la muñeca.
	I have pain in this knee.	Yo tengo dolor en esta rodilla.

	english	spanish
	It hurts to move my elbow.	Me duele mover el codo.
	I am dizzy.	Estoy mareado (a).
	I have chest pain.	Tengo dolor en el pecho.
	I have headaches.	Tengo dolores de cabeza.
	I have trouble breathing.	Tengo falta de respiración.
	I am pregnant.	Estoy embarazada.
	I am nauseated.	Siento náuseas.
	I am weak.	Estoy débil.
Past medical history	Are you being treated for any chronic health problem?	¿Está siendo tratamiento para algún otro crónico problema médico?
	Do you have a history of...	¿Tiene un pasado medico de...
	anemia	anemia
	asthma	asma
	cancer	cáncer
	cirrhosis	cirrosis
	diabetes	diabetes
	epilepsy	epilepsia o convulsiones
	hypertension	hipertension/ la presión alta
	thyroid disease	enfermedad de la tiroides
	heart problems	enfermedad de corazón
	hepatitis	hepatitis
	tuberculosis	tuberculosis
	HIV/AIDS	SIDA
	What date did you start taking HIV medicine?	¿Cuándo comenzó a tomar las medicina para la SIDA?
	What was the date of your last CD4?	¿Cuándo fue de su última examen de CD4?
	What was the result of your last CD4?	¿Cuál fue el resultado de su último examen de CD4?
	Have you had pneumonia or meningitis?	¿Ha tenido neumonía o menigitis? (Una infección de los pulmones o del cerebro).
Past surgical history	Have you had surgery in the past?	¿Ha tenido cirugía en el pasado?
	What type of surgery was done?	¿Cuáles son los tipos de cirugía que ha tenido?
	What year was the surgery done?	¿En qué año fue la cirugía?
Medications	Do you take medication at home?	¿Tomas algún medicamento en casa?
	What is the name of the medication?	¿Cómo se llama el mdicamento?
	Can you show me the medication bottle?	¿Me puede mostrar el recipiente (la botella) del medicamento?
	Have you taken illegal drugs?	¿Has tomado drogas (ilegales) recientemente?

5

	english	spanish
	Are you taking bactrim?	¿Está tomando Bactrim?
Allergies	Have you had reactions to medications?	¿Tiene alergias a algunas medicinas?
Family history	Is your mother living?	¿Su madre todavia vive?
	Is your father living?	¿Su padre todavia vive?
	Do your brothers/sisters have health problems?	¿Tiene hermanos o hermanas con problemas de salud?
Social history	Do you drink alcohol?	¿Tóma alcohol o cerveza?
	How many drinks per day?	¿Cuántos vasos de alcohol tomas por dia?
	Do you drink alcohol every day?	¿Tóma alcohol diariamente?
	Do you smoke?	¿Fuma cigarrillos?
Review of systems	Do you have skin problems?	¿Tiene problemas de la piel?
Skin	Do you have any blisters or sores?	¿Teine algunas apollas o llagas?
Lymphatic	Do you have lymph node enlargement or pain?	¿Tiene hinchazon o dolor en los ganglios linfaticos?
Bone	Do you have bone pain?	¿Tiene dolor en los huesos?
	Do you have joint pain?	¿Tiene dolor en las articulaciones o conjuturas?
	Do you have joint swelling?	¿Tiene inflamación de las articulaciones o conjuturas?
	Do you have pain in the back or neck?	¿Tiene dolor en la espalda o en el cuello?
Blood	Do you have bleeding problems?	¿Tiene problemas de sangrados?
Endocrine	Do you urinate frequently?	¿Orina con mucha frecuencia?
	Are you frequently thirsty?	¿Tiene sed frecuentemente?
	Has your weight decreased?	¿Ha perdido peso?
Head	Have you suffered from a head trauma in the past?	¿Ha tenido algún trauma de la cabeza en el pasado?
	Do you have vertigo, syncope?	¿Te sientes mareado? ¿Te has desmayado?
Eyes	Do you have vision loss?	¿Tiene perdida de visión?
	Do you have double vision?	¿Tiene doble visión or vez doble?
	Do you have blurred vision?	¿Vez borroso?
	Do you have pain in bright light?	¿Sufres de dolor en los ojos con luz brillante?
Ears	Have you had a hearing problem recently?	¿Has tenido algun problema con los oidos?
	Do you have drainage from the ears?	¿Tiene secreciones de los oidos?
	Have you had gradual hearing loss in only one ear?	¿Está usted perdiendo gradualmente la audición solamente en un oído?
Nose	Do you have frequent nosebleeds?	¿Sangra frecuentemente su nariz?

6

	english	spanish
Mouth	Do you have a toothache?	¿Tiene dolor de los dientes?
	Do you have pain in just one tooth?	¿Tiene usted dolor que afecta a un sólo diente?
	Do you have a chipped or broken tooth or one that is loose in the socket?	¿Se ha roto o desportillado un diente, o tiene el diente flojo dentro del alvéolo (la cavidad donde está insertado ese diente) dental?
	Do you have pain in a tooth when you eat or drink cold food or liquids?	¿Siente dolor cuando come o toma alimentos o líquidos fríos?
	Do you have lumps or swelling in your mouth?	¿Tiene alguna protuberancia o hinchazón en la boca?
Throat	Do you have hoarseness? (Have you had a change in your voice?)	¿Has tenido la voz ronca? (¿Has tenido un cambio en la voz?)
	Do you have a sore throat?	¿Tiene dolor de lagarganta?
Neck	Do you have neck stiffness?	¿Siente rígido el cuello? (¿Tiene dolor en le cuello?)
Breast	Have you noticed breast lumps?	¿Haz notado alguna bolita en sus senos?
	Do you have nipple discharge?	¿Tiene secreciones de los pezones?
	Do you have swelling around or below your nipples?	¿Tiene usted hinchazón debajo o alrededor, o debajo y alrededor de uno o de ambos pezones?
Respiratory	Do you have difficulty breathing?	¿Tiene usted sensación de falta de aire?
	Do you sit up at night to breathe?	¿Tiene que sentarte para respirar en la noche cuando duermes?
	Do you have pain when you take a deep breath?	¿Tiene dolor cuando respiras profondamente?
	Do you have wheezing?	¿Tiene respiración sibilante?
	Do you have a cough?	¿Tiene usted una tos?
	How long have you had the cough?	¿Por cuanto tiempo has tiendo la tos?
	Do you have a lot of sputum?	¿Tiene muchas flemas?
	Have you recently started spitting up blood or bloody sputum?	¿Hace poco que usted comenzó a toser sangre o a tener flemas con sangre?
	What color is your sputum?	¿De que color es la flema?
	Have you had tuberculosis?	¿Has tenido tuberculosis?
Cardiovascular	Do you have chest pain?	¿Tiene dolor en el pecho?
	Do you have palpitations?	¿Tiene palpitaciónes?
	Do you have leg edema?	¿Has tenido hinchazon en la peirnas?
	Have you been weak?	¿Se has sentido debil?
Gastrointestinal	Do you have abdominal pain? (Do you have pain in your belly?)	¿Tiene dolor de pansa?

7

english	spanish
...after you eat, with certain foods?	...después de comer? ...con algunas comidas en particular?
When did this problem start?	¿Cuándo comenzo este problema?
Has it been weeks, months, years?	¿Ha sido por semanas, meses, años?
Are you in pain now?	¿Siente dolor ahora?
Touch the spot.	Enséñame dónde le duele.
Is the pain better than yesterday?	¿El dolor esta mejor que ayer?
Do you have ...fever?	¿Tiene...fiebre?
...night sweats?	...sudor en la noche?
...chills?	...escalofrios?
How is your appetite?	¿Cómo está su apetito?
Have you vomited?	¿Haz vomitado?
Are you nauseated? (past tense)	¿Siente nauseas? (¿Haz sentido nauseas?)
Did you have a stool today?	¿Haz hecho popó noy? (excremento = formal term; popó is common term)
When was your last stool?	¿Cuándo fue la ultima rez que defecaste or hisiste popó?
Do you have constipation?	¿Sufre de estrieñimento?
Do you have diarrhea?	¿Tiene diarrea?
How many times have you had diarrhea today?	¿Cuántas veces ha tenido diarrea hoy?
Is your stool black?	¿Est negro su excremento o su popó?
Is your stool bloody?	¿Tiene sangre su excremento?
Have you recently traveled outside the country?	¿Ha viajado recientemente a otro país?
What color was the stool?	¿Qué color era el excremento?
Do you have itching around the anus even when you are not having a bowel movement?	¿Tiene comezón (picor) alrededor del recto incluso cuando no está teniendo una evacuación intestinal (defecando haciendo popó)?
Do you have pain with swallowing?	¿Tiene dolor cuándo traga?
Do you have difficulty swallowing?	¿Tiene dificuldad al tragar?
Do you have burning pain in the stomach?	¿Siente que te quema algo en el estómago?
Have you had a gastroscopy in the past? (A camera that passes through your mouth to see your stomach)	¿Ha tenido una gastroscopía en el pasado? (Una camara que pasa por su boca para ver su estómago.)
Genitourinary Do you have burning on urination?	¿Tiene dolor o sensación de ardor al orinar?
Have you had penile discharge?	¿Le sale una secreción de la punta del pene?
Do you have sores on the penis?	¿Tiene úlceras en la pene?
Is your urine cloudy?	¿La orina suya es túrbida?

english	spanish
Do you have sharp pains in your back or groin?	¿Tiene dolores intensos y agudos como en puñalada en la espalda o en la ingle?
Do you have an aching pain under your scrotum?	¿Tiene un dolor debajo del escroto?
Do you have difficulty starting to urinate?	¿Tiene dificultad para comenzar a orinar?
How often do you void at night?	¿Cuántas veces tiene que ir al baño durante de la noche?
Do you have the urge to void after just urinating and are you urinating only small amounts?	¿Siente usted necesidad de orinar justo después de haber ido al baño, y está usted orinando tan sólo pequeñas cantidades a la vez?
Is the urine stream slow?	¿Está despacio el flujo de su orina?
Do you leak urine when you cough or sneeze?	¿Que deja escapar gotitas de orina cuando tose o estornuda?
Do you have blood in the urine?	¿Tiene sangre en la orina?
Have you ever passed a kidney stone?	¿Ha expulsado piedras de los riñones?

Women's health

english	spanish
Are you pregnant?	¿Está embarazada?
Are your periods regular?	¿Es normal su menstruación?
Are your periods painful?	¿Su ciclos menstruales se han vuelto dolorosos?
Do you have heavy periods?	¿Tiene mucho sangrado con sus menstruaciones?
When did your last period start?	¿Cuándo comenzó su última menstruación?
How long do your periods last?	¿Cuántos días le dura su menstruación?
Do you have vaginal itching?	¿Le pica lavagina?
Do you vaginal pain?	¿Tiene dolor en su vagina?
Do you have unusual discharge from the vagina?	¿Tiene secreciones anormales de su vagina?
...a lot or a little?	...muchas secreciones o pocas?
How many times have you been pregnant?	¿Cuántas veces ha estado embarazada?
How many children do you have?	¿Cuántos hijos tiene?
Do you know your blood type?	¿Sabe su tipo de sangre?
What is it?	¿Cuál es?
Are you in labor?	¿Está dando luz?
When did your labor start?	¿Cuándo empezó su parto?

Peripartum/ neonatal

english	spanish
Is this your first baby?	¿Es este su primer hijo?
Do you feel the baby move?	¿Siente que se mueve su bebe?

english	spanish
When did your water break?	¿Cuándo se rompío su fuente de agua?
Were you ill before the delivery or during the pregnancy?	¿Estaba enferma antes del parto o durante del embarazado?)
What was the baby's birth weight?	¿Cuánto fue el peso de su bebe al nacer?
Is the baby nursing well?	¿Está amamantando bien su bebe?
Has the baby had any convulsions?	¿Ha tenido convulsiones su bebe?
Apgar at 1 minute.	¿Cuánto eran los apgar en un minuto?
Apgar at 5 minutes.	a cinco minutos?
Moro reflex.	Reflejo del abrazo.
Fontanelle.	Fontanela

Amniotic fluid

english	spanish
clear fluid	fluido cloro
colored fluid (What color was the amniotic fluid?)	¿De que color era la fuente?
meconium stained	¿De color verde?

Pediatrics

english	spanish
Is he (she) drinking ok?	¿Está tomando líquidos bien?
Is he (she) eating ok?	¿Está comiendo bien?
Have you seen worms in the vomit or the stool?	¿Ha visto gusanos en el vomito o en el excremento?

Neurologic

english	spanish
Do you have: facial weakness?	¿Tiene...debilidad de la cara?
facial numbness?	durmencimiento la cara?
leg weakness?	debilidad en las piernas?
leg numbness?	durmencimiento de las piernas?
arm weakness?	debilidad de los brazos?
arm numbness?	durmencimiento de los brazos?
Have you ever been unconscious?	¿Ha perdido en conocimiento en el pasado?
Have you had tremors? (Do your hands shake or other parts of your body?)	¿Ha tenido tremores? ¿Le tiemblan las manos o otros partes de su cuerpo?)
Have you had recent vision loss in one eye?	¿Ha perdido recientemente la visión en un ojo?
Have you had problems with your balance?	¿Ha tenido problemas con su equilibrio?
Do you walk without problems?	¿Camina sin dificultad?
Do you have pain in your back that travels to your buttock and down the back of your leg?	¿Tiene dolor en la parte posterior de su cadera que comienza en la parte baja de la espalda y que se extiende hacia las nalgas o hacia la pierna?

Psychiatric

english	spanish
Do you have anxiety?	¿Sientes anciedad?
Do you have depression?	¿Sufre de depresión?

	english	spanish
Extremities	Is the ankle pain so severe you cannot walk on it?	¿El dolor es tan intenso que usted es incapaz de caminar apoyando el tobillo?
	Do your have a grinding pain in your knee? Do you have the knee lock up occasionally?	¿Usted todavía tiene una sensación de desgaste en la articulación o el conjunto? ¿Alguna vez se le traba la rodilla incluso después de que ya está mejor?
	Do you have pain in your calf when walking that is better with rest?	¿Le duelen las pantorrillas después de caminar y se alivia usted del dolor con el descanso?
	Do you feel pain when you move your shoulder?	¿Siente dolor al mover el hombro?
	Do you have pain or numbness in your hand, wrist or fingers, especially when flexing your wrist?	¿Tiene durmencimiento o dolor en los dedos, mano, muñeca o brazo, especialmente cuando flexiona la muñeca?
	Do you have pain when gripping a doorknob and does the pain go from the outside of the elbow to your wrist?	¿Le cuesta trabajo agarrar la manija (perilla) de la puerta, y le comienza el dolor en la parte externa de su codo y el dolor se extiende a lo largo de su brazo hasta la muñeca?
Physical exam	appearance, height	apariencia, estatura
General	pulse bp resp temp weight (in pounds/ kilograms)	pulso, presión arterial, respiración temperatura, peso (en libras/ kilogramos)
	skin	piel
HEENT	visual acuity	agudez visual
	conjunctiva, sclera	conjunctiva, esclerotica
	pupils	pupilas
	optic disc	disco optico
	ear canal, tympanic membrane	canal auditivo externo, timpano
	nasal mucosa	mucosa nasal
	sinuses	senos
	teeth	dientes
	mouth, gums, dental, uvula "open your mouth"	boca, encias, dientes, uvula "abre la boca"
	"Stick out your tongue."	"Saca la lengua."
	"Say ahh."	"Dí ahhh."
Pulmonary	auscultation "Breathe deep."	"Respira profundamente."
	percussion	percusión
Back	"Lie down on your back, please."	"Recuéstese en la espalda, por favor."
	"Lie on your left side."	"Acuestase en su lado izquirdo."
	"Lie on your right side."	"Acuestase en su lado derecho."
	tenderness "Does it hurt here?"	sensibilidad"¿Tiene el dolor aquí?"

	english	spanish
	cva tenderness	ángulo costovertbral
Cardiovascular	heart rate, rhythm "Breathe normally."	ritmo cardiaco, "Respira normalmente."
	heart murmur?	¿soplo en el corazon?
	carotid "Hold your breath."	carótida "Manten su respiración."
	jugular venous distention	distensión pulso yugular
Breasts	nipple discharge	secreciones de sus pesones
	tenderness "Does it hurt here?"	¿Tiene el dolor aquí?"
	mass	masas o bolitas
Vascular	carotid, radial, aortic pulsation	carótida, radial, aórtico pulsación
	femoral, dorsalis pedis, posterior tibial	femoral, dorsal del pie, posterior tibial
	leg edema	hinchazon de las pierras
Abdomen	"Lie down."	"Acuéstase."
	"Does it hurt here?"	¿Tiene el dolor aquí?"
	umbilicus	ombligo
	hernia, inguinal	hernia, ingle
	palpation	palpación
	auscultation	auscultación
	fluid wave, superficial abdominal veins?	ondo de fluido, vena superficial abdominal
Maternal/gyn	uterine height (cm)	altura del utero
	Fetal heart rate	pulso fetal
	urine sample	una muestra de orina
	presentation	presentación
	head presentation	presentación cefálica
	breech presentation	presentación de nalgas
	transverse presentation	presentación transversa
	speculum exam	examen con el espéculo
	vaginal exam	examen vaginal
	gestational age	tiempo de gestación
	amniotic fluid	fluido amniotico
Genitourinary; male	circumcised?	¿circoncisión?
	genital herpes?	¿herpes genitales?
	testicles	testículos
Rectal exam	hemorrhoids, nodules, prostate?	hemorroides, nódulo, próstata
	"I want to check your rectum (for hemorrhoids), bend over please."	"Quiero revisar su recto para alas hemorroides. Inclinarse, por favor."
	guaiac; positive or negative	positivo, negativo
Neurologic	N1 olfactory: coffee, peppermint?	N1 olfatorio: cafe, menta?

	english	spanish
Cranial nerves	N2 optic: snellen, confrontation "Follow my finger with your eyes, without moving your head."	N2 óptico:"Siga mi dedo con sus ojos sin mover la cabeza."
	N3,4, 6, oculomotor, trochlear, abducens: EOM's "Follow my finger"	N3,4,6 motor ocular común, patético, abducente: "Siga mi dedo con sus ojos sin mover la cabeza."
	N5 trigeminal	N5 trigémino
	"Clench your jaw."	"Presiona su mandíbula o quijada."
	"Move your jaw back and forth."	"Mueve su mandíbula lateralmente."
	forehead (ophthalmic), cheek(maxillary), chin (mandibular) "Do you feel this?"	frente (oftálmico), mejilla (maxilar), mentón (mandibular) "¿Siente eso?"
	N7 facial: "Raise your eye brows." ("Do like this.")	N7 facial "Levante sus cejas." ("Haz le asi.")
	"Close your eyes tightly, smile big."	"Cierra sus ojos, sonries."
	N8 acoustic: whisper, Rinne	N8 auditivo: susurro, Rinne
	"Can you hear this?"	"¿Escucha esto?"
	"Tell me when you can't feel vibration"	"Díme cuando no puede sentir la vibración."
	N9 glossopharyngeal: swallow, (hoarseness), "Swallow now."	N9 glosofaríngeo: trago (ronquera), "Traga ahora."
	N10 vagus: swallow, soft palate, gag reflex	N10 neumogástrico: trago, paladar blando, reflejo nauseoso
	"Stick out your tongue."	"Saca la lengua."
	N11 spinal acessory nerve: "Turn your head, shrug your shoulders."	N11 espinal :"Voltea su cabeza y levanta sus hombros."
	N12 hypoglossal: tongue midline	N12 hipoglosal: lengua saliente línea media del boca.
Glasgow coma score	opens eyes to: spontaneous (4),to speech (3), to pain (2), none (1)	Apertura ocular: espontánea (4), respuesta a la voz (3), respuesta al dolor (2), sin respuesta (1)
	best motor "Hold up 2 fingers." obeys commands (6), localizes (5), withdraws (4), abnormal flexion (3), abnormal extension (2), none (1)	Respuesta motora: "Enséñame dos dedos." obedece (6), localiza (5), flexiona (4), flexión anormal (3), extensión anormal (2), sin respuesta (1)
	best verbal: clear (5), confused (4), inappropriate (3), garbled (2), none (1)	respuesta verbal: oriented (5), desorientada (4), palabras inusuales (3), sonidos incomprensibles (2), sin repuesta (1)
Motor	Motor function	Función motor
	biceps brachii, elbow flexion	bíceps braquial, flexión codo
	"Pull your arm up."	"Jale su brazo."
	wrist extensors	extensor carpo
	"Bend your wrist up."	"Doble su muñeca arriba."
	triceps brachii, elbow extension	tricéps braquial, extensión codo

english	spanish
"Straighten your arm out."	"Estira su brazo."
finger flexors, distal phalanx middle finger	flexor digitorum profundus
"Bend the tip of this finger."	"Doble la punta de este dedo."
finger abduction, little finger	abductor digiti minimi manus
"Hold the small finger tightly" (don't let me squeeze your fingers.)	"Mantenga su dedo chiquito firmamente" (no me puede apretar sus dedos).
iliopsoas, hip flexors	iliopsoas
"Move your knee to your chest."	"Mueve su rodilla hasta su pecho."
quadriceps, knee extensors	quadriceps femoris
"Straighten your leg out."	"Estira su pierna."
tibialis anterior, ankle dorsiflexors	tibialis anterior
"Pull your foot up." (point your foot up)	"Tira su pie arriba." (apunta su pie arriba)
extensor hallucis longus, long toe extension	extensor hallucis longus
"Raise your toe up."	"Eleva el dedo de su pie arriba."
gastrocnemius, ankle plantar flexors	gastrocnemius
"Push your foot down."	"Empuja su pie abajo."

Sensory

english	spanish
Sensation "Say 'yes' if you can feel this"	"Di 'si' si puede sentir esto?"
C-4 (top of acromioclavicular joint)	C-4 (encima de la articulación acromioclavicular)
C-5 (lateral side of antecubital fossa)	C-5 (aspecto lateral de fosa antecubital)
C-6 (thumb)	C-6 (aspecto dorsal, falange proximal del pulgar)
C-7 (middle finger)	C-7 (aspecto dorsal, falange proximal del dedo medio)
C-8 (little finger)	C-8 (aspecto dorsal, falange proximal del dedo meñique)
T-4 (nipple line)	Th-4 (línea del pezón)
T-10 (umbilicus)	Th-10 (ombligo en línea clavicular medio)
L-2 (mid-anterior thigh)	L-2 (muslo anteromedial)
L-3 (medial femoral condyle)	L-3 (cóndilo medial de fémur)
L-4 (medial malleolus)	L-4 (maléolo medial)
L-5 (dorsum of the foot, at third MTP joint)	L-5 (aspect dorsal de pie en articulación metatarsofalángico trecer)
S-1 (Lateral heel)	S-1 (aspecto lateral del talón)
S-2 (popliteal fossa of the knee, in the midline)	S-2 (fosa poplítea)

	english	spanish
	S-3 (ischial tuberosity)	S-3 (tuberosidad isquiática)
	S4-5 (perianal area)	S4-5 (area perianal)
reflex	Reflexes	Reflejo
	triceps right and left	tríceps, derecho y izquierdo
	biceps, right and left	bíceps, derecho y izquierdo
	brachialradial, right and left	braquiorradial, derecho y izquierdo
	patella, right and left	rotuliano, derecho y izquierdo
	ankle, right and left	tobillo, derecho y izquierdo
	Babinski, right and left (great toe extension= positive)	Babinski, derecho y izquierdo
screen	Tandem walk	Marcha tándem
	"Walk like this, one foot in front of other." (Or, say walk like this and demonstrate.)	"Camina asi, con un pie en frente del otro."
	heel walk, toe walk	marcha talón, caminar de puntillas
	"Walk on your heels."	"Camina en sus tacones."
	"Walk on your toes."	"Camina en los dedos de sus pies."
	Romberg "Stand up, hold your arms out, close your eyes."	Romberg "Levantate, estira tus brazos, cierra los ojos."
Coordination	rapid alternating movement (2nd finger, thumb) "Do this, fast".	"Haz esto, rápido."
	heel-shin "Move your right heel from your left knee to the ankle with your eyes shut."	talón-espinilla "Mueve su talón derecho desde su rodilla izquierda hasta su tobillo con los ojos cerrados."
	finger nose finger "Touch my finger with your finger then touch your nose."	dedo-con-dedo "Toca mi dedo con tu dedo, depués toca su nariz."
Discriminative	stereognosis (key, pencil, cup) "Close your eyes; what is this in your hand?"	estereognosis "Cierra los ojos. ¿Qué es esto en su mano?"
	graphesthesia (draw #3 in hand) "Close your eyes, what is the number written in your hand?"	grafestesia "Cierra los ojos. ¿Qué numero está escrito en su mano?"
	point localization: "Close your eyes, tell me what part of your body is being touched."	"Cierra los ojos. ¿Qué parte de su cuerpo estoy tocando?"
	two point discrimination "Do you feel one or two points of contact?"	"¿Siente uno o dos?"
Memory	SLUMS Examination	SLUMS Examination
	Saint Louis University Mental Status Examination	Saint Louis University Mental Status Examination
SLUMS	What day of the week is it? (1)	¿Qué día de la semana es hoy?
SLUMS	What is the year? (1)	¿En qué año estamos?
SLUMS	What state are we in? (1)	¿En qué estado estamos?

	english	spanish
SLUMS	Please remember these five objects. I will ask you what they are later. Apple Pen Tie House Car	Por favor, recuerde los cinco objetos que le voy a nombrar. Mas tarde, le preguntaré nuevament por ellos. Manzana Lapiz Corbata Perro Casa
SLUMS	You have $100 and you go to the store and buy a dozen apples for $3 and a tricycle for $20. How much did you spend? (1) How much do you have left? (2)	Usted tiene ciento dolares, y en la tienda compra una docena de manzanas por tres dolares y una bicicleta por veinte dolares. Cuánto dinero gastó? Cuánto dinero le queda?
SLUMS	Please name as many animals as you can in one minute. (0) 0-4 animals, (1) 5-9 animals, (2) 10-14 animals, (3) 15+ animals	Por favor en un minuto nombre todos los animales que pueda.
SLUMS	What were the five objects I asked you to remember? Apple Pen Tie House Car. One point for each correct answer.	Cuáles fueron los 5 objectos que le dije que recordara? Manzana Lapiz Corbata Perro Casa.
SLUMS	I am going to give you a series of numbers and I would like yoiu to give them to me backwards. For example, if I say 42, you say 24. (0) 87, (1) 649, (2) 8537	Voy a decirle una serie de números. Me gustaría que usted me los dijera al revés. Por ejemplo, si yo digo 42, usted debe decir 24. (0) ocho siete, (1) seis cuatro nueve, (2) ocho cinco tres siete
SLUMS	This is a clock face. Please put in the hour markers and the time at ten minutes to elevel o'clock. (2) Hour markers correct? (2) Time correct?	Este círculo representa un reloj. Por favor escriba los números de las horas y las manecillas señalando las once menos diez.
SLUMS	Place an X in the triangle. □△◇, (1) Which of the figures is the largest? (1)	Por favor, señale el triángulo con una equis. Cuál de estas figuras es la mas grande?
SLUMS	I am going to read you a story. Please listen carefully because afterwards, I'm going to ask you some questions about it. Jill was a very successful stockbroker. She made a lot of money on the stock market. She then met Jack, a devastatingly handsome man. She married him and had three children. They lived in Chicago. She then stopped work and stayed at home to bring up her children. When they were teenagers, she went back to work. She and Jack lived happily ever after.	Voy a contarle una historia. Por favor, escuche cuidadosament, porque al terminar le voy a hacer unas preguntas sobre esta historia. María era una abogada muy exitosa y ganaba mucho dinero en la compañía donde trabajaba. Ella conoció a Carlos, un hombre muy apuesto, y, al cabo del tiempo, se casaron, tuvieron tres hijos y vivían en Chicago. Ella dejo de trabajar para criar a sus hijos y cuando estos fueron adolescentes ella volvió al trabajo. Ella y Carlos vivieron felices por siempre.
SLUMS	What was the female's name? (2)	Cuál era el nombre de la mujer?
SLUMS	What work did she do? (2)	Que profesión tenía ella?
SLUMS	When did she go back to work? (2)	Cuando volvió a trabaja?

	english	spanish
SLUMS	What state did she live in? (2)	En que estado vivía?
SLUMS	Add total score, with high school education: 27-30 normal, 21-26 mild cognitive disorder, 1-20 dementia. Without high school education: 25-30 normal, 20-24 mild cognitive disorder, 1-19 dementia.	escuela secundaria: 27-30 normal, 21-26 deterio cognición un poco, 1-20 demencia. Sin escuela secundaria: 25-30 normal, 20-24 deterio cognición un poco, 1-19 demencia.
Counseling	You need to go for an x ray.	Necesita una radiografia.
	Do you understand?	¿Entiende usted?
Pulmonary	I have the result of your sputum.	Tengo el resultado de su muestra de flema.
	You have...	Tiene...
	tuberculosis	tuberculosis
	pneumonia	neumonia
	Your lungs are...	Sus pulmones son...
	one is affected, the other is healthy.	un pulmon está enfermo, el otro esta sano.
	Your illness can be healed.	Su enfermedad se puede curar.
Gastroenterology	There is an ulcer in your stomach.	Tiene una ulcera en su estómago.
	You need to quit drinking beer completely.	Tiene que dejar de tomar cerveza completamente.
Surgery	You need to have an operation today.	Necesita una cirugia/operación hoy.
	We need to sew up (suture) this wound.	Necesitamos cerrar esa herida con suturas.
	When did you last eat and drink?	¿Cuándo fue la ultima vez que injeriste alimentos o liquidos?
	You need to rest at the hospital a few days.	Necesita descansar en el hospital por unos días.
Pharmacy	You take this medicine two (one, three, four)times per day.	Toma este medicina dos (una, tres cuatro) veces por día.
	Do not stop this medication!	No suspendas esta medicina!
	Take this medication only if you want to.	Toma este medicina solo si quieres.
	Take this medication before eating.	Toma este medicamento antes de comer.
	Take this medication with food.	Toma este medicamento con alimentos.
	Take this medication after meals.	Toma este medicamento después de comidas.
Maternity	The nurse is on her way.	La enfermera está en camino/ahorita viene.
	She will help with the delivery.	Ella la ayudará en el parto.

17

	english	spanish
Laboratory/ imaging	I need a... 1) urine sample 2) stool sample 3) blood sample 4) sputum specimen.	Necesito una 1) muestra de orina 2) muestra de excremento 3) nuestra de sangre 4) muestra de flemas
Procedures	I need to put this tube in your nose.	Necesito poner este tubo en su naríz.
	I need to start an IV.	Necesito ponerle suero intravenoso.
	I need to give you a shot 1) in the arm 2) in the leg.	Necesito ponerle una injección 1) en el brazo 2) en la pierna.
General	The situation is grave.	La situación es grave.
	Treatment is not usually needed.	Por lo general no se requiere tratamiento.

English	Spanish
abasia *Inability to walk due to impaired coordination.*	abasia, movimiento incierto
abdomen *The portion of the body bordered by the diaphragm and the pelvis.*	abdomen, vintre
abdominal girth	circunferencia abdominal
abdominal reflex *Elicited by stroking the abdomen lightly from mid-axillary line to umbilicus. A normal response is contraction of the umbilicus toward the stimulated side.*	reflejo abdominal
abdominocentesis *Puncturing of the abdominal wall for drainage purposes.*	abdominocentesis, punción abdominal
abducens nerve *A motor nerve (6th cranial nerve) that controls the lateral rectus muscle of the eye.)*	nervio abducens
abducent *Abducting or to separate.*	abducente
abductor pollicis brevis *Abducts the thumb.*	músculo abductor corto del pulgar
abductor pollicis longus *Abducts and flexes the thumb.*	músculo abductor largo del pulgar
aberrant *Different than normal.*	aberrante Desviado del curso normal.
ablatio placentae *Abruption or detachment of the placentae.*	ablatio placentae
ablation *Surgical removal or amputation.*	ablación
abnormal	anormal
ABO system *The system using human blood antigens to determine blood type.*	determinación del grupo sanguíneo
abortion *Premature expulsion of the fetus from the uterus.*	aborto Expulsión prematura.
above	antecedente
abrupt	abrupto, abrupta
abruptio placentae *The premature detachment of a normally implanted placenta resulting in maternal decompensation.*	abruptio placentae
abscess *A localized collection of pus.*	absceso
absence	ausencia
absolute	absoluto
absorption (intestinal absorption)	absorción (absorción entérica)
abuse	abuso
acalculia *The inability to perform mathematical calculations.*	acalculia
acanthoma *An adult cornifying squamous carcinoma.*	acantoma
acanthosis *Hypertrophy of the prickle cell layer of the skin.*	acantosis
acanthosis nigricans *A skin disorder characterized by dark, thick, velvety skin in the body folds and creases.*	acantosis pigmentaria
acapnia *A condition of lower than normal carbon dioxide level in the blood.*	acapnia
acariasis *Mite infestation.*	acariasis
acaricide *A treatment for mite infestation.*	acaricida
acarus *A mite.*	acarus
acatalasia *A condition characterized by the congenital absence of the enzyme catalase.*	acatalasia
acathisia *The inability to sit quietly or to have motor restlessness.*	acatisia

English	Spanish
accelerate *(To accelerate the healing process).*	acelerar (Acelerar la cura.)
access	ataque, acceso
accessory *Complimentary or concomitant.*	accesorio, accesoria
accessory nerve (XI) *Supplies motor innervation to the sternocleidomastoid and trapezius.*	nervio accesorio
accident	accidente
acclimatization *The process of becoming adapted to a new environment.*	aclimatación
accommodation *A term used to describe the ability of the eye to adjust to various distances.*	acomodación
accomplish	acabar, realizar
according to	según
accretion *The expected growth of tissue from the intake of nutrients.*	aumento, acrecentamiento
acephalous *A absence of a head.*	acéfalo
acetabular *Referring to the acetabulum.*	acetabular
acetabulum *The cup-shaped cavity with which the head of the femur articulates.*	acetabulo
acetaminophen *Mild analgesic drug used for pain relief.*	acetaminofeno
acetonemia *The presence of acetone in the blood.*	acetonemia
acetonuria *The presence of acetone in the urine.*	acetonuria
acetylcholine *A reversible acetic acid ester of choline.*	acetilcolina
acetylsalicylic acid *The chemical name for common aspirin.*	ácido acetilsalicílio
achalasia *Inability to relax the smooth muscle fibers of the gastrointestinal tract. In the case of esophageal achalasia one has dilatation and hypertrophy of the esophagus.*	acalasia
achieve	llevar a cabo, realizar
Achilles tendon reflex *The normal response to tapping the achilles tendon with a reflex hammer is the plantar flexion of the foot.*	reflexo del tendón de Aquiles
achilliodynia *Pain around the calcaneal tendon.*	aquilodinia
achillobursitis *Inflammation around the calcaneal tendon.*	aquilobursitis
achlorhydria *The absence of hydrochloric acid in gastric secretions.*	alorhidria
acholia *The lack of bile.*	acolia
achondroplasia *A congenital inadequacy of enchondral bone formation resulting in a type of dwarfism.*	acondroplasia
achromatic spindle *The threads between the poles of the spindle in karyokinesis.*	huso acromático
achromatopsia *Inability to differentiate yellow, blue, red or their intermediates.*	acromatopsia
achylia *The absence of chyle.*	aquilia
acid phosphatase *A phosphate derived chemical that is optimally active in an acidic environment.*	fosfatasa ácida
acid *Substance with a pH less than 7.*	ácido
acid-base balance *The equilibrium of the electrolytes in the body.*	equilibrio ácido-base
acidemia *A lower than normal pH in the blood.*	acidemia
acidity *Referring to an acid state.*	acidez
acinitis *The inflammation of the acini.*	acinitis
acne *Inflamed or infected sebaceous glands.*	acné
acne rosacea *A chronic disease characterized by the presence of flushing of the skin of the nose, forehead and cheeks.*	acné rosácea

20

English	Spanish
acne vulgaris *Chronic acne occurring on the face, chest and back of youth.*	acné vulgar o común
acorea *The absence of the pupil of the eye.*	acorea
acoustic crest *A prominence on ampulla of the semicircular ducts.*	cresta acústica
acoustic neuroma *A nonmalignant tumor that can cause deafness, tinnitus and vertigo.*	neuroma acústica
acoustic *Referring to the auditory system.*	acústico, acústica
Acquired Immunodeficiency Syndrome (AIDS) *Presence of an AIDS defining illness or having a CD4 of less than 200/mm3.*	síndrome de inmunodeficienia adquirida (SIDA)
acrocephaly *A condition characterized by a pointed head.*	acrocefalia
acrocyanosis, Raynaud's disease *A benign condition in which the feet and hands are cyanotic, cold and sweating.*	acrocianosis, enfermedad de Raynaud
acrodermatitis *Inflammation of the skin of the hands and/or feet.*	acrodermatitis
acrodynia *An infantile condition exhibited by swollen bluish-red extremities and later polyarthritis..*	acrodinia
acromegaly *Hyperplasia of the nose, jaw, fingers and toes.*	acromegalia
acromioclavicular *Referring to the junction of the acromion and clavicle.*	acromioclavicular
acromion *The flattened process extending laterally from the spine of the scapula which forms the most prominent point of the shoulder.*	acromión
acrophobia *The morbid fear of heights.*	acrofobia
acrotic *Referring to the surface.*	acrótico
actin *A protein in the muscle that, along with myosin, facilitates muscle contraction and relaxation.*	actina
actinic dermatosis *A skin disease caused by exposure to radiation from the sun, ultraviolet waves or gamma radiation.*	dermatosis actínico
actinomycosis *A chronic bacterial infection that effects the face and neck and is caused by Actinomyces israelii. In rare cases it can cause a pulmonary infection.*	actinomicosis
actinon *A radioactive element, radon-219.*	radón 219
action potential *The alteration in electrical potential associated with the movement along a nerve cell.*	potencial de acción
activity	actividad
actomyosin *Myosin and actin complex present in muscles.*	actomiosina
acuity *1. Relating to accuracy of hearing, as in hearing acuity. 2. Severity of illness as in, "What is the patient's acuity?"*	agudeza, precisión
acupuncture *Traditionally an aspect of Chinese medicine involving insertion of needles into the skin.*	acupuntura
acute *Abrupt onset.*	agudo, aguda
acyesis *Feminine sterility.*	esterilización
adactylia *A congenital condition exhibited by the absence of toes and fingers.*	adactilia
Adam's apple *A prominence on the anterior neck caused by the thyroid cartilage of the larynx.*	nuez de Adán
Adams-Stokes Syndrome *Characterized by bradycardia, syncope and convulsions.*	enfermedad de Adams-Stokes
add, to	añadir
addiction	adicción
Addison's disease *A disease of the adrenal gland exhibited by anemia, hypotension and a bronze tone to the skin.*	enfermedad de Addison
adduction *To bring toward the midline.*	aducción
adductor *A muscle that brings a part to the midline.*	músculo aductor

English	Spanish
adenectomy *The removal of a gland.*	adenectomía
adenitis *The inflammation of a gland.*	adenitis
adenocanthoma *Malignant tumor comprised of glandular tissue.*	adenoacantoma
adenocarcinoma *Cancer from glandular tissue.*	adenocarcinoma
adenofibroma *Connective tissue with glands that form a tumor.*	adenofibroma
adenohypophysis *The anterior portion of the pituitary gland.*	adenohipófisis
adenoid *Referring to a gland.*	adenoideo
adenoidectomy *Removal of the adenoids.*	adenoidectomía
adenoiditis *Inflammation of the adenoids.*	adenoiditis
adenoids *Pharyngeal tonsils.*	adenoides
adenolymphoma *A salivary gland tumor, also called Warthin's tumor.*	adenolinfoma
adenomyoma *A tumor characterized by the overgrowth of endometrial and uterine muscle tissue.*	adenomioma
adenomyosis *A condition characterized by the overgrowth of endometrial and uterine muscle tissue.*	adenomiosis
adenopathy *Generally referring to a condition of the lymphatic glands.*	adenopatía
adenosine triphosphate (ATP) *A chemical that represents the energy reserve of the muscle.*	adenosina trifosfato
adenosine diphosphate *A product of hydrolysis of ATP.*	adenosina difosfato
adenosine monophosphate *A nucleotide, it is produced when ATP is converted to ADP.*	adenosine monofosfato
adenovirus *A type of a virus that can cause upper respiratory tract infections.*	adenovirus
adephagia *Insatiable hunger.*	bulimia
adequate	adecuado,adecuada
adherence	adherencia
adhesion *The abnormal adherence of tissue exposed to inflammation or after surgery.*	adesión
adhesive capsulitis *Also known as frozen shoulder.*	capsulitis adhesiva
adhesive tape *Tape used to secure dressings or intravenous lines to the body.*	cinta adhesiva
adiadochokinesia *The inability to perform rapid alternating movements.*	adiadococinesia
Adie's pupil *Characterized by a weak light reaction and a strong but slow near response.*	pupila de Adie
adipose *Referring to fat.*	adiposa
adipsia *Absence of thirst which can be caused by SIADH, hydrocephalus or injury/tumor to/of the hypothalamus.*	adipsia
aditus *The entrance to an organ or part.*	aditus
adjust	ajustar
adjustment	ajuste
adjuvant *Term used to describe the medical treatment after initial therapy, as in adjuvant radiation therapy after initial chemotherapy.*	adjutor
admission	admisión
adnexa *The appendages, for example, of the uterus are the ovaries, fallopian tubes and the ligaments of the uterus.*	anejos
adolescence	adolescenia
adrenal *Referring to being near the kidney.*	suprarrenal
adrenal cortex *The outer layer of the adrenal gland.*	corteza suprarrenal
adrenal gland *A gland located on the superior aspect of both kidneys.*	glándula suprarrenal
adrenal medulla *The innermost part of the adrenal gland.*	médula suprarrenal

English	Spanish
adrenalectomy *Excision of the adrenal gland.*	adrenalectomía
adrenaline (epinephrine) *A hormone secreted by the adrenal glands and a synthetic medication used for treatment of allergic reactions and cardiac arrest.*	adrenalina
adrenergic *That which is activated or transmitted by epinephrine.*	adrenogénico
adrenocorticotrophic hormone (ACTH) *A hormone that influences the cortex of the adrenal glands.*	adrenocorticotropina
Adson maneuver *A test used to screen for thoracic outlet syndrome.*	maniobra de Adson
advanced	avanzado
adventitia *Outermost.*	adventicia
adverse effect *In reference to medication use, it is an undesirable consequence of the drug.*	efecto adverso
advise, to	advertir, recomendar
aerobe *An organism that grows in the presence of oxygen.*	aerobio
aerodontalgia *The dental pain that occurs with low atmospheric pressure, like during airflight.*	aerodontalgia
aerophagy or aerophagia *A condition associated with hysteria in which one swallow repeatedly swallows air and then belches.*	aerofagia
afebrile *Absence of fever.*	afebril
affect	afectar
affected	afectado, afectada
affective disorders *Manic-depressive psychosis.*	trastornos afectivo (a)
afferent loop syndrome *The obstruction of the duodenum or jejunum after gastrojejunostomy, resulting in duodenal distention.*	síndrome de asa aferente
afferent *Moving toward the center.*	aferente
affinity *To have a natural liking for.*	afinidad
afibrinogenemia *Marked deficiency of fibrinogen in the blood.*	afibrinogenemia
aflatoxin *A toxin produced by Aspergillus flavus.*	aflaxotin
after-load *Referring to the amount of pressure the heart needs to pump against. If one has left heart failure it is beneficial to reduce after-load.*	poscarga
after-pains *The pain experienced after childbirth caused by uterine contractions.*	entuertos
after-taste	permanencia dela sensación del gusto
afterbirth *The tissue expelled after the birth of a child that includes the placenta and allied membranes.*	secundinas
agar *Media used for bacterial cultures.*	agar
age	edad
agenesis *The absence of an organ.*	agénesis
agglutination *The process of adherence of a mass.*	aglutinación
aggression	agresión
aging	envejecimiento
agitation	agitación
aglutition *The inability to swallow.*	aglutición
agnathia *Congenital abnormality characterized by the absence of the mandible.*	agnatia
agnosia *A condition exhibited by the loss of sensory stimuli.*	agnosia
agonist *A synthetic compound that activates cells normally activated by natural chemicals.*	agonista
agony *Anguish or torment.*	agonía

English	Spanish
agoraphobia *The fear of being in a large open space.*	agorafobia
agranulocytosis *A condition characterized by leukopenia and neutropenia.*	agranulocitosis
agraphia *The inability to express one's thoughts in writing.*	agrafia
agreement	acuerdo, pacto
ague *A term used to describe recurrent fever typically associated with malaria.*	ague
Aicardi syndrome *A rare genetic anomily in which the corpus collosum is absent or insufficient. It is characterized by seizures, microphthalmos, coloboma and developmental delays.*	síndrome de Aicardi
AIDS *Aquired Immunodeficiency Syndrome*	SIDA
air	aire
air embolism *The blockage of an artery or vein by an air bubble.*	embolia gaseosa
air flow	fliujo aire
air hunger	falta de aire
akathisia *A condition exhibited by motor restlessness and inability to sit quietly.*	acatisia
akinesia *An absence of movement or sparsity of movement.*	aquinesia
akinesthesia *Lack of perception of movement.*	aquinestesia
albinism *Congenital absence of pigment in the eyes, skin and hair.*	albinismo
albino *A person who lacks pigment in the eyes, skin and hair.*	albino, albina
albumin *A protein that is soluble in water and coagulates if heated.*	albúmina
albuminuria *The presence of albumin in the urine.*	albuminuria
alcohol	alcohol
alcoholic	alcohólico, alcohólica
alcoholism *An addiction to alcohol.*	alcoholismo
aldehyde *A substance derived by oxidizing and containing a CHO group from alcohol.*	aldehído
aldosterone *A steroid secreted by the adrenal cortex that regulates electrolytes.*	aldosterona
aldosteronism *A condition characterized by the excessive secretion of aldosterone.*	aldosteronismo
alert	alerta
alexia *Inability to read due to a central brain lesion.*	alexia
algae	algas
algid *cold*	álgido, álgida
algogenic *Pain causing.*	algogénico
algorhithm *Any procedure designed to solve a problem in a step-by-step or mechanical fashion.*	algoritmo
alimentary	alimenticio, alimenticia
alkali *A class of compounds that form soluble carbonates.*	álcali
alkaline *Referring to something with properties of an alkali.*	alcalino
alkalinuria *The urine in an alkaline state.*	alcalinuria
alkaloid *Plant derived nitrogenous organic compound.*	alcaloide
alkalosis *A condition in which the pH is increased.*	alcalosis
alkaptonuria *A condition exhibited by the urine turning dark upon standing because of the presence of alkapton bodies in it.*	alcaptonuria
all over the body	por todo el cuerpo
allantois *A posterior portion of the hind-gut of an embryo.*	alantoides
allele *A type of a gene; in humans there are two alleles per chromosome pair.*	alelo
allergens *Compounds that cause an allergic reaction.*	alérgenos

English	Spanish
allergy *An immune response by the body to a compound it is hypersensitive to.*	alergia
alleviate	aliviar
allograft *A tissue transplant of from someone of the same species but different genotype.*	aloinjerto
allopathy *Treatment of disease with minute amounts of natural substances.*	alopatía
alopecia *The absence of hair in areas where it normally exists.*	alopecia
alpha wave *Electroencephalographic waves with a frequency of 8-13 per second.*	onda alfa
alpha-fetoprotein *A glycoprotein that has a high serum level in hepatocellular and nonseminomatous germ cell tumors.*	alfa-fetoproteína
alteration	alteración
altitude sickness *A general term used for an illness that occurs at high altitude.*	anoxia por altitud
alveolar *Referring to the alveolus.*	alveolar
alveolus *A small sac like structure commonly used for the pulmonary alveolus.*	alvéolo
Alzheimer's disease *A dementia of unknown cause or pathogenesis.*	enfermedad de Alzheimer
amalgam *An alloy that includes mercury as one ingredient.*	amalgama
amalgamate *To make an amalgam by dissolving a metal in mercury.*	amalgamar
amastia *A development condition exhibited by the absence of breasts.*	amastia
amaurosis *Blindness that occurs without an ocular lesion but may include the optic nerve.*	amaurosis
amaurosis fugax *This transient monocular blindness is considered a sign of an impending stroke.*	amaurosis fugax
amaurotic pupil *A pupil that will not respond to light when directly exposed but will respond when the other eye is exposed to light.*	pupilo amaurótica
ambidextrous *Ability to use both hands equal ability.*	ambidextro, ambidextra
ambisexual *Referring to both sexes.*	ambisexual
amblyopia *Decreased vision without an ocular lesion.*	ambliopía
ambulation *A walk.*	paseo
ambulatory electrocardiographic monitoring *A continuous recording of the electrocardiogram used to detect occult dysrhythmias.*	monitor de Holter para 24 horas
ambulatory *Referring to one's ability to walk.*	ambulatorio, ambulatoria
ameba *A one-celled protozoan.*	ameba
amebiasis *A condition in which one is infected with amebae, mostly commonly Entamoeba histolytica.*	amebiasis
amebic liver abscess *A pus filled fluid collection within the liver caused by amoebe.*	absceso hepático amebiano
amebicide *A compound used to treat amebiasis.*	amebicida
ameboma *A mass caused by inflammation as seen in amebiasis.*	ameboma
amelia *A congenital anomaly exhibited by the absence of limbs.*	amelia
ameliorate	mejorar
amenorrhea *The absence of menses.*	amenorrea
amentia *The absence of mental ability.*	amencia
ametria *Congenital absence of the uterus.*	ametria
ametropia *Abnormal refractive ability of the eyes resulting in hypermetropia, myopia or astigmatism.*	ametropía
amino acid *A compound containing a carboxyl and an amino group.*	aminoácido

25

English	Spanish
ammonia *A colorless alkaline gas.*	amoníaco
amnesia *The inability to remember past events.*	amnesia
amnesia, antegrade *The inability to remember events which occurred after the insult that caused the condition.*	amnesia anterógrada
amnesiac stroke *Cerebral infarct exhibited by loss of memory.*	accidente cerebrovascular con amnesia
amniocentesis *Transabdominal aspiration of amniotic fluid.*	amniocentesis
amniography *X-ray of the gravid uterus after insertion of opaque dye.*	amniografía
amnion *The membrane lining the placenta which produces the amniotic fluid.*	aminos
amniotic fluid *The fluid surrounding the fetus.*	fluido amniótico
amorphous *A fetus with no heart and no definitive shape.*	amorfo, amorfa
amount	cantidad
ampulla *The dilated end of a duct.*	ampolla
ampulla chyli *Also called cisterna chyli; it is a dilated area of the thoracic duct that collects lymph from several areas.*	ampolla del quilo
amygdala *Any almond shaped structure such as the tonsil*	amígdala
amylase *An enzyme involved in the hydrolysis of starch.*	amilasa
amyloidosis *The accumulation of amyloid in body tissues.*	amiloidosis
amyotonia *A condition associated with the lack of muscle tone.*	amiotonía
amyotrophic lateral sclerosis *A progressive neurodegenerative disorder.*	atrofia muscular progresiva
amyotrophy *Atrophy of muscle tissue.*	amiotrofia
anabolism *The formation of molecules in organisms from simpler molecules.*	anabolismo
anacrotic *Referring to a prominent bulge on the ascending portion of a pulse recording.*	anacrótico
anaerobe *An organism that lives in the absence of oxygen.*	anaeróbico
anal	anal
anal fistula *An opening in the skin that tracts to the anal canal thus causing some fecal material to leak from the opening in the skin.*	fístula anal
analeptic *A medication used as a stimulant to the central nervous system.*	analéptico
analgesia *The absence of pain.*	analgesia
analgesic *A medication used to remove pain.*	analgésico
analogous *To resemble or be similar to.*	análogo
anaphase *A stage in mitosis following metaphase.*	anafase
anaphoresis *Reduced activity of the sweat glands.*	anaforesis
anaphylaxis *An exaggerated response to a foreign substance.*	anafilaxis
anaplasia *The loss of normal differentiation of tumor cells.*	anaplasia
anastomosis *Surgical formation of a connection between two previously separate parts.*	anastomosis
anatomical chart *A pictorial diagram of part of the anatomy.*	gráfico anatómico (a)
anatomical dead space *The area between the mouth and pulmonary alveoli.*	espacio muerto anatómico
anatomical *Referring to the anatomy.*	anatómico, anatómica
anatomical snuff-box *The area on the back of the hand near the base of the thumb that is between the extensor pollicus longus and extensor pollicus brevis.*	tabaquera anatómica
anatomy *The study of body structure.*	anatomía
ancylostomiasis *A type of nematode parasite, also called hookworm.*	anquilostomiasis

English	Spanish
androgen *A compound that produces masculinizing characteristics.*	andrógeno
androgynous *Referring to a female pseudohermaphroditism (a genetic female with masculine characteristics).*	androginoide
android pelvis *A pelvis shaped like a man's.*	pelvis androide
androsterone *A hormone excreted in the urine of men and women.*	androsterona
anemia *Lower than normal red blood cell count.*	anemia
anencephaly *The congenital absence of the cranial vault and cerebral hemispheres.*	anencefalia
aneroid *The absence of liquid.*	aneroide
anesthesia *Loss of sensation.*	anestesia
anesthetic *A chemical that produces anesthesia.*	anestésico
anesthetist *A person who administers anesthesia.*	anestestista
aneurysm *A condition exhibited by the dilatation of the walls of an artery or vein to form a blood-filled sac.*	aneurisma
angiectasia *Dilation of a blood or lymph vessel.*	angiectasia
angina pectoris *Exercise induced myocardial ischemia.*	angina de pecho
angioedema *Also called angioneurotic edema, it is caused by a histamine reaction. It can produce welts in mild cases but in severe cases can cause swelling of the lips and tongue.*	angioedema
angiogram *Radiologic imaging of blood vessels.*	angiograma
angiography *Roentgenographic imaging of blood vessels.*	angiocardiografía
angioma *A tumor comprised of blood or lymph vessels.*	angioma
angioneurotic *Caused by a neurosis affecting the blood vessels, like vasospasm.*	angioneurótico
angioneurotic edema *A condition exhibited by sudden edema of skin and mucous membranes.*	edema angioneurótico
angioplasty *Surgical alteration of blood vessels.*	angioplastia
angiosarcoma *A sarcoma comprised of blood vessels.*	angiosarcoma
angiospasm *A spasm of a blood vessel.*	angioespasmo
angiotensin *A blood protein that increases aldosterone secretion.*	angiotensina
angiotensin converting enzyme inhibitors (ACEI) *A class of medicines that prevent conversion of angiotension I to angiotensin II, a potent vasoconstrictor.*	angiotensina
angitis or angiitis *The inflammation of a lymph or blood vessel.*	angiitis
anguish	angustia
anhidrosis *A condition exhibited by reduced quantity of sweat.*	anhidrosis
anhidrotic *Something the reduces the quantity of sweat.*	anhidrótico
anhydrous *Lacking water.*	anhidro
aniseikonia *A condition in which the ocular image of an object is viewed differently by each eye.*	aniseiconía
anisocoria *Pupillary diameter inequality.*	aniscoria
anisocytosis *Variation in size of erythrocytes.*	anisocitosis
anisomelia *Unequal size of arms or legs.*	anisomelia
anisometropia *Refractive power inequality between the two eyes.*	anisometropía
ankle	tobillo
ankle clonus *An abnormal response exhibited by alternating plantar- and dorsiflexion noted after the examiner rapidly dorsiflexes the foot.*	clono tobillo
ankle edema or dependent edema	edema dependiente
ankle joint	articulación tobillo
ankle support (device)	soporte tobillo

English	Spanish
ankle swelling	tobillo chichón
ankyloglossia *Limitation of tongue motion because of a short frenulum.*	anquiloglosia
ankylosing spondylitis *A type of arthritis found in the spine that is exhibited by bony fusion.*	espondilitis anquilosante
ankylosis *Abnormal immobility of a joint.*	anquilosis
annular *Referring to a ring.*	anular
anomia *Inability to name or recognize familiar objects.*	anomia
anonychia *Congenital absence of fingernails or toenails.*	anoniquia
anoperineal *Referring to the anus and perineum.*	anoperineal
anorchous *The absence of testicles.*	agenesia gonadal
anorectal *Referring to the anus and rectum.*	anorrectal
anorexia nervosa *A mental disorder characterized by the desire to avoid eating and to lose weight.*	anorexia nervosa
anorexia *The loss of appetite.*	anorexia
anorrectal abscess *A localized collection of pus in the anorrectal region.*	absceso anorrectal
anosmia *Lack of the sense of smell.*	anosmia
anovulation *Lack of ovulation.*	anovulación
anovulatory cycle *A menstrual cycle in which no ovum is released.*	ciclo anovulatorio
anoxemia *Reduction in blood oxygen concentration.*	anoxemia
anoxia *Reduced oxygen levels in body tissues.*	anoxia
antacid *A medication, usually with a calcium or magnesium base that binds with acid in the stomach.*	antiácido
antagonist *A muscle or agent that acts in counteract to effects of another muscle or agent.*	antagonista
antemetic *A medication used to control nausea.*	antiemético
antemortem *Refers to: before death.*	antemortem
antenatal *Refers to events before birth.*	antenatal
anterior root *A motor nerve root that is in the anterior part of the spinal cord between the anterior and lateral funiculi.*	raíz anterior
anterior *Toward the front.*	anterior
anterograde *Moving forward.*	anterógrado
anteroinferior *Toward the front and lower part.*	anteroinferior
anterolateral *Toward the front and away from the midline.*	anterolateral
anteromedian *Toward the front and toward the midline.*	anteromediano
anteroposterior *From front to the back. (An AP x-ray has the beam directed from the front to the back.)*	anteroposterior
anterosuperior *Toward the front and the upper part.*	anterosuperior
anteversion *The forward leaning of an organ.*	anterversión
anthelmintic *An agent used to destroy worms.*	antihelmíntico
anthracosis *Pneumoconiosis caused by coal dust.*	antracosis
anthrax *An infectious disease caused by Bacillus anthracis; there are cutaneous, inhalation and gastrointestinal syndromes.*	àntrax
anti-inflammatory agents *Medications used to reduce inflammation.*	agentes antiinflamatorios
antibiotic *A medication that inhibits or kills microorganisms.*	antibióticos
antibody *A protein that combines with and counteracts foreign substances.*	anticuerpo
anticholinergic *Parasympathetic blocker.*	anticolinérgico, anticolinérgica

English	Spanish
anticholinesterase *Cholinesterase blocker.*	anticolinesterasa
anticoagulant *Medication used to inhibit coagulation.*	anticoagulante
anticodon *A series of three nucleotides that form a unit of genetic code for transfer RNA.*	anticodón
anticonvulsant *Medication used to treat seizures.*	anticonvulsivo
antidepressant *Medication used to treat depression.*	antidepresivo
antidiuretic hormone *Vasopressin.*	antidiurético
antidote *A medication that neutralizes a toxin.*	antidoto
antigen *A foreign substance, like bacteria, that induces an immune response.*	antigeno
antiglobulin test (Coombs' test) *Test used to detect erythroblastosis fetalis.*	prueba de antiglobinemia
antihemophilic factor *Also called factor VIII. A deficiency of the factor causes hemophilia.*	factor antihemofílico
antihistamine *Medication used to treat conditions exhibited by a histamine response*	antihisamina
antilymphocyte *A serum globulin that has antibodies to lymphocytes.*	antilimfocite
antilymphocyte globulin *The gamma globulin portion of antilymphocyte serum.*	globulina antilimfocite
antimalarial *Medication used to treat malaria.*	antipalúdico
antimetabolite *A substance that impedes metabolism.*	antimetabolito
antimigraine *Medication used to treat headaches.*	para tratar los síntomas de la migraña
antimitotic *Impeding mitosis.*	antimitótico
antimycotic *Inhibition of fungal growth.*	antimicótico
antinuclear factor *Also called antinucleic antibody (ANA); it is found in conditions such as lupus and rheumatoid arthritis.*	factor antinuclear
antiperistaltic *An agent that impedes normal peristalsis.*	antiperistáltico
antipruritic *Medication used to treat pruritus.*	antipruriginoso, antipruriginosa
antipyretic *Medication used to treat fever.*	antipirético, antipirético
antiseptic *A substance that inhibits microorganism growth.*	antiséptico
antiserum *A substance that contains antibodies to specific antigens.*	antisuero
antispasmodic *Medication used to treat muscle spasm.*	antiespasmódico
antithrombin *A substance that inhibits thrombin, thus decreasing the body's ability to coagulate.*	antitrombina
antithyroid *A substance inhibiting the effect of the thyroid.*	antitiroideo
antitoxin *A substance that inhibits the effect of a toxin.*	antitoxina
antitussive *Medication used to diminish a cough.*	calmante para la tos
antivenin *An antitoxin formulated for various types of snake bites.*	antiveneno
antrotomy *To cut open the antrum.*	antrotomía
antrum *Referring to a cavity or chamber.*	antro
anuria *The lack of urine excretion.*	anuria
anus *The body opening distal to the rectum.*	ano
anxiety *Nervousness or unease.*	ansiedad
anxiety neurosis *Abnormal presence of anxiety.*	neurosis de ansiedad
anxious *Experiencing nervousness or unease.*	ansioso, ansiosa
aorta *The large artery originating at the left ventricle and going to the pelvis where it bifurcates.*	aorta

29

English	Spanish
aortic insufficiency *A dysfunction of the aortic valve allowing backflow of blood into the heart.*	insuficiencia aórtico (a)
aortic *Referring to the aorta.*	aórtico, aórtica
aortic stenosis *Narrowing of the aortic orifice.*	estenosis o estrechamiento
aortic valve *The valve situated between the left ventricle and the aorta.*	válvula aórtica
apart	aparte
apathy	apatia
aperistalsis *Lack of intestinal peristalsis.*	aperistalsis
aperture *An opening or hole, as in the hole the light passes through in a camera.*	apertura
apex *The highest point of something.*	apex
apex of heart *Normally found 8cm to the left of the midsternal line in the 5th intercostal space.*	vértice del corazón
Apgar score *A scoring system for newborns that utilizes heart rate, respiratory effort, muscle tone, responsiveness and skin color.*	Apgar, test de
aphagia *The lack of eating.*	afagia
aphakia *The congenital absence of the lens of the eye.*	afaquia
aphasia *Diminished ability to communicate via speech or writing.*	afasia
aphid *A minute insect that feeds on plants.*	afido
aphonia *The loss of voice.*	afonía
aphthous stomatitis *Grouped small lesions that occur on the tongue or in the mouth.*	estomatitis aftosa
apicetomy *Removal of the apex of the petrous portion of the temporal bone.*	apiceotomía
aplastic anemia *Bone marrow failure causing a decrease in all types of blood cells.*	anemia aplásica
apnea *Absence of respiration.*	apnea
apocrine gland *A gland that releases some of its cytoplasm in secretions; an example is axillary sweat glands.*	glándula apocrina
aponeurosis *A tendinous expansion that connects with muscle to move a part.*	aponeurosis
apophysis *Generally a bony outgrowth that forms a process or tubercle.*	apófisis
apoplexy *Extravasation of blood within an organ.*	apoplejía
appearance	apariencia
appendectomy *Surgical excision of the appendix.*	apendectomía
appendicitis *Inflammation of the appendix.*	apendicitis
appendix *An appendage of the cecum.*	apéndice
apperception *The ability to interpret sensory impressions.*	apercepión
application	aplicación
applicator	aplicador
appointment	cita
apprehension *A fear that something unpleasant will happen.*	aprehensión
approval	aprobasión
approximate	aproximado, aproximada
approximately	aproximadamente
apraxia *The inability to carry out intentional movements when paralysis is not present.*	apraxia
apron	delantal

English	Spanish
apt *Suitable in the circumstances.*	apto
aptitude *A natural talent for something.*	aptitud
aptyalism *Diminished or absence of saliva.*	aptialismo
aquaint	dar a conocer
aqueous humor *The fluid between the cornea and lens, anterior to the globe.*	humor acuoso (a)
aqueous *Use of water as a solvent or medium.*	acuoso, acuosa
arachnodactyly *A condition exhibited by abnormally long and slender fingers.*	aracnodactilia
arachnoid *Refers to that which resembles a spider web.*	arachnoides
arbovirus *Virus that is transmitted by arthropods; responsible for diseases such as Yellow fever and dengue fever.*	arbovirus
arcuate nucleus *Small masses of gray matter found on the medulla oblongata.*	núcleo arqueados
arcus *Narrow opaque band.*	arcus
areola *The pigmented skin surrounding a nipple.*	areóla
argininosuccinicaciduria *Presence of arginosuccinic acid in the urine; associated with mental retardation.*	argininosuccinicoaciduria
argue, to	argumentar
Argyll Robertson symptom *Presence of small pupils that do not react to light but will constrict when the person focuses on a near object.*	signo de Argyll Robertson
argyria *The greyish discoloration of the skin and conjunctiva.*	argiria
arm	brazo
around	cerca de
arousal *Awaken an emotion.*	excitación
arrhenoblastoma *An ovarian tumor that results in masculine secondary sex characteristics.*	arrenoblastoma
arrhythmia *An abnormal heart rhythm.*	arritmia
arterial blood gas *Measurement of the arterial concentration of carbon dioxide and oxygen.*	tensión de gases en sangre arterial
arterial *Referring to an artery.*	arterial
arteriectomy *Surgical excision of an artery.*	arteriectomía
arteriography *Roentgenography of an artery after infusion of contrast media.*	arteriografía
arterioplasty *Surgical repair of an artery.*	arterioplastia
arteriosclerosis *Hardening and thickening of arterial walls.*	arterioesclerosis
arteriotomy *Creation of an opening in an artery.*	arteriotomía
arteriovenous malformation *A sac like structure created by the abnormal communication of an adjacent artery and vein.*	arteriovenoso malformaciones
arteritis *Inflammation of an artery.*	arteritis
artery *Vessel that carries oxygenated blood from the heart to the periphery.*	arteria
arthralgia *Joint pain.*	artralgia
arthritis *Joint inflammation.*	artritis
arthrodesis *Surgical fusion of a joint.*	artrodesis
arthrodynia *Joint pain.*	artrodinia
arthrography *Joint roentgenography.*	arthrografía
arthroplasty *Plastic surgery involving a joint.*	artroplasia
arthroscopy *Viewing of the inside of a joint with a specially designed scope.*	artroscopia
arthrotomy *Surgical opening of a joint.*	artrotomía
articular *Referring to a joint.*	articular
artifact *An aberration from the normal.*	artefacto

English	Spanish
artificial *Not natural produced.*	artificial
arytenoid *Referring to the cartilage in the posterior larynx.*	aritenoideo
asbestos *A heat resistant silicate material.*	asbesto
asbestosis *Lung disease caused by the inhalation of asbestos.*	asbestosis
ascaricide *Agent that destroys ascaris.*	ascaricida
ascaris *A nematode from genus intestinal lumbricoid parasite, also called round worm.*	Ascaris
ascending colon *The portion of the colon between the cecum and the right colic flexure.*	colon ascendente
ascertain, to *Synonym of "to determine".*	determinar
ascites *Serous fluid in the abdominal cavity.*	ascitis
ascorbic acid *Commonly known as vitamin C; a deficiency of this vitamin causes scurvy.*	ácido ascórbico
asepsis *Lack of infection.*	asepsia
aseptic *Being free of septic matter.*	aséptico, aséptica
asexual *Without sex or sex organs.*	asexual
asleep	dormido
Asperger's syndrome *A condition characterized by disturbed social interaction; if was named after the Austrian scientist who first described it.*	Asperger, sindrome de
aspermia *Absence of sperm.*	aspermia
asphyxia *A condition exhibited by a lack of oxygen and subsequent loss of consciousness or death.*	asfixia
aspiration *Taking air or matter into the lungs. Removal of fluid from a cavity.*	aspiración
aspirator *A device used to remove fluid from a cavity.*	aspirador
aspirin *Common name for acetylsalicylic acid.*	aspirina
assay *A procedure for measuring the activity of a biological sample.*	ensayo
assessment *An evaluation.*	evaluación
assistance	asistencia
assisted ventilation *The act of helping one breathe through artificial means.*	respiración asistido
asteatosis *A condition exhibited by diminished sebaceous secretion.*	asteatosis
astereognosis *Lack of ability to recognize objects by touching them.*	astereognosía
asterixis *Commonly known as a flapping tremor, it is characterized by involuntary jerking movements of the hands and is seen commonly in hepatic encephalopathy.*	temblor de aleteo Asterixis.
asthenia *Diminished strength and energy.*	astenia
asthenopia *Visual fatigue accompanied by ocular pain.*	astenopía
astragalus *Synonym of talus.*	astrágalo
astringent *An agent causing contraction of the skin.*	astringente
astrocytoma *A tumor comprised of astrocytes.*	astrocitoma
astroglia *The neurologic tissue which is composed of astrocytes.*	astroglia
asymmetry *Lack of symmetry.*	asimetría
asymptomatic *The absence of symptoms.*	asintomático, asintomática
asynclitism *Oblique presentation of the head during delivery.*	asinclitismo
at random	al azar
atavism *The inheritance of characteristics from remote rather than immediate ancestors.*	atavismo
ataxia *Lack of muscular coordination.*	ataxia

32

English	Spanish
atelectasis *Incomplete expansion or collapse of a lung.*	atelectasis
atherogenic *Something that causes atheromatous lesions in arterial walls.*	aterogénico
atheroma *Degenerative arteriosclerosis.*	ateroma
athetosis *An involuntary symptom exhibited by continuous slow, writhing movements, mostly in the hands.*	atetosis
athlete's foot *Common term for tinea pedis.*	pie de atleta
atlas *The first cervical vertebra.*	atlas
atomizer *A device for propelling a fine mist.*	atomizador
atony *Absence of normal muscle tone.*	atonía
atresia *Closure of a body orifice as in atresia ani in which there is a congenital imperforate anus.*	atresia
atrial flutter *Sawtooth waves on an electrocardiogram with atrial rate of 250-330 per minute.*	aleteo auricular
atrial natriuretic factor *A chemical secreted by the right atrium that promotes sodium excretion in the urine.*	factor natriurético auricular
atrial *Referring to the atrium.*	auricular
atrial septal defect *An abnormal communication between the atria of the heart.*	defecto septal atrial
atrio-ventricular block *An interruption of the electrical conduction at the atrio-ventricular node.*	bloqueo atrioventricular
atrioventricular bundle *Also called bundle of His.*	fascículo auriculoventricular
atrioventricular *Referring to the atrium and ventricle.*	atrioventricular
atrium *Referring to a chamber used as an entrance, as in the entrance to the heart.*	atrio, atria
atrophic *Referring to atrophy.*	atrófico
atrophy *A diminution in the size of a part.*	atrofia
atropine *A parasympathetic agent derived from Atropa belladonna.*	atropina
attack *A fit or paroxysm.*	ataque
atypical *Not usual.*	atipico, atipica
audiogram *The recording of a one's hearing in decibels.*	audiograma
audiologist *A specialist in the field of hearing.*	audiólogo, audióloga
audiometer *A device used to measure hearing.*	audiómetro
auditory *Referring to hearing.*	auditivo, auditiva
aural *Referring to the ear.*	aural, auricular
auricle *The external portion of the ear.*	auricula
auricular *Referring to the auricle.*	aural, auricular
auriculotemporal *The area of the ear and temple.*	auriculotemporal
auscultation *The act of listening to sounds emanating from the body.*	auscultación
autism *A mental condition exhibited by difficulty in forming relationships, communicating and uses abstract thought.*	autismo
autistic *Referring to autism.*	austistico, autistica
autoantibody *An antibody that acts against the organism's own tissue.*	autoanticuerpo
autoantigen *A normal tissue constituent that prompts a cell-mediated response.*	autoantígeno
autoclave *A device used for sterilization with the use of steam under pressure.*	autoclave
autogenous *Self-generated.*	autogena
autograft *Grafting tissue from one part of person to another part of the same person.*	autoinjerto
autohypnosis *Self-hypnosis.*	autohipnosis

33

English	Spanish
autoimmunization *The body's ability to promote an immune response without external resources.*	autoinmunización
autolysis *A state of self destruction of cells within a body.*	autólisis
autonomic nervous system *Responsible for regulation of cardiac muscle, smooth muscle and glandular activity.*	sistema nervioso autonómico (a)
autopsy *Examination of a body post-mortem in an attempt to determine cause of death.*	autopsia
autosomal *Referring to an autosome.*	autosómico
autotransfusion *The reinfusion of one's own blood.*	autotranfusión
availability	disponibilidad
available	disponible
avascular *An area with no blood supply.*	avascular
avascular necrosis	necrosis avascular
avian flu *A viral disease found in birds and fowl that can be transmitted to humans; it is exhibited by respiratory and gastrointestinal symptoms but can lead to encephalitis.*	gripe de las aves
avian *Referring to birds.*	aviario
avitaminosis *A state of vitamin deficiency.*	avitaminosis
avoidable	evitable
awakening	despertamiento
away from	ausente
axilla *The hollow beneath the arm.*	axila
axillary *Referring to the axilla.*	axilar
axis *The second cervical vertebra.*	axis
axon *The structure along which nerve impulses are transmitted from the cell body to other cells.*	axon
azo itch *A pruritis noted in people who use azo dyes.*	prurito azoico
azoospermia *The absence of spermatozoa in the semen.*	azoospermia
Azorean disease *A form of hereditary ataxia found in peoples of Azorean descent. Also called Machado-Joseph disease or Portuguese-Azorean disease.*	enfermedad de Azores
azotemia *Prerenal disease.*	azotemia
azoturia *An excess of urea in the urine.*	azoturia
Babinski's sign *A reflex that occurs when the plantar surface of the foot is stimulated. The great toe turns upward- normal in infancy but when it turns upward in an adult it means there is central nervous system injury.*	reflejo plantar (reflejo de Babinski)
baby	bebé
baby-scale	balanza bebé
bacillary *Referring to bacilli.*	bacilar
bacillus *A rod-shaped bacterium.*	bacilo
back pain	lumbalgia
bacteremia *The presence of bacteria in the blood.*	bacteriemia
bacteria *Plural for any organism of the order Eubacteriales.*	de bacterium
bacterial *Referring to bacteria.*	bacteriano, bacteriana
bactericidal *An agent that destroys bacteria.*	bactericida
bacteriostatic *An agent that impedes bacterial growth.*	bacteriostático
bacteriuria *The presence of bacteria in the urine.*	bacteriruia
bagassosis *A pulmonary disorder contracted from inhalation of the waste of sugar cane (bagasse dust).*	bagazosis

English	Spanish
Baker cyst *A synovial fluid collection in the popliteal fossa.*	quiste de Baker
balanitis *Inflammation of the glans of the penis.*	balanitis
ballottement *Presence of movement of a floating object by palpation.*	peloteo
balm	bálsamo
bandage	vendaje
banding *The process of encircling with a thin piece of material.*	vendaje circular
barber's itch *Ringworm that is transmitted by contaminated shaving equipment.*	foliculitis de la barba
barium enema *Administration of barium into the rectum followed by roentgenography to check for rectal or colon abnormalities.*	enema de bario
Barretts's esophagus *A condition characterized by varying degrees of esophageal injury from gastric acid.*	síndrome de Barrett
Bartholin's cyst or abscess *This is a purulent fluid collection in the Bartholin cysts which are located in the perivaginal area.*	absceso o quiste de Bartolino
basal ganglia *Structures adjacent to the thalamus that are involved with coordination of movement.*	ganglios basales
basal *Referring to the base.*	basal
basilar *Referring to the base or lower segment.*	basilar
basilic vein *A vein in the hand that joins the brachial veins to form the axillary vein.*	veno basílica
basin	palangana
basophil *A polymorphonuclear granulocyte.*	basófilo
bear, to *To endure or resist.*	soportar, resistir
bear, to *To give birth to a child.*	dar a luz
bearing down *As in during labor.*	pujar
beat *As in heart beat.*	latido, pulsación
bed	cama
bed rest	guardo cama
bedbug Cimex lectularius. *A small insect that is parasitic and hides in clothing or bedding.*	chinche
bedpan	bacin
bedridden	postrado en cama
bee sting	picdura de abeja
beforehand	antes
behavior disorder *An abnormal mental state.*	desarreglo emocional
Bell's palsy *Unilateral facial paralysis related to dysfunction of the seventh cranial nerve.*	parálisis de Bell
below	abajo de
belt	cinturón
benign *Not harmful.*	propicio
bereavement *The sorrow one feels with the loss of a loved one.*	pérdida de un ser querido
berylliosis *A lung exhibited by granulomas and caused by inhalation of beryllium.*	berilosis
best	mejor
betablocker *A substance that inhibits adrenergic stimulation. It is used to reduce pulse, blood pressure and to treat angina.*	beta bloqueador
beyond	más allá de

English	Spanish
bezoar *A concretion composed of either hair, vegetable/fruit fibers or hair and vegetable/fruit fibers that is found in the stomach.*	bezoar
biased *Prejudiced.*	tendencioso
biceps *A muscle with two heads usually referring to the biceps brachii which is used for forearm flexion.*	biceps
biceps reflex *The biceps brachii tendon is hit with a reflex hammer and results in flexion of the forearm as a normal response. This assesses the C5-C6 region.*	reflejo biceps
bicuspid *Having two points as in bicuspid valve or a premolar tooth.*	bicúspide
bifid *Presence of two branches.*	bífido
bifurcate ligament *A ligament on the dorsum of the foot that includes the calcaneonavicular and calcaneocuboid ligaments.*	ligamento bifurcado
bifurcate *When one branch divides into two branches.*	bifurcarse
bilateral *Referring to both sides.*	bilateral
bile *An alkaline fluid secreted by the liver to aid digestion.*	bilis
bile ducts *The structures that are conduits for passage of bile from the liver and gallbladder to the duodenum.*	conductos biliares
bile pigments *The golden brown or green-yellow color associated with bile.*	pigmentos biliares
bile salts *Normally occurring salts of bile acids.*	ácidos biliares
Bilharzia *Historical name of a genus of flukes or nematodes now known as Schistosoma.*	Bilharzia
biliary *Referring to bile, bile ducts or gallbladder.*	biliar
bilious *Something that contains bile.*	bilioso, biliosa
bilirubin *A pigment found in bile that is responsible for the yellow color seen in patients with elevated serum levels of bilirubin.*	bilirrubina
biliuria *The presence of bile in the urine.*	bilirubinuria
biliverdin *A green pigment formed by oxidation of bilirubin.*	biliverdina
bill	cuenta
Bill maneuver *During childbirth, use of forceps at midpelvis to help extract the head.*	maniobra de Bill
bimanual *Use of two hands, as in bimanual pelvic examination in which the right hand touches the cervix uteri and the left hand presses above the mons pubis.*	bimanual
binaural *Referring to both ears.*	biauricular
binocular *Referring to both eyes.*	binocular
binovular *Derived from two different ova.*	biovular
bioassay *A laboratory test determination as compared to normal.*	bioensayo
bioavailability *The portion of a drug that is able to be utilized by the body after it is introduced to the body.*	biodisponsibilidad
biochemistry *The study of chemistry and physiochemical processes in living organisms.*	bioquímica
biology *The study of living organisms.*	biologia
biopsy *The removal and examination of bodily tissues or fluids.*	biopsia
biotin *A vitamin involved in the synthesis of fatty acids and glucose.*	biotina
birth	nacimiento
birth control *Any method of limiting contraception.*	control de la natalidad
birth defect *A congenital anomaly.*	anomalía congénito
birth rate *The number of live births per 1000 of a given population per year.*	natalidad
bistoury; scalpel *A surgical knife.*	escalapo, bisturí

English	Spanish
bitemporal hemianopsia *A visual defect seen commonly in pituitary tumors in which the visual defect is in the temporal portion of each eye.*	hemianopsia bitemporal
bitter	amargo
black	negro
black fly *From the family Simuliidae, a gnat that can cause disease in humans; also called buffalo fly.*	jején de búfalo
black stools *Common term for melena.*	melena
blackout *Common term for loss of consciousness.*	desmayo
blackwater fever *A term used to describe the fever associated with malaria when the urine is reddish-black.*	fiebre del agua negra
bladder	vejiga
blast injury *Trauma from a wave of air pressure.*	atentados con explosivos
blastomycosis Infection caused by organisms of genus Blastomyces.	blastomicosis
bleach	lejía
bleeding	sangrado
bleeding time *The time of bleeding after a controlled standardized puncture of the earlobe.*	tiempo de sangrado
blemishes	manchas
blennorrhea *Discharge from the mucous membranes, usually referring to gonorrhea.*	blenorrea
blepharitis *Inflammation of the eyelids.*	blefaritis
blepharospasm *A spasm of the orbicularis oculi muscle that causes closure of the eyelid.*	blefaroespasmo
blind	ciego, ciega
blind loop syndrome *A condition in which there is a non-functional section of the bowel that is thought to be responsible for malabsorption and Vitamin B12 deficiency.*	síndrome de asa ciego
blind spot *An area of insensitivity to light located at the point of entry of the optic nerve on the retina.*	punto ciego
blindness	ceguera
blinking	parpadeo
blister *Common term for bulla.*	ampolla
bloated *Sensation of having an abnormally large amount of air in the viscera.*	aventado, aventada
blood	sangre
blood alcohol level *A quantitative measurement of the amount of alcohol in the blood.*	concentración de alcohol en la sangre
blood bank	banco de sangre
blood brain barrier *A matrix of capillaries that move blood between the blood and brain, as well as, limiting some substances from passing.*	barrera hematoencefálica
blood cell	célula sangre
blood clot	coágulo de sangre
blood grouping *Testing blood to determine which type should be used for transfusion.*	determinación de grupos sanguineos
blood pressure *Written as the measurement in mmHg at the time of systole of the left ventricle over the time of diastole.*	presión arterial
blood sedimentation rate (ESR) *The settling time of erythrocytes in a prepared sample. This is a measure of the abnormal concentration of substances that are associated with pathological states.*	indice de sedimentación de eritrocito

English	Spanish
blood stream *Common term or the arterial or venous systems.*	torrente sanguíneo
blood tubing *(used for infusion of blood)*	de tubos de sangre
blood type *Determined and listed in the ABO system.*	grupo sanguíneo
blood volume	volumen sanguíneo
blue	azul
blunt	despuntado, despuntada
blurred vision	visión borroso
blurt out, to *To speak without considering the repercussions.*	soltar
blush, to *To have an increased volume of blood flow to one's face causing a red tint to the skin.*	sonroharse
body surface area *Dubois formula is: (weight in kilograms)to the 0.425th power x (height in centimeters) to the 0.725th power x 0.007184.*	superficie corporal
body weight	peso corporal
bolus *A fluid bolus is a phrase used for rapid infusion of fluid.*	bolo
bone	hueso
bone graft *The transfer of bone to aid in the healing of a complex fracture.*	injerto óseo
bone marrow *The soft material filling the cavity of bones.*	medula óseo
bone marrow puncture *The aspiration of marrow to look for pressure of disease.*	aspiración médula ósea
bone scan *Bone imaging using technetium 99m (99mTc) diphosphate.*	tomografía de los huesos
bonesetter *A person who sets bones without being a physician.*	técnico ortopédico
border; margin	borde, margen
born	nacido, nacida
bottle	botella
bougienage *Passage of a bougie through a body orifice with the goal of increasing the diameter of the orifice.*	bougienage
brace	braguero
brace; splint	corsé
brachial artery *A continuation of the axillary artery and branches into the radial and ulnar among others.*	arteria braquial
brachial plexus *A cluster of nerves coming off the last four cervical and first thoracic spinal nerves form the nerve supply the the chest and arms.*	plexo braquial
brachial plexus neuropathy *Characterized by acute arm or shoulder pain followed by focal muscle weakness.*	neuropatía del plexo braquial
brachial *Referring to the arm.*	braquial
brachium cerebelli *Synonym of pedunculus cerebellaris superior (upper portion the cerebellum).*	brachium conjunctivum cerebelli
Bracht maneuver *Delivery of a fetus in a breech position.*	maniobra de Bracht
brachycephaly *The presence of a short broad skull.*	braquicefalia
bracing	abrazadera
bradycardia *Lower than normal cardiac rate measured in beats per minute.*	bradicardia
bradykinin *A peptide that causes contraction of smooth muscle and dilation of blood vessels.*	bradicinina
brain *A common term for cerebrum.*	cerebro
brain death *Cessation of cerebral functioning.*	muerte cerebral
brain stem *An organ that consists of the medulla oblongata, pons and midbrain.*	tallo encefálico

English	Spanish
brainstem herniation *Movement of the brainstem into the incisura because of increased intracranial pressure.*	hernia cerebral
branchial *Referring to or resembling the gills of a fish.*	branquial
break	fractura
breast	pecho, seno
breast feeding	lactancia materna
breath	respiración
breath sounds *The noise heard upon auscultation with a stethoscope.*	ruidos respiratorios
breath test (for alcohol)	alcohómetro
breech birth *Delivery with the feet or buttocks coming first.*	presentación de nalgas
bregma *Located at the convergence of the coronal and sagittal sutures.*	bregma
bright	brillante
bring, to	traer
brisk	rápido, rápida
broad ligament of uterus *Supports the uterus on both sides.*	ligamento ancho del útero
Brodie's knee *Also referred to as chronic hypertrophic synovitis of the knee.*	rodilla de Brodie
broken (arm)	brazo fracturado
bromidrosis *Foul smelling perspiration.*	bromhidrosis
bromism *Poisoning caused by excessive intake of bromine.*	bromismo
bronchial carcinoma *A general term for a malignancy of the bronchi.*	carcinoma broncogénico
bronchial *Referring to the bronchus.*	bronquial
bronchiectasis *The presence of abnormally wide bronchi or branches.*	bronquiectasia
bronchiole *A small branch that a bronchus divides into.*	bronquiolo
bronchiolitis *Inflammation of the pulmonary bronchioles.*	bronquiolitis
bronchitis *Inflammation of the mucous membranes of the bronchioles that causes bronchospasm and cough.*	bronquitis
bronchogenic *Referring to the bronchi.*	broncogénico (a)
bronchography *Roentgenography of the bronchi after administration of contrast media.*	broncografía
bronchopneumonia *Pneumonia that starts in the distal bronchioles.*	bronconeumonía
bronchoscopy *Use of a scope to visualize the bronchi.*	broncoscopía
bronchospasm *Bronchial smooth muscle spasm.*	bronceospasmo
bronchus *The major air channels that bifurcate from the distal trachea.*	bronquio
brow presentation *The term used to describe which part of the body (forehead) is being delivered first in childbirth.*	presentación frontal del feto
brown	café
Brown-Séquard syndrome *Unilateral spinal cord lesions, proprioception loss and weakness occur ipsilateral to the lesion, while pain and temperature loss occur contralateral.*	síndrome de Brown Séquard
brucellosis *A gram-negative bacteria in cattle that causes persistent fever in humans.*	brucelosis
bruise	contusión
bruit *An abnormal sound heard through a stethoscope indicating turbulent blood flow.*	ruido
brush	cepillo
bubo *An inflamed, swollen lymph node in the axilla or inguinal region.*	bubón

English	Spanish
bubonic plague *A form of plague exhibited by the formation of buboes.*	peste bubónica
buccal *Referring to the cheek.*	bucal
buccinator *A thin, flat muscle in the cheek wall.*	buccinador
buccinator muscle *Pulls the mouth posteriorly.*	músculo buccinador
bug	bicho
bulbar palsy *Paralysis due to changes in the motor center of the medulla oblongata.*	parálisis bulbar progresiva
bulging	protuberancia
bulimia *Pathologic increase in hunger.*	bulimia
bulky	voluminoso
bulla *A large cutaneous serous filled vesicle.*	ampolla
bullous pemphigoid *A benign disease of the aged characterized by large bullae forming on the torso and extremities.*	penfigoide ampollar
Bumke's pupil *Dilation of the pupil in response to anxiety.*	pupilo de Bumke
bundle branch block *A cardiac dysrhythmia produced by a blockage of a branch of the bundle of His.*	bloque de rama
bundle of His *The atrial contraction rhythm is facilitated by this bundle to the ventricles.*	manojo de His
bunion *Swelling of the bursa of the metatarsal head of the first metatarsal.*	bunio
burn	quemadura
burr	abrojo
burr hole *A treatment of subdural hematoma that involves drilling a hole into the cranium to release the hematoma.*	agujero de buril
bursitis *Inflammation of the bursa.*	bursitis
burst, to	reventar
buttocks	nalgas
Buzzard maneuver *Testing of the patellar reflex while the client firmly touches the floor with their toes in a sitting position.*	maniobra de Buzzard
bypass	baipás
byssinosis *A disease caused by inhalation of cotton dust; a type of pneumoconiosis.*	bisinosis
cachexia *Generalized weakness and severe wasting.*	caquexia
cadaver *A dead body.*	cadáver
caduceus *An ancient herald's wand with two serpents twined around that is a symbol of the medical arts.*	caduceo
caisson disease *Decompression sickness.*	enfermedad de los cajones
calcaneal spur *A bony protrusion on the calcaneus.*	espolón calcáneo
calcaneus *Commonly called the heel bone.*	calcáneo
calcareous *Referring to something containing lime or calcium.*	calcáreo
calcemia *The presence of an abundance of calcium in the blood.*	calcemia
calciferol *It is formed when egesterol is exposed to ultraviolet light; a D vitamin.*	calciferol
calcification *Deposition of calcium salts causing hardening of an organic tissue.*	calcificación
calcitonin *A thyroid hormone that lowers serum calcium levels.*	calcitonina
calcium *A chemical element that is an essential component in teeth and bone.*	calcio

40

English	Spanish
calcium channel blocker *A medication used to treat angina, supraventricular arrhythmias and hypertension; it works by blocking calcium influx into myocytes and vascular smooth muscle cells.*	bloqueador de los canales de calcio
calculus *A stone of minerals that can lead to the blockage of the bile duct or ureters.*	cálculo
calf	pantorrilla
calibrate, to *To adjust an instrument using a standard.*	calibrar
calibration *The process of calibrating an instrument.*	calibrado
callosity *Callus; thickened hardened skin.*	callosidad
callus *Thickened hardened skin.*	callo
calorie *A unit of heat.*	caloría
calvaria *The portion of the skull that is composed of the superior aspects of the occipital, parietal and frontal bones.*	calvaría
calvaria *The superior portions of the frontal, parietal and occipital bones.*	bóveda craneal
calyx *A cup shaped organ or cavity.*	calyx
canaliculus *A term for various small channels.*	canalículo
cancel, to	cancelar
cancellous *A bony mesh-like structure with many pores.*	cancellus
cancellous bone *Describing the cancellous interior of bone.*	hueso cancellus
cancer; carcinoma *A disease of uncontrolled abnormal cell growth.*	cáncer
cancroid *A tumor occurring in the stomach, small or large bowel.*	cancroide
cancrum oris *Gangrenous stomatitis.*	cancrum oris
candle	candela
canine teeth *Located between the incisors and premolars.*	canino dientes
canker sore *An ulceration, usually of the mouth or lips.*	afta
cannabis *A plant from the Cannibidaceae family that is known for its psychotropic effects.*	canabis
cannula *A tube inserted into the body.*	cánula
cantering rhythm *Gallop rhythm.*	ritma de galope
capillary *A vessel that connects arterioles to venules.*	capilar
capillary fragility test *Application of a blood pressure cuff high enough to restrict venous return and after five minutes count the number or petechiae produced.*	prueba de capilar fragilidad
capillary nevus *A growth of skin that involves the capillaries.*	nevo capilar
capitate bone *The bone at the base of the palm that articulates with the third metacarpal.*	capitado
Caplan nodules *These are pulmonary nodules noted in people with rheumatoid arthritis who were exposed to coal dust.*	nódulo de Caplan
capsule	cápsula
capsulitis *Inflammation of a capsule.*	capsulitis
capsulotomy *Incision of a capsule as in with eye surgery.*	capsulotomía
caput *The head.*	caput
caput succedaneum *Edema that occurs in the scalp of an infant during child-birth.*	caput succedaneum
carbohydrate *A group of organic compounds including sugar and starch.*	carbohidrato
carbon dioxide gas	dióxido de carbono
carbon monoxide poisoning *This tasteless, odorless gas causes constitutional symptoms but can lead to death upon inhalation.*	tóxico monóxido de carbono

41

English	Spanish
carboxyhemoglobin *A compound formed from hemoglobin when it is exposed to carbon monoxide.*	caboxihemoglobina
carcinogenic *That which causes cancer.*	carcinogénico, carcinogénica
carcinoid *A tumor occurring in the stomach, intestine and colon.*	carcinoide
carcinoma *A malignant growth.*	carcinoma
carcinomatosis *Dissemination of cancer throughout the body.*	carcinomatosis
cardia *The superior aspect of the stomach at the opening of the esophagus.*	cardias
cardiac *Referring to the heart.*	cardíaco, cardíaca
cardiac arrest *Cessation of function of the heart.*	paro cardíaco
cardiac failure *Decreased cardiac output of the heart.*	insuficiencia cardíaca
cardiac output *Amount of blood pumped by the heart in liters per minute.*	rendimiento cardíaco
cardiac pacing *Electromechanical stimulation of the heart.*	estimulación artificial
cardiology *A specialty of medical practice involve treatment and prevention of heart disease.*	cardiología
cardiomyopathy *Chronic cardiac muscle disease.*	cardiomiopatía
cardiorespiratory assistance *Use of artificial means to support respiration and circulation.*	rusucitación cardiopulmonar
cardiovascular *Referring to the heart or circulatory system.*	cardiovascular
carditis *Inflammation of the heart.*	carditis
caregiver	asistente de salud
caries *Referring to decay or death of a tooth.*	caries
carina *The protrusion of the lowest tracheal cartilage.*	carina
carneous *Synonym of fleshy.*	cárneo
carotene *A hydrocarbon that can be converted to vitamin A.*	caroteno
carotid body *Carotid artery receptors that are sensitive to blood chemistry changes.*	glomo carotídeo
carotid bruit *An abnormal noise heard over the carotid artery that may be a sign of stenosis or aortic valvular disease.*	ruido carotídeo
carotid sinus syncope *Dizziness and syncope that results from hyperactivity of the carotid sinus reflex.*	síncope del seno carotídeo
carotid *Referring to the large artery on each side of the neck.*	carótida
carpal tunnel syndrome *Paresthesia that results from compression of the median nerve.*	síndrome del tunel del carpio
carpometacarpal *Referring to the carpus and metacarpus.*	carpometacarpiano
carpopedal spasm *A spasm of the carpus and the foot.*	espasmo carpopedal
carpus *The joint between the hand and wrist.*	carpo
caruncle *A small fleshy protuberance.*	carúncula
casein *The principal protein in milk, a phospholipid.*	caseína
Casoni's test *Hydatid fluid is injected intradermally; subsequent formation of a larger papule indicates hydatid disease.*	prueba intradérmica de Casoni
cast; plaster cast	vaciado; vaciado de yeso
castor bean *A bean that can yield the poisonous compound ricin.*	ricino
castration *Excision of the gonads.*	castriación
casualty	victima de accidente
cat cry syndrome *A hereditary congenital disorder exhibited by microcephaly, hypertelorism, and cognitive deficits.*	síndrome del maullido de gato

English	Spanish
cat scratch fever *An infectious disease characterized by local inflammation a the site of the scratch, local lymph adenopathy and fever.*	enfermedad causada por rasguño de gato
catabolism *The reduction of complex molecules to more simple ones in living organisms.*	catabolismo
catalepsy *A condition exhibited by rigidity and the person maintains the same position if he is moved by another.*	catalepesia
cataphoresis *The use of an electric field to move charged particles in fluid.*	cataforesis
cataplexy *A condition exhibited by rigidity and immobility.*	cataplejía
cataract *An opacity of an eye lens or the capsule.*	cataracta
catarrh *Inflammation of a mucous membrane.*	catarro
catatonia *Seen in schizophrenia, it is a state of stupor or excitability and abnormal movements.*	catatonía
catch a cold	constipado
catharsis *The act of cleansing or purging, usually referring to thought.*	catarsis
cathartic *To be cleansed or evacuated, referring to thought or the cleansing of the bowels.*	catártico
catheter *A flexible tube inserted into the body.*	catéter, sonda
cat's eye pupil *A pupil in the shape of an oval.*	pupilo de ojo de gato
cauda equina *The roots of the lower spinal nerves.*	cola equina
caudal *Referring to a cauda.*	caudal
caudate *Referring to the caudate nucleus.*	caudado
causative	causativo
caustic *Abrasive or corrosive.*	cáustico, cáustica
cautery *Application of an electric current to cut something.*	cauterio
cavernous hemangioma *A tumor composed of connective tissue with blood filled areas.*	hemangioma cavernosa
cavernous sinus *Large venous sinus located adjacent to the sphenoid bone and posterior to the petrosal sinuses.*	sino carvernoso
cavernous sinus thrombosis *A blood clot in the base of the brain.*	trombosis del seno cavernoso
cavity *Pouch or chamber.*	cavidad
cecum *The portion of the bowel between the ileum and and the ascending colon.*	ciego
celiac *Referring to the abdominal cavity.*	celíaco
cell body	cuerpo celular
cell membrane *The semipermeable structure surrounding the cytoplasm of a cell.*	membrana celular
cell *The smallest functional unit of an organism.*	célula
cell wall	pared celular
cellulitis *Infection characterized by diffuse, subcutaneous inflammation.*	celulitis
cellulose *A polysaccharide that occurs naturally in fibrous products.*	celulosa
center	centro
centigrade *A scale with 100 gradations, usually referring to a temperature scale.*	centígrado
centimeter *One hundredth of a meter.*	centímetro
central nervous system (CNS) *The brain and spinal cord.*	sistema nervioso autonómico (a)
centrifuge *Machine used to separate substances of different weights.*	centrifugadora
centripetal *The movement toward the center.*	centrípeto, centrípeta

43

English	Spanish
cephalic *Towards the head.*	cefálico, cefálica
cercaria *Larval trematode worm that live in a molluscan.*	cercaria
cerebellum *The part of the brain in the posterior portion of the skull that controls muscle coordination and movement.*	cerebelo
cerebral malaria	paludismo cerebral
cerebral palsy *A condition exhibited by motor incoordination and speech changes that is the result of brain injury occurring ante-, intra- or post- partum.*	parálisis cerebral
cerebral *Referring to the cerebrum.*	cerebral
cerebration *Operating activity of the cerebrum.*	cerebración
cerebrospinal fluid (CSF) *The fluid between the pia mater and arachnoid membrane.*	liquido cerebroespinal
cerebrovascular accident (stroke) *A decrease in level of consciousness and paralysis caused by a cerebrovascular thrombosis, hemorrhage or vasospasm.*	cerebrovascular accident
cerumen *Waxy substance found normally in the external ear canals.*	cerumen
Cervical insufficiency (formerly incompetent cervix) *Painless changes in the cervix that result in recurrent second semester pregnancy loss.*	incompetencia del cuello uterino
cervical pleura *The dome-like cap of the pleura.*	capo del cuello uterino
cervical *Referring to the neck or the cervix.*	cervical
cervicectomy *Excision of the cervix uteri.*	cervicectomía
cervicitis *Inflammation of the cervix.*	cervicitis
cervix uteri *The narrow end of the uterus.*	cuello del útero
cesarian section *Incision of the abdominal and uterine walls in order to deliver a fetus when natural delivery is not possible.*	cirugía de parto
cestode *A class of parasitic flatworms.*	cestodo
chancre *The initial ulcer that is the source of entry for a pathogen.*	chancro
chancroid *A sexually transmitted disease caused by Haemophilus ducreyi that is exhibited by ulcers without indurated margins.*	chancroide
check for, to	examinar para
cheek	mejilla
chelating agent *A compound used to bind with metal typically used in the treatment of poisoning.*	agente quelación
chelilitis *Inflammation of the lip.*	queilitis
chemoreceptor *A sense organ that responds to stimuli.*	quimiorreceptora
chemosis *Swelling of conjunctival tissue adjacent to the cornea.*	quemosis
chemotaxis *The response of an organism to chemical agents.*	quimiotaxis
chemotherapy *Use of medication (chemical agents) in the treatment of disease. This term is commonly used to refer to the treatment of cancer patients with medication.*	quimioterapia
chest	tórax, pecho
chest leads	deviación precordiales
chest wall	pared torácica
chest x-ray *Roentography of the thorax.*	rayos X de pecho
chew, to	masticar
Cheyne-Stokes respirations *A breathing pattern characterized by alternating apnea with hyperpnea.*	síndrome de respiración de Cheyne -Stokes
chiasma *The optic chiasma is the area inferior to the hypothalamus where the optic nerves cross.*	quiasma

English	Spanish
chicken pox, varicella *A viral disease characterized by extremely pruritis blisters over the entire body.*	varicella
chigger *A parasitic mite of the genus Trombicula.*	nigua
child	niño
childbirth	parto
childhood	infancia
chill	enfriamiento
chimera *A mixture of genetically distinct tissues.*	quimera
chin	mentón
chiropodist *A doctor trained in the treatment of feet.*	quiropodista
chiropractic *Referring to the medical practice of adjusting malaligned joints.*	quiropráctica
chiropractor *A medical practitioner who is involved with the treatment of disease by manipulating malaligned joints.*	quiropráctico
chlamydiosis *A disease caused by the species Chlamydia.*	clamidiasis
chloasma *Brown or black macula that occur on the face during pregnancy or when there is ovarian dysfunction.*	cloasma
chloroform *A colorless, sweet smelling liquid formerly used as a general anesthetic.*	chloroformo
chloroma *A malignant tumor associated with myelogenous leukemia.*	cloroma
choanae *The two openings between the nasal cavity and the nasopharynx.*	coana
choanal atresia *A congenital condition characterized by blockage of the nasal passages by tissue.*	atresia coanal
choice	elección
choke, to	atragantarse
cholagogue *A compound used to stimulate flow of bile from the liver.*	colagogo
cholangiogram *Radiologic imaging of the gallbladder and bile ducts.*	colangiografía
cholangitis *Inflammation of the bile ducts.*	colangitis
cholecystectomy *Surgical excision of the gallbladder.*	colecistectomía
cholecystenterostomy *Creation of a surgical anastomosis between the intestine and the gallbladder.*	colecistenteronotomía
cholecystitis *Inflammation of the gallbladder.*	colecistitis
cholecystolithiasis *The presence of gallstones in the gallbladder.*	colecistolitiasis
choledocholithotomy *Creation of an incision in the bile duct for the purpose of removing a stone.*	coledocolitomía
cholelithiasis *Presence or creation of gallstones.*	colelitiasis
cholemia *Bile or bile products in the blood.*	colemia
cholera *An infectious disease exhibited by vomiting and diarrhea and caused by Vibrio cholerae.*	cólera
cholestatis hepatitis *Liver inflammation caused by obstruction of bile flow from the liver to the duodenum.*	hepatitis colestática
cholesteatoma *A cystic mass that has a lining made of keratinizing material and cholesterol.*	colesteatoma
cholesterol *A compound or its derivatives are found in cell membranes and precursors to hormones but high levels can cause atherosclerosis.*	colesterol
cholinergic *Referring to the stimulation, activation or transmission of acetylcholine.*	colinérgico
cholinesterase *An esterase used to cleave acetylcholine into choline and acetic acid.*	colinesterasa

45

English	Spanish
choluria *Term indicating the presence of bile in the urine.*	coluria
chondralgia *Cartilaginous pain.*	condralgia
chondritis *Cartilaginous inflammation.*	condritis
chondroma *Cartilaginous hyperplastic growth.*	condroma
chondromalacia *Excessive softening of the cartilages.*	condromalacia
chondromalacia of the patella *Softening of the articular cartilage of the patella.*	condromalacia rotuliana
chondrosarcoma *Cartilaginous tumor which exhibits rapid growth.*	condrosarcoma
chorda *A cord or sinew.*	cuerda
chordee *Downward bending of the penis.*	encordamiento
chorditis *Inflammation of a vocal or spermatic cord.*	corditis
chorea *Involuntary, continuous rapid, jerking movements.*	corea
chorionic villus *Cord-like projections of a fertilized ovum.*	vellosidad coriónicas
choroid *Similar to the chorion (fertilized ovum or zygote)*	coroides
choroiditis *Inflammation of the choroid.*	coroiditis
choroidocyclitis *Inflammation of the ciliary processes and choroid.*	coroidocilitis
chromatin *A desocyribose nucleic acid that carries the genes of inheritance.*	cromatina
chromosome *A structure in the nucleus of living cells that carries genetic information.*	cromosoma
chronic *When referring to an illness, it means recurring or persistent.*	crónico, crónica
chyle *A combination of lymph fluid and fat that enters the blood via the thoracic duct.*	quilo
chylomicron *A one micron particle of emulsified fat.*	quilomicrón
chylous *Referring to chyle.*	quiloso, quilosa
chyme *The gruel produced by gastric digestion.*	quimo
cicatricial *Referring to cicatrix.*	cicatrizal
cicatrix (scar) *New tissue in a healed wound.*	cicatriz
cilia *The hairs growing on the eyelid or a motile extension of a cell surface.*	cilio
ciliary body *The connection between the iris and the choroid.*	cuerpo ciliar
cinchonism *The toxic effects induced by ingestion of cinchona bark; it is exhibited by tinnitus, deafness and cognitive changes.*	cinconismo
circadian *Referring to a 24 hour period.*	circadiano
circadian rhythm *Naturally recurring fluctuations in a 24 hour period.*	ritmo circadiano
circumcision *Surgical excision of the foreskin.*	circuncisión
circumference *The distance around an object or part.*	circunferencia
circumflex nerve *The axillary nerve that has an origin in the posterior branch of the brachial plexus.*	nervio circunflejo
circumscribe *To have well defined borders.*	circunscribir
cirrhosis *A liver disease characterized by destruction of liver cells and increased connective tissue.*	cirrosis
cirsoid *Similar to a tortuous vein, artery or lymph vessel.*	cirsoide
cisternal puncture *A trans-occipitoatlantoid ligament puncture of the cisterna magna so CSF can be obtained.*	punción cisternal
clasp	cierre
clasp knife reflex *The lengthening of the extensor muscles resulting in flexion.*	rigidez en navaja
claudication *Intermittent claudication is a phrase used to describe pain experienced in the leg from arterial insufficiency.*	claudicación

English	Spanish
claustrophobia *An unreasonable fear of being in an enclosed environment.*	claustrofobia
clavicle *A bone that articulates with the sternum and scapula.*	clavícula
clavus *A corn or horny protrusion.*	clavio
clawhand *A hand deformity caused by ulnar nerve palsy exhibited by the hyperextension of the metacarpophalangeal joints and flexion of the interphalangeal articulations.*	mano en garra
clean catch urine specimen *A urine specimen obtained by having a patient cleanse the perineal area prior to voiding in a collection device.*	muestra de orina limpia
clear	claro, clara
clear one's throat, to	carraspear
clearance	aclaramiento
cleavage *A sharp division or demarcation.*	segmentación
cleft lip *A congenital abnormal opening of the lip.*	labio leporino
cleft palate *A congenital abnormal opening in the palate.*	paladar hendido
cleidocranial dysostosis *A congenital condition exhibited by abnormal ossification of the cranial bones and absence of clavicles.*	disostosis cleidocraneal
cleidotomy *A procedure used in difficult deliveries in which the clavicle is broken to facilitate childbirth.*	cleidotomía
click *A sound heard by the sudden closure of a heart valve.*	clic
clinic	clínica
clinical record	hoja clínica
clinical signs *Physical assessment data.*	cuadro clínico
clitoris *A small erectile body in the anterosuperior aspect of the vulva.*	clítoris
clockwise	dirección de las manecillas del reloj
clonic *Referring to a spasm that alternates in rigidity and relaxation.*	clónico
closed	cerrado, cerrada
closed reduction of fractures *The realignment of a fracture without use of surgery.*	reducción cerrada de fracturas
clot *A thrombus or embolus.*	coágulo
clubbing *Increase in the mass of the soft tissue of the terminal phalanges.*	dedo en palillo de tambor
cluster headache *A unilateral, severe, recurrent headache.*	cefalagia de Horton
cnemial *Referring to the shin.*	cnemial
coaching (during labor)	coche durante parto
coagulation *The formation of a clot.*	coagulación
coarctation *A stricture, as in narrowing of the aorta with coarctation of the aorta.*	coartación
coated tablet	comprimido recubierto
cobalt *A metal that with causes polycythemia with increased ingestion.*	cobalto
cocaine *A highly addictive opiate derivative.*	cocaína
cocaine addiction *Physical habituation to cocaine.*	adicción cocaína
coccus *A spherical shaped bacterium.*	coco
coccydynia *Coccygeal pain.*	coccidinia
coccyx *The small bone formed by the natural fusion of rudimentary vertebrae.*	cóccix
cochlea *The essential organ of hearing which is in a spiral form.*	cóclea
cock-up splint *A splint used to maintain the wrist in dorsiflexion; used for carpal tunnel syndrome.*	férula muñeca

English	Spanish
cockroach	cucaracha
cod	bacalao
codeine *A morphine derived analgesic.*	codeína
codon *A series of three nucleotides that form a unit of genetic code.*	codón
coffee-ground emesis	vómito en borra de café
cog wheel *As in cogwheel rigidity which is a jerky passive movement after there was increased tone.*	rigidez en rueda dentada
cognition *The process of acquiring thought or understanding.*	cognición
cognitive disorders *Any disease process that involves altered cognition.*	trastornos cognitivo
coitus *Sexual intercourse between members of the opposite sex.*	coito
cold *Having a sense of being cold.*	frío
cold sore *A perioral blister caused by herpes simplex.*	úlcera de herpes simple
cold *Viral upper respiratory tract infection.*	resfrío
colectomy *Surgical removal of part of the colon.*	colectomía
colic *Acute abdominal pain.*	cólico
colitis *Inflammation of the colon.*	colitis
collagen *The principal supportive protein bone, skin, tendon and cartilage.*	colágeno
collapse	postración
collarbone *Common term for the clavicle.*	clavícula
collodion *A product of the breakdown of colloid.*	colodión
colloid *A solution used for infusion, such as albumin or hetastarch, that are more likely to remain in the intravascular space than crystalloids.*	coloide
coloboma *A congenital defect that involves a fissure of the eye.*	coloboma
colon *The portion of the large intestine that goes from the cecum to the rectum.*	colon
colonoscopy *Inspection the color, ideally to the cecum, with a lighted scope.*	colonoscopía
color blindness *The inability to distinguish colors.*	incapacidad para distinguir colores
color chart	guía colorimétrica
color of conjunctiva *A point of assessment to check for pallor.*	conjunctivo coloración
colostomy bag *A pouch attached to the skin with a mild adhesive that collects stool emitted from a colostomy.*	bolsa de colostomía
colostomy *Surgically creating an opening in the colon that is extended to outside the abdominal wall.*	colostomía
colostrum *The fluid secreted by the mammary glands a few days around parturition.*	colostro
colpitis; *vaginitis Inflammation of the vagina.*	colpitis
colpocele *A hernia into the vagina.*	colpocele
colporrhaphy *A surgical procedure that involves suturing the vagina.*	colporrafia
colposcope *A scope used to visualize the vagina.*	colposcopio
colposcopy *Use of a scope to visualize the vagina and cervix.*	colposcopía
coma *A state of unconsciousness.*	coma
comatose *Referring to a coma.*	comatoso, comatosa
comb	peine
comedones *The medical term for blackheads.*	comedón
commensal *Living in or on another organism without being a detriment.*	comensal
comment	comentario
common *That which is usual.*	común

48

English	Spanish
compatible *To coexist without problems.*	compatible
compendium *A concise summary about a subject.*	compendio
complaint	queja
complement fixation test *A laboratory test for the presence of an antibody in the serum that involves inactivation of the complement in the serum.*	prueba de fijación del complemento
complete blood count *An assay that includes white blood cell, red blood cell, platelet count, hemoglobin, hematocrit and white blood cell differential.*	recuento sanguíneo completo
compliance *The act of going along with a plan.*	conformidad
comply, to	cumplir
compound	compuesto
compound fracture *Open fracture.*	fractura compuesta
comprehension *Understanding.*	comprensión
compression	compresión
concavity *The state of being concave.*	concavidad
concentration	concentración
concentric *Referring to circles or arcs that share the same center.*	concéntrico
conception *The act of an egg being fertilized by sperm.*	concepción
concha *A part of the body that is spiral shaped. Nasal concha are the small bones in the sides of the nasal cavity.*	cornete
concretion *A hard solid mass.*	concreción
concussion *Head trauma resulting in temporary loss of consciousness.*	concusión, conmoción cerebral
condom *A covering for the penis or the vagina (female condom) used during sexual intercourse that is meant to reduce the chance of pregnancy or infection.*	condón
condyle *A rounded protrusion of a bone.*	cóndilo
condyloma *A warty papule near the anus or vulva.*	condiloma
cone	cono
confabulation *The fabrication of experiences to compensate for memory loss.*	confabulación
confidence	confianza
confinement	restricción
conflict	conflicto
confusion	confusión
congenital *A disease or anomaly present from birth.*	congénito, congénita
congenital heart disease *A cardiac disorder present prior to birth.*	anomalía congénito cárdiaca
congenital syphilis *Passed to the child in utero, the child may have failure to thrive, fever and a flattened bridge of the nose.*	sífilis congénita
congestive	congestivo, congestiva
congestive heart failure *A diminished cardiac output leading to passive engorgement.*	insuficiencia cardíaca congestiva
conjugate diameter *A pelvic inlet measurement used to determine whether a woman is capable of delivering a fetus vaginally.*	diámetro conjugado del estrecho inferior de la pelvis
conjunctiva *The membrane that lines the eyelid.*	conjuntiva
conjunctivitis *Inflammation of the conjunctiva.*	conjuntivitis
consanguinity *The relationship by blood.*	consanguinidad
conscious *Being award and being able to respond to one's surroundings.*	consciente
conservative	conservativo

49

English	Spanish
consistent	consistente
consolidation *An area of fixed secretions in the lung.*	consolidación
constipation *A condition exhibited by difficulty in having a bowel movement due to hard stools.*	estreñimiento
constriction	constricción
contact	contacto
contact lenses	lentes de contacto
contagious *Description of a disease that can be spread by direct or indirect contact.*	contagioso, contagiosa
contaminate, to	contaminar
content	contenido
contraceptive *A device or medication used to prevent pregnancy.*	contraceptivo
contradictory	contradictorio
contraindication	contradicción
contusion *An area of broken capillaries in the skin causing discoloration; commonly called a bruise.*	contusión
convenient	conveniente
conversion *When referring to a psychiatric condition it is the exhibition of physical symptoms as a manifestation of mental disease.*	trastorno de conversión
convex *Having an exterior curved the outside of a sphere.*	convexo, convexa
convulsion *An involuntary series of tonic and clonic movements.*	convulsión
cool	frío
cope with, to	poder con
copper	cobre
copra itch *A pruritis noted in people working with copra (dried kernel from a coconut).*	prurito por copra
copulation *Sexual relations.*	copulación
cor pulmonale *Heart disease that is secondary to lung disease.*	cor pulmonale
coracoid *A prominence on the scapula to which the biceps is attached.*	coracoides
cord compression *Pressure being applied to the spinal cord.*	compresión de la médula espinal
core	centro
cornea *The transparent segment located at the anterior part of the eye.*	córnea
corneal *Referring to the cornea.*	corneal
corneal transplant *Surgical replacement of a cornea with a donor cornea.*	trasplante corneal
coronal suture *The line of intersection of the frontal bone and the two parietal bones.*	sutura coronal
coronary angiography *Roentgenographic visualization of the coronary vessels after injection of dye.*	angiografía coronaria
coronary occlusion *A blockage in a coronary artery.*	oclusión coronaria
coronary vessel *Referring to a coronary artery.*	arteria coronaria
coroner *A person who investigates sudden or suspicious deaths.*	médico forense
coronoid *Crown-shaped.*	coronoide
corpulence *Fatness.*	obesidad
corpus callosum *A point of connection between the two cerebral hemispheres.*	cuerpo calloso
corpus luteum *A structure that is discharged from an ovary; it degenerates if it is not impregnated.*	corpus luteum
corpuscle *A red or white blood cell.*	corpúsculo

English	Spanish
cortex *An external layer.*	corteza, córtex
cortical *Referring to the cortex.*	cortical
corticosteroid *A hormone developed in the adrenal cortex.*	corticoesteroide
corticotropin *A hormone of the adrenal cortex.*	corticotropina
cortisol *An adrenal cortical hormone, also called hydrocortisone.*	cortisol
cortisone *An adrenal cortical hormone responsible for carbohydrate regulation.*	cortisona
coryza *An acute condition exhibited by copious nasal discharge.*	coriza
cost	costo
costochondritis *Inflammation of the rib and or its cartilage.*	costocondritis
cotton wool	algodón
cough	tos
coughing fit	tos seca recurrente
count, to	contar
cowpox; vaccinia *A viral disease of cows that was used for an original smallpox vaccine.*	viruela bovina
cow's milk	leche de vaca
coxalgia *Pain in the hip.*	coxalgia
crab louse *Phthirus pubis is formal name for a louse that infests pubic hair and causes intense itching.*	ladilla
crack one's knuckles	tronarse los nudillos
cradle	cuna
cramp	calambre
cranial mononeuropathy III *Dysfunction of the third cranial nerve causes double vision and eyelid drooping.*	mononeurapatía del III par craneal
cranial mononeuropathy VI *A disorder of the sixth cranial nerve causes double vision.*	mononeuropatía del VI par craneal
cranial *Referring to the skull.*	craneal
cranioclast *An instrument used to crush a fetal skull.*	craneoclasto
craniopharyngioma *A tumor that originates in the hypophyseal stalk.*	craneofaringioma
craniosynostosis *Closure of the sutures of the skull that occurs prematurely.*	craneosinostosis
craniotabes *Softening of the skull bones causing widened sutures; this occurs in rickets.*	craneotabes
craniotomy *Surgical creation of a hole in the skull.*	craneotomía
cranium *The skeleton of the head.*	cráneo
craving	ansia
craw-craw *A pruritic papular skin eruption sometimes caused by Onchocerca.*	kra-kra
creatine *A compound involved with muscle contraction.*	creatina
creatinine *A compound excreted in the urine that is produced by the metabolism of creatine.*	creatinina
Credé's maneuver *Manual pressure over the bladder to assist in expression of urine in an atonic bladder.*	maniobra de Credé
crenotherapy *A form of treatment from mineral springs.*	crenoterapia
crepitus *A noise heard when one auscultates the lungs that is similar to the sound of rubbing hair between one's fingers. It is also considered the sound of two broken bones rubbing together.*	chasquido crujido
cretinism *A chronic condition caused by diminished thyroid hormone secretion.*	cretinismo
crevice *A narrow opening.*	grieta

English	Spanish
cribriform *Like a sieve; the olfactory nerves pass through the cribriform plate of the ethmoid bone.*	cribiforme
cricoid *The ring-shaped cartilage of the larynx*	cricoideo
cripple	lisiado, lisiada
crisis *Seizure.*	ataque convulsivo
Crohn's disease *An inflammatory bowel disease.*	Crohn, enfermedad de
cross-infection *Transfer of infection between individuals, each with a different organism.*	infección cruzada
cross-matching (blood) *Evaluation of blood to determine compatibility between the donor and recipient prior to transfusion.*	pruebas sanguíneas cruzadas
cross-section	sección transversal
croup *An acute laryngeal condition that is accompanied by a hoarse, barking cough.*	crup
cruciform *Shaped like a cross.*	cruciforme
crural; femoral *Referring to the femur or leg.*	crural
crush syndrome *Rhabdomyolysis occurring as a result of muscle injury from mechanical stress.*	síndrome de aplastamiento
crust	costra
crutches	muletas
cryesthesia *Abnormal sensitivity to cold.*	criestesia
cryosurgery *The application of extreme cold to destroy tissue.*	criocirugía
cryotherapy *The use of cold for therapeutic purposes.*	crioterapia
cryptococcal meningitis *A meningeal infection associated with AIDS.*	menitgitis criptocóccica
cryptorchism *A condition characterized by the failure of the testes to descend into the scrotum.*	criptorquismo
cryptosporidiosis *A parasitic related diarrhea seen in AIDS.*	criptosporidiosis
crystalloid *A substance that can pass through a semipermeable membrane; not a colloid.*	cristaloide
crystalluria *The presence of crystals in the urine.*	cristaluria
CSF *Abbreviation for cerebrospinal fluid.*	LCR líquido cefalorraquídeo
CT scan *Computerized axial tomography.*	tomografía axial computarizada
cubic millimeter *A unit of volume.*	mililitro cúbico
cubitus *1. The bend at the elbow. 2. Ulna.*	cubitus
cuffed tube *A cannula that has an balloon on the tip that can be inflated with air or fluid.*	tubo balón Inflable esférico utilizado para retenertubos o catéteres.
culdoscopy *Examination of the female pelvic viscera with a scope inserted through the posterior vaginal fornix.*	culdoscopía
culture *The growth of bacteria in artificial medium.*	cultivo
culture broth *A medium used to grow bacteria.*	medio de cultivo
cumulative effect *A consequence of successive additions.*	efecto acmulativo
cuneiform *The three bones between the navicular bone and the metatarsals.*	cuneiforme
curare *A toxic botanical substance used at one time in poison darts in South America.Curare derivatives have been used in general anesthesia.*	curare
curative *A remedy capable of healing completely.*	curativo
cure	curación

English	Spanish
curettage *Removal of tissues from a cavity.*	curetaje
curette *The instrument used during a curettage.*	cureta
current	corriente
currently	actualmente
Cushing's syndrome *Characterized by trunkal obesity, moon face, acne, abdominal striae, hypertension, decreased carbohydrate tolerance, protein catabolism, psychiatric disturbances, and osteoporosis.*	síndrome de Cushing
cushion	cojinete
cut	cortada
cutaneous *Referring to the skin.*	cutáneo, cutánea
cuticle *The dead skin at the base of the toenail or fingernail, also called the eponychium.*	cuticula
cyanocobalamin *Also called B12; used to treat pernicious and other macrocytic anemias.*	cianocobalamina
cyanosis *Bluish discoloration of the skin and mucous membranes.*	cianosis
cyclical vomiting *Periods of recurrent vomiting with no apparent pathologic cause and the person has a normal state of health between the episodes.*	vómito psicógeno
cyclitis *Inflammation of the ciliary body.*	ciclica
cyclodialysis *The surgical creation of a communication between the anterior chamber of the eye and the suprachorodial space for the purpose of treating glaucoma.*	ciclodiálisis
cycloplegia *Paralysis of the ciliary muscle.*	cicloplejía
cyclothymia *Manic-depressive tendencies.*	ciclotimia
cyclotomy *Surgically creating an opening in the ciliary body.*	ciclotomía
cystadenoma *Adenoma associated with cysts of neoplastic origin.*	cistadenoma
cystectomy *Surgical removal of a cyst or the bladder.*	cistectomía
cystic *Referring to a cyst.*	cistico, cistica
cystic duct *The duct connecting the gallbladder to the common bile duct.*	conducto cistico
cystic fibrosis *A congenital disorder exhibited by abnormal thick mucous which leads to problems in the intestines, pancreas and lungs.*	fibrosis cistica
cysticercosis *The state of being infected with a type of tapeworm.*	cisticercosis
cystinosis *A congenital disorder of increased cystine that leads to renal insufficiency, rickets and dwarfism.*	cistinosis
cystinuria *The presence of cystine in the urine.*	cistinuria
cystitis *Inflammation of the urinary bladder.*	cistitis
cystocele *Protrusion of the urinary bladder through the vaginal wall.*	cistocele
cystography *Roentgenographic visualization of the urinary bladder after insertion of contrast media.*	cistografía
cystolithiasis *Presence of a calculus in the urinary bladder.*	cistolitiasis
cystoscope *A device used to visualized the urinary bladder.*	cistoscopio
cystoscopy *Direct visualization of the urinary bladder with a cystoscope.*	cistoscopía
cytology *The study of cells, their function and structure.*	citología
cytoplasm *The protoplasm of the cell except for the nucleus.*	citoplasma
cytotoxic *Referring to being harmful to cells.*	citotóxica
cytotoxin *That which is harmful to cells.*	citotoxina
dacryoadenitis *Inflammation of the lacrimal gland.*	dacriadenitis
dacryocystitis *Inflammation of a lacrimal sac.*	dacriocistitis

English	Spanish
dacryocystorhinostomy *Surgical reaction of a communication between the lacrimal sac and nasal cavity.*	dacriocistorrinostomía
dacryolith *A stone in the lacrimal sac or duct.*	dacriolito
dandruff *Dead skin found in the hair.*	caspa
dark adaptation *Adjustment to low light by reflex dilation of the pupil.*	adaptacióna la oscuridad
date of admission	día de ingreso
date of birth	fecha de nacimiento
daughter	hija
De Quervain tenosynovitis *Inflammation of the tendons of the wrist including the abductor pollicis longus and extensor pollicis brevis.*	tendinitis de De Quervain
dead	muerto, muerta
dead space *The area in the respiratory tract where air is not exchanged.*	espacio muerto
deadline	fecha
deaf	sordo, sorda
deaf-mute	sordomudo, sordomuda
deafness	sordera
death	muerte
debility *Physical weakness.*	debilidad
debridement	desbridamiento
decade	década
decapitation *The physical separation of the head from the body.*	decapitación
decerebrate rigidity *Rigid extension of the arms which is an abnormal posture associated with increased intracranial pressure.*	rigidez de descerebración
decerebrate *The removal of the brain.*	descerebrado
decibel *A unit used in the measurement of sound.*	decilbelio
decidua *The mucous membrane lining the uterus during pregnancy.*	decidua
deciduous teeth *The first teeth.*	primera dentición
decline	declinación
decompensation *The inability of an organ to respond to functional overload.*	descompensación
decompression *The surgical procedure relieving pressure on a part.*	descompresión
decrease	disminución
decubitus ulcer *A wound caused by laying in one position for too long; also referred to as a pressure ulcer.*	úlcera por decúbito
decussation *An area of intersection.*	cruzamiento
deep	profundo, profunda
deep tendon reflex *Reflexes exhibited by the stretching of a tendon.*	reflejo tendinoso profundo
deep vein thrombosis (DVT) *A blood clot that forms within a vein, typically in the lower extremities.*	trombosis venosa profunda (TVP)
deer tick	garrapata de venado
defecation *The discharge of feces from the rectum.*	defecación
defect	defecto
defibrillator *A device used to convert an abnormal cardiac rhythm (ventricular fibrillation) into a normal rhythm with use of electrical stimulation.*	desfibrilador
deficiency	deficiencia
deformity	deformidad

English	Spanish
deglutition *The process of swallowing.*	deglución
dehydration	deshidratación
delirium *An acute mental state exhibited by altered thought processes and restlessness.*	delirium
delirium tremens *A condition seen when alcohol is withdrawn which is exhibited by restlessness, hallucinations and tremors.*	delirium tremens
deliver, to (as in, to give birth)	partear
deltoid *A term referring to "three". The deltoid muscle has its origin at three areas: clavicle, acromion, and spine of the scapula.*	deltoideo, deltoidea
delusion *A belief that is contradictory to rational thought.*	delirio
delusional *Referring to a delusion.*	delusorio
demanding	exigente
demarcation *Having a fixed boundary.*	demarcación
dementia *A chronic brain disorder exhibited by memory loss, personality changes and faulty reasoning.*	demencia
demography *The study of the structure of human populations.*	demografía
demulcent *Something that relieves irritation or inflammation.*	demulcente
demyelinating disease *A condition characterized by the loss of myelin.*	enfermedad desmielinizante
dendrite *Impulses are transmitted along a dendrite to a nerve cell body.*	dendrita
denervated *To remove nerve supply.*	desnervado
dengue *A mosquito-borne viral disease exhibited by fever and joint pain.*	dengue
density *The denseness of an object.*	densidad
dental *Referring to teeth.*	dental
dental calculus *Calcium phosphate and carbonate adhered to the teeth.*	cálculo dentario
dental caries *Decay of teeth.*	caries dentales
dentatum *Also referred to as nucleus dentatus.*	dentado
dentist *A professional capable of treating diseases of the teeth and gums.*	dentista
dentition *The natural teeth.*	dentición
denture *A frame that holds artificial teeth.*	dentadura
deny, to	negar
deoxyribonucleic acid (DNA) *The carrier of genetic information.*	ácido desoxirribonucleico
depilatory *An agent used to remove hair.*	depilatorio
depressed	deprimido, deprimida
depression *A medical condition exhibited by profound despondency.*	depresión
deprivation *The lack of a necessity.*	depravación
dermatitis *Non-specific inflammation of the skin.*	dermatitis
dermatography *A description of the skin.*	dermatografía
dermatologist *A physician specializing in dermatology.*	dermatólogo
dermatology *The medical profession involving the treatment of skin conditions.*	dermatología
dermatome *The area of sensation of the skin supplied by a single posterior spinal root.*	dermatoma
dermatomycosis *An infection of the skin by Trichophyton, Microsporum or Epidermophyton fungi.*	dermatomicosis
dermatomyositis *Inflammation of the skin, subcutaneous tissue and adjacent muscle.*	dermatomiositis
dermatophyte *A fungal parasite living on the skin.*	dermatófito

English	Spanish
dermatosis *Any skin disease.*	dermatosis
dermis *The "true skin" that lies beneath the epidermis.*	dermis, piel
dermographia *A raised, pale line with hyperemic borders is elicited upon scratching the skin with a dull instrument, in this condition.*	dermografía
dermoid cyst *An abnormal growth containing hair follicles, skin and sebaceous glands.*	quiste de secuestración
descending	descendente
desensitize, to *To gradually expose a person to an offending agent to prevent an abnormal response upon a secondary exposure.*	desensibilizar
desiccation *The act of drying up.*	desecación
desmoid *A tumor typically found in the abdomen which contains. muscle and connective tissue.*	desmoide
despite	despecho
desquamation *The shedding of skin in flakes or sheets.*	descamación
deterioration	deterioración
detoxification *The process of removing toxins from the body.*	destoxificación
detrimental *Harmful.*	perjudicial
detritus *Particulate matter produced by the decomposition of an organic substance.*	detrito
detrusor urinae *Smooth muscle fibers that extend from the urinary bladder to the pubis.*	detrusor urinario
deuteranomaly *Abnormal color vision sometimes called "green weakness".*	deuteranomalía
deviated septum *Characterized by deviation of the nasal septum.*	tabique nasal desviado
deviation *Away from the norm.*	desviación
dexter; *right; straight; erect*	diestro
dextran *A high glucose polymer used as a plasma substitute.*	dextráa
dextrocardia *Location of the heart in the right hemithorax.*	dextrocardía
dhobie itch *So called because the contact dermatitis is caused by the soap used by laundry workers in India who are called "dhobie".*	prurito dhobie Tiña cruris
diabetes insipidus *Caused by a deficiency in vasopressin, it is exhibited by great thirst and large volume urine output (and normal blood sugar).*	diabetes insípidia nefrógena
diabetes mellitus *A disease exhibited by a deficiency of the pancreatic hormone insulin.*	diabetes mellitus
diabetic *A person who has diabetes mellitus.*	diabético, diabética
diabetic neuropathy	neuropatía diabética
diagnostic *A specific symptom or characteristic.*	diagnóstico
diapedesis *The outward passage of blood elements through an intact vessel wall.*	diapédesis
diaper	pañal
diaper rash	eritema de los pañales
diaphoretic *Exhibited by profuse perspiration.*	diaforético
diaphragm *The muscular separation between the thoracic and abdominal cavities.*	diafragma
diaphragmatic hernia *Protrusion of visceral contents through the diaphragm.*	hernia diafragmática
diaphysis *The central part of a long bone.*	diáfisis
diarrhea *Increase in frequency and a loose consistency of the stools.*	diarrea
diarthrosis *An articulation allowing free movement.*	diartrosis
diastase *Amylase.*	diastasa

English	Spanish
diastole *The period of dilatation of the heart; between the first and second heart sounds.*	diástole
diathermy *The use of heat produced from high-frequency electric currents to medically or surgically treat someone.*	diatermia
diathesis *A medical tendency to develop a specific condition.*	diástesis
die, to	morir
diet	dieta, régimen
dietitian *A professional who works with diet and nutrition.*	dietista
differential *A term used to refer to the various options for diagnoses.*	diferencial
differential diagnosis *A list of possible alternative diagnoses for a patient who is ill.*	diagnóstico diferencial
differential leukocyte count *The percentage of different types of leukocytes.*	recuento sanguíneo diferencial de glóbulos blancos
digestion *The process of enzymatic breakdown of food in the alimentary canal.*	digestión
digit *Finger.*	dedo
digitalis *Cardiac medication derived from the leaf of Digitalis purpurea.*	digitalis
dilatation *The process of becoming wider or larger.*	dilatación
dilator *An instrument that dilates.*	dilatador
dilution *The process of making a weaker solution.*	dilución
dimercaprol *A medication used as a binding agent for heavy metal poisoning.*	dimercaprol
dioptre *Referring to refraction or transmitted and refracted light.*	dioptría
dioxide *A compound containing two oxygen atoms.*	dióxido
diphtheria *A contagious bacterial disease characterized by a grey membrane on the pharynx along with respiratory or cutaneous symptoms; caused by Corynebacterium diphtheriae.*	difteria
diplegia *The paralysis of both arms or both legs.*	diplejía
diplococcus *A bacterium that occurs in pairs including pneumococcus and Neisseria gonorrhoeae and Neisseria meningitidis.*	diplococo
diploid *A nucleus containing two complete sets of chromosomes.*	diploide
diplopia *Double vision.*	diplopía
dipsomania *Twins that are joined at some part of their bodies.*	dipsomanía
dirty	sucio, sucia
disability	incapacidad
disaccharide *A type of sugar that yields two monosaccharides upon hydrolysis.*	disacárido
disappearance	desaparecimiento
disarticulation *The separation or amputation of a joint.*	desarticulación
discharge date	fecha de alta
discomfort	incomodidad
discrete	discreto
disease	enfermedad
disease outcome *The response obtained from treatment.*	resultado clínico
disequilibrium *The absence of stability.*	desequilibrio
disinfectant *A substance that kills bacteria.*	desinfectante
dislocation *The displacement of a bone when referring to an articulation.*	luxación, dislocación
disorder *Impairment.*	desarreglo
disorientation *Mental confusion.*	desorientación

English	Spanish
displacement *Movement from normal position.*	desplazamiento
disrobe, to	desnudar
dissecting aneurysm *A condition in which blood is present between the layers of an artery.*	aneurisma di-secante
dissection	disección
dissemination *To be spread or dispersed widely.*	diseminación
dissolution *Disintegration.*	disolución
distal *Situated away from the center of the body.*	distal
distended bladder *Urinary bladder filled beyond the normal capacity.*	distensión vesical
distension *Swollen.*	distención
distichiasis *Presence of two rows of eyelashes on one eyelid which are turned inward toward the globe.*	distiquia
distribution	distribución
diuresis *Increased excretion of urine.*	diuresis
diuretic *Medication which causes an increased excretion of urine.*	diurético
diurnal *Occurring during the day.*	diurno, diurna
diverticulitis *Inflammation of the diverticulum.*	diverticulitis
diverticulosis *Presence of diverticulum.*	diverticulosis
diverticulum *A sac or pouch created by herniation of a mucous membrane in the alimentary canal.*	divertículo
diving	buceo
dizygotic twins *Twins from two separate zygotes (non-identicle twins).*	gemelos dicigóticos
dizziness *Sensation of losing one's balance.*	mareo
DNA Deoxyribonucleic acid. *The hereditary material in humans and almost all other organisms.*	ácido desoxirribonucleico
DNR Do not resuscitate. *The term used to indicate a person should not have life sustaining measures taken if they were to have cardiopulmonary arrest.*	NR no resucitar
donor *Referring to a person who donates tissue or an organ.*	persona contribuyente
dopa reaction *A dopa-oxidase reaction, changing dopa into melanin.*	reacción dopa
dopamine *An intermediate product in the creation of norepinephrine.*	dopamina
dorsal *Referring to the back or back surface.*	dorsal
dorsal root *A description of the site of ganglion found on the dorsal root of each spinal nerve.*	raíz dorsal
dorsiflexion *Backward bending of the foot or hand.*	dorsiflexión
dorsum *The back part.*	dorso
dosage *The frequency and amount of a medication.*	dosis
dose regimen *The amount, frequency and length of treatment of a medication.*	régimen medicina
dose *The quantity of a medication.*	dosis
dosing interval *The number of times per unit a medication is given.*	intervalo medicina
double	doble
douche *Cleansing of a canal; unless otherwise specified it refers to cleansing of the vaginal canal.*	ducha
Douglas' pouch *A recess in the peritoneum between the rectum and the uterus. Also called the rectouterine pouch.*	excavació rectouternia
down	abajo
Down's syndrome *A congenital chromosomal defect (trisomy 21) that caused diminished intellectual function, short stature and a broad face.*	síndrome de Down
drainage tube *A cannula used to allow outflow of fluids.*	tubo de drenaje

58

English	Spanish
drape *The fabric used as a sterile covering in the OR.*	campo
drawsheet *The topsheet of a bed.*	zalea
dream	sueño
dressing *The gauze applied to a wound.*	vendaje, apósito
dribble	goteo
drill	taladro
drink, to	beber
drinking water	agua potable
drop	gota
drop by drop	gota a gota
drop foot gait *A gait characterized by dragging the foot, as there is no ankle dorsiflexion.*	marcha pie caído
drop foot *The symptom in a person with a nerve injury causing impaired ankle dorsiflexion.*	pie caído
dropper *A device used to administer medicines one drop at a time.*	gotero
drops per minute	gota por minuto
drowning	ahogamiento
drowsiness	sopor
drug	droga
drug dependence *Addiction to a substance.*	abuso de drogas
drug eruption *A diffuse rash caused by a medication.*	erupción por drogas
drug reaction	reacción por drogas
drunk *Inebriated.*	borracho
dry	seco
dual diagnosis *Term used to describe the presence of alcohol/drug addiction associated with a psychiatric diagnosis such as depression.*	diagnóstico doble
duct	conducto
ductus arteriosus *A fetal artery that communicates between the pulmonary artery and the descending aorta.*	conducto arterioso permeable
dumping syndrome *Characterized by rapid bowel evacuation after eating in patients with prior gastric surgery.*	síndrome de vaciamiento gástrico demasiado rápido
duodenal *Referring to the duodenum.*	duodenal
duodenal ulcer *A defect in the lining of the first portion of the small bowel, typically caused by H. pylori.*	úlcera duodenal
duodenectomy *Excision of the duodenum.*	duodenectomia
duodenitis *Inflammation of the duodenum.*	duodnitis
duodenum *The portion of the small bowel between the stomach and jejunum.*	duodeno
duplication	doblez
Dupuytren's contracture *A disease of the palmar fascia causing a flexion contracture of the fourth and fifth fingers.*	contractura de Dupuytren
dura mater *The outermost covering of the brain and spinal cord.*	duramadre
dust	polvo
dwarf *Abnormally small person.*	enano
dysaphia *Altered sense of touch.*	disafia
dysarthria *Difficulty in articulation of speech.*	disartria
dysbarism *Condition caused by a change in pressure, noted most commonly among scuba divers.*	disbarismo

English	Spanish
dyschezia *Pain experienced during defecation.*	disquecia
dyschondroplasia *The formation of cartilaginous and bony tumors near the epiphyses.*	discondroplasia
dyscoria *A discordance in pupillary reaction.*	discoria
dyscrasia *An abnormal condition, mostly referring to the blood.*	discrasia
dysdiadocokinesia *The inability to arrest one motor response and substitute its opposite.*	disdiadococinesia
dysentery *A severe form of diarrhea with blood and mucous in the stool.*	disentería
dysesthesia *1. Impairment of the sense of touch. 2. The presence of persistent pain upon receiving a light touch.*	disestesia
dysfunction	desorden
dyshidrosis *Disregulation of sweating*	dishidrosis
dyshidrotic eczema *A dermatitis characterized by vescicobullous lesions.*	eczema dishidrosis
dyskinesia *Abnormal movement.*	discinesia
dyslalia *The absence of comprehensible speech articulation.*	dislalia
dyslexia *Difficulty in learning or reading written language with no effect on intelligence.*	dislexia
dysmenorrhea *Pain during menstruation.*	dismenorrea
dyspareunia *Pain during sexual intercourse.*	dispareunia
dyspepsia *Indigestion.*	dispepsia
dysphagia *Difficulty in swallowing.*	disfagia
dysphasia *Difficulty in speaking caused by cerebral dysfunction.*	disfasia
dysplasia *The increase in organ size due to an increase in the number of abnormal cell types.*	displasia
dyspnea *Difficult breathing.*	disnea
dystocia *Difficult birth caused by fetal position, narrow pelvis or lack of opening of the cervix.*	distocia
dysuria *Difficulty or pain upon urination.*	disuria
ear	oído
ear infections	infecciones de los oídos
ear, external	auris externa
ear, inner	auris interna
ear-drum *Common term for tympanic membrane.*	timpano del oído
earache	dolor de oído
eat, to	comer
eating disorder *General term for pathologic eating habits.*	trastorno alimenticio
ecchondroma *Hyperplastic growth of cartilage on the surface of other cartilage.*	excondroma
ecchymosis *Skin discoloration caused by bleeding beneath the epidermis.*	equimosis
Echinococcus *A tapeworm of the family Taeniidae that can cause hydatid cysts.*	Equinococo
echocardiography *The use of ultrasound waves to visualize the heart and its structures.*	ecocardiografía
echoing sounds	repetición de sonidos
echolalia *The meaningless repetition of the words spoken by another person.*	ecolalia
eclampsia *A maternal condition characterized by convulsions and hypertension that can lead to maternal and fetal death.*	eclampsia
ecmnesia *Memory loss for recent events but retained memory of remote events.*	ecmnesia
ectasia *Expansion or distension.*	ectasia

60

English	Spanish
ectoderm *The outermost layer of the three layers of the embryo.*	ectodermo
ectopic *Abnormal position.*	ectópico
ectopic pregnancy *A pregnancy that is not intrauterine.*	embarazo ectópico
ectrodactylia *A congenital anomaly exhibited by absence of one digit or part of a digit.*	ectrodactilia
ectropion *Eversion of the eyelid, usually the lower lid.*	ectropión
eczema *A medical condition exhibited by pruritic, red, scaly patches on the scalp, cheeks and extensor surfaces.*	eczema
edema *Extravascular fluid accumulation.*	edema
edematous *Referring to the presence of edema.*	edematoso
education	educación
effector *An organ that responds to a stimulus.*	efector
efficacious *Effective.*	eficaz
effort	esfuerzo
effusion *The accumulation of fluid in a body cavity.*	efusión
egg	huevo
egocentric *Thinking of self without considering the feelings or thoughts of others.*	egocéntrico
ehrlichiosis *A tickborne infectious disease.*	erliquiosis
ejaculation *The emission of semen at the moment of sexual climax in a male.*	ejaculación
elastic bandage *A stretch gauze used for compression of an extremity.*	vendaje elástico
elastin *A connective tissue-based glycoprotein.*	elastina
elbow	codo
elderly	de avanzada edad
elective *Non-urgent and not life-saving.*	electivo
electrocardiogram *Display of a person's heart beat that can be used in the diagnosis of cardiac disorders.*	electrocardiograma
electroconvulsive therapy (ECT) *The electrical stimulation of the brain to treat mental disorders.*	terapéutica de choque
electrode *A device used to facilitate conduction of electricity to or from a body.*	electrodo
electroencephalogram (EEG) *A display of brain waves used in the diagnosis of brain disorders, especially epilepsy.*	electroencefalograma
electrolyte *The ionized constituents including potassium, sodium, chloride and others.*	electrolito
electromyography *The display of the electrical activity of muscle.*	electromiografía
electron microscope *A device that uses electron beams and lenses to give high magnification.*	microscopio electrópio
electrophoresis *The movement of charged particles in a fluid that is under the influence of an electric field. This is used in testing for various maladies in the form of serum protein electrophoresis.*	electroforesis
elephantiasis *A condition caused by nematode parasites leading to lymphatic obstruction and limb or scrotal swelling.*	elefantiasis
elixir *A medical solution.*	elixir
emaciation *Abnormally thin and weak.*	extenuación
embolectomy *The removal of an embolus.*	embolectomie
embolus *A blood clot, air bubble or fatty deposit that cause obstruction of a vessel.*	embolismo

English	Spanish
embryo *The term used to describe a fertilized ovum in the first 8 weeks of development.*	embrión
embryology *The study of the embryo.*	embriología
emergence *Coming into prominence.*	salida
emergency *An urgent, life-threatening situation.*	aprieto, emergencia
emergency room	sala de emergencia
emesis *Vomiting.*	vómito
emetic *An agent that induces vomiting.*	emético
emmetropia *The normal correlation between eye refraction and the axial length of the eyeball.*	emetropía
emollient *Having softening or soothing qualities.*	emoliente
emotion *An intense feeling.*	emoción
empathy *To be concerned for and share the feelings of another.*	empatía
emphysema *Abnormal enlargement of the airspaces distal to the terminal bronchioles.*	enfisema
empty	vacío
empyema *A collection of purulent material in a body cavity, usually referring to a thoracic empyema.*	empiema
emulsion *The dispersion of one liquid into another, but it is not dissolved.*	emulsión
enarthrosis *The type of joint in which a spherical bone is set into the socket of another bone.*	enartrosis
encephalic *Referring to the brain.*	encefálico
encephalitis *Inflammation of the brain.*	encefalitis
encephalocele *The protrusion of the brain through a defect in the skull.*	encefalocele
encephalography *Roentgenography of the brain.*	encefalograma
encephalomacia *Abnormal softness of the brain.*	encefalomalacia
encephalomyelitis *Inflammation of the brain and spinal cord.*	encefalomielitis
encephalopathy *Degeneration of cerebral function.*	encefalopatía
enchondroma *An abnormal increase in cartilage growth on the inside of bone or of other cartilage.*	encondroma
encopresis *Involuntary defecation.*	encopresis
end organ *The encapsulated end of a sensory nerve.*	órgano terminal
end point *The last stage of a process.*	punto terminal
end stage *Terminal stage. End stage cancer means there is no cure possible and death is imminent.*	fase terminal
endarteritis *Tunica intima inflammation.*	endarteritis
endemic *When a disease is commonly found in a location or in a people group.*	endémico
endocarditis *Inflammation of the endocardium.*	endocarditis
endocervicitis *Inflammation of the mucosal lining of the cervix.*	endocervicitis
endocrine glands *Glands that secrete hormones and other substances into the blood.*	glándulas endocrinas
endocrine *Referring to glands that secrete hormones and other chemicals into the blood.*	endocrino
endocrinology *The study of endocrine glands and hormones.*	endrocrinología
endoderm *The innermost layer of the embryonic germ cell layers.*	endodermo
endogenous *Originating from within.*	endógeno
endolymph *The fluid collection the labyrinth of the ear.*	flúido endolinfático
endometrioma *An isolated benign mass containing endometrial tissue.*	endometrioma

English	Spanish
endometriosis *Presence of uterine mucosal tissue in the pelvis in abnormal locations.*	endometriosis
endometritis *Inflammation of the endometrium.*	endometritis
endometrium *The mucous membrane lining of the uterus.*	endometrio
endoneurium *The tissue in a peripheral nerve that separates the individual nerve fibers.*	endoneurio
endoplasmic reticulum *A framework of tubules within the cytoplasm of eukaryotic cells.*	retículo endoplasmático
endorphins *Hormones secreted that activate the body's opiate receptors and act as analgesics.*	endorfinas
endoscope *A device used to view the interior of a hollow organ (sigmoidoscope, gastroscope)*	endoscopio
endothelioma *A mass that propagates from the endothelium of blood vessels, lymphatics or serous cavities.*	endotelioma
endotracheal *Within the trachea.*	endotraqueal
endow	dotar
enema *A procedure involving insertion of fluid into the rectum.*	enema
enkephalins *Peptides found in the brain that have similar effects as the endorphins.*	encefalinas
enlargement *Becoming bigger.*	aumento
enophthalmos *Posterior displacement of the eyeball in the orbit.*	enoftalmia
enormous *Very large.*	enorme
enostosis *The abnormal bony growth inside a bone or on the cortex.*	enostosis
ensure, to *To make certain of.*	asegurer
ENT *Abbreviation for ears, nose and throat.*	ONG oído nariz y garganta
enteral feeding *Nutrition supplied via the alimentary canal.*	entérico intestino
enterectomy *Surgical resection of part of the intestine.*	enterectomie
enteric *Referring to the intestines.*	entérico
enteritis *Inflammation of the intestines.*	enteritis
enterobiasis *An infection caused by worms from the genus Enterobius.*	enterobiasis
enterococcus *A gram positive cocci that occurs naturally in the intestine but is pathogenic elsewhere in the body.*	enterococo
enterolith *A calculus of the intestine.*	enterolito
enteroptosis *Inferior displacement of the intestines in the abdomen.*	enteroptosis
enterotomy *A surgical opening of the intestines.*	enterotomía
entrapment neuropathy *Weakness or numbness caused by compression of a peripheral nerve.*	neuropatía de atrapamiento
enucleation *Surgical removal of a globe.*	enucleación
enuresis *Involuntary urination.*	enuresis
enzyme *A compound that acts as a catalyst for reactions within cells as assists with digestion outside of cells.*	enzima
eosinophil *A cell with eosin stain used to designate a type of leukocyte that is elevated during allergic reactions.*	eosinófilo
eosinophilia *An increased number of eosinophils in the blood.*	eosinofilia
ependyma *The glial lined covering of the cerebral ventricles and the central portion of the spinal cord.*	epéndimo
ependymoma *A tumor composed of cells that line the ventricles of the brain.*	ependimoma

English	Spanish
ephedrine *A chemical used to treat asthma because it expands bronchial passages and used to control spinal anesthesia associated shock because it constricts blood vessels.*	efedrina
ephelis *Medical term for the common freckle.*	efelis
epiblepharon *A condition exhibited by the eyelashes pressing against the eyeball.*	epibléfaron
epicardium *The serous membranous, innermost lining of the pericardium.*	epicardio
epicondyle *A protrusion at the distal end of the humerus.*	epicóndilo
epicondylitis *Inflammation of the epicondyle.*	epicondilitis
epicranium *The skin, fibrous layer (aponeurosis), and muscles lining the scalp.*	epicráneo
epidemic *Ubiquitous development of an infectious disease.*	epidemia
epidemiology *The study of the incidence, development and control of disease.*	epidemiología
epidermis *The skin cells overlying the dermis.*	epidermis
epidermophytosis *A fungal skin infection caused by an organism from the genus Epidermophyton.*	epidermofitosis
epididymitis *Inflammation of the duct that moves sperm from the testis to the vas deferens.*	epididimitis
epididymo-orchitis *Inflammation of the epididymis and the testis.*	epididimoorquitis
epidural *The space around the dura of the spinal cord.*	epidural
epidural analgesia *Medication into this space produces analgesia for surgical procedures.*	analgesia espinal
epidural hematoma *Formation of a collection of blood outside the dural layer of the brain; usually caused by trauma.*	hematoma epidural
epigastrium *The section of the abdomen that overlies the stomach.*	epigastrio
epiglottis *Tissue at the base of the tongue that covers the trachea when one swallows.*	epiglotis
epilation *Removal of hair and the roots.*	epilación
epilepsy *A condition associated with abnormal brain activity and exhibited by sudden, recurrent convulsions, sensory disturbances and loss of consciousness.*	epilepsia
epileptic seizure *A convulsion related to abnormal brain activity (as opposed to being precipitated by hypoglycemia.)*	ataque epiléptico
epileptiform *Being similar to epilepsy.*	epileptiforme
epileptogenic *That which induces seizures.*	epileptogénico
epinephrine *A hormone secreted by the adrenal gland.*	epinefrina
epiphysis cerebri *A small structure situated on the mesencephalon between the two sections of the thalamus.*	epífisis cerebral
epiphysitis *Inflammation of the end of a long bone that is separated from the shaft by a cartilaginous disc.*	epifisitis
episcleritis *Inflammation of the tissue lying above the sclera.*	epiescleritis
episiotomy *A surgical incision of the vagina used to aid childbirth.*	episiotomía
epispadias *A congenital condition characterized by the urethral meatus being at the superior aspect of the penis*	epispadius
epistaxis *Bleeding emanating from the nose.*	epistaxis
epithelial *Referring to the epithelium.*	epitelial
epithelial cast *Debris found in the urine composed of columnar renal epithelium.*	cilindro epitelial
epithelioma *A malignant tumor composed of epithelial cells.*	epitelioma
epithelium *The tissue lining the skin and the gastrointestinal tract that is derived from the embryonic ectoderm and endoderm..*	epitelio

English	Spanish
epitrochlea *The medial condyle of the humerus.*	epitróclea
equal	igual
equilibrium *When opposing forces are in balance.*	equilibrio
equipment	equipo
ergometer *A device that measures energy expenditure.*	ergómetro
ergonomics *The study of workplace design that focuses on reducing work-related injuries.*	ergonomía
ergosterol *A compound converted to vitamin D2 upon exposure to ultraviolet light.*	ergosterol
erosion *The gradual destruction of surface tissue.*	erosión
error	error, falta
eructation *A belch or burp.*	eructación
erysipelas *An acute infection caused by Streptococcus pyogenes that causes fever along with swelling and inflammation. The infection frequently effects the face or one leg.*	erisipelas
erythema mutliforme *A skin condition exhibited by purpuric lesions and bullae usually on the distal parts of extremities but can affect the face and trunk.*	eritema multiforme
erythema nodosum *The presence of red or purple nodules on the pretibial area.*	eritema nudoso
erythroblast *A nucleus containing immature erythrocyte.*	eritroblasto
erythroblastosis fetalis *A hemolytic disease of the newborn.*	eritroblastosis
erythrocyanosis *A condition exhibited by purple patches with asymmetric swelling, pruritis and burning.*	eritrocianosis
erythrocyte *Called a red blood cell, it transports oxygen and carbon dioxide to and from the tissues.*	eritrocito
erythrocytopenia *Low level of erythrocytes in the blood stream.*	ertitrocitopenia
erythrocytosis *A higher than normal level of erythrocytes in the blood stream.*	eritrocitosis
erythropoiesis *The production of red blood cells.*	eritropoyesis
eschar *Dry, hard, dead tissue commonly seen with a chronic pressure ulcer or anthrax.*	escara
eserine *Physostigmine.*	eserina
esophageal *Referring to the esophagus.*	esofágico
esophagectomy *Surgical removal of the esophagus.*	esofagectomía
esophagitis *Inflammation of the esophagus.*	esofagitis
esophagoscopy *Visual inspection the esophagus utilizing a scope.*	esofagoscopia
esophagus *The muscular tube that connects the throat to the stomach.*	esófago
esotropia *Medial deviation of the eye at primary gaze.*	esotropia
Esotropia *Commonly called "cross-eyed", characterized by a convergent gaze.*	estrabismo convergente
essential	esencial
estrogen *A hormone involved with developing and maintaining female sexual characteristics.*	estrógeno
ethanol *Synonym for ethyl alcohol.*	etanol
ethmoid *A bone at the root of the nose which has perforations for the olfactory nerves to transit.*	etmoides
etiology *The underlying cause of a problem.*	etología
eunuch *A man who has been castrated.*	eunuco
euthanasia *Killing someone painlessly who is thought to have a terminal condition.*	eutanasia

English	Spanish
evacuation *The emptying of an organ of fluids or gas.*	evacuación
evaluation	evaluación
eventration *Protrusion of the intestines from the abdomen.*	evantración
eversion *To turn outward.*	eversión
every	todo
every day	todos los días
every other day	cada dos días
evident *Obvious.*	evidente
evisceration *The removal of bowels from the body.*	evisceratión
evoked potential *Electrical impulses that can be noted after stimulation of sensory organs.*	potential evocada
evulsion *Forcible extraction.*	evulsión
exacerbation *Worsening of an existing problem.*	exacerbación
examination	examen
exanthema *A rash that accompanies a disease or fever.*	exantema
excess	exceso
exchange transfusion *Treatment of hyperbilirubinemia in neonates.*	ex-sanguinotransfusión
excipient *An inactive substance used to deliver an active substance.*	excipiente
excisional biopsy *Surgical removal of tissue for pathologic examination.*	biopsia por extracción
excoriation *Superficial loss of skin.*	excoriación
excrement *Feces.*	excretmento
excreta *Fecal material.*	excreta
exenteration *Complete surgical removal of an organ.*	extenteración
exercise-induced dyspnea	disnia por esfuerzo excesivo
exercised induce angina *Chest pain noted during exertion related to coronary artery disease.*	angina de esfuerzo
exfoliation *The shedding of scales.*	exfoliación
exhumation *The process of removing a dead body from a grave.*	exhumación
exogenous *Referring to external factors.*	exógeno
exomphalos *Umbilical hernia.*	exomphalos
exostosis *A bony prominence growing from the surface of a bone.*	exóstosis
exotoxin *A toxin released from a living cell.*	exotoxina
exotropia *A type of strabismus that is characterized by the eyes turned outward.*	exotropía
expansion	expansión
expect, to	esperar
expectorant *A substance that promotes the secretion of sputum.*	expectorante
expectoration *The presence of sputum that has been coughed out.*	expectoración
expiration date	fecha de vencimiento
expiratory *Referring to exhalation of air from the lungs.*	expiratorio
expiratory reserve volume *Amount of air left in the lung after a maximal exhalation, in liters.*	volumen de reserva espiratorio
expulsion *Evacuation or elimination.*	expulsión
expulsion of placenta	expulsión de la placenta
extend	extender
extension *Going from a bent to straight position.*	extensión

English	Spanish
extensor plantar response *Great toe extension indicating a positive Babinski sign.*	reflejo plantar (reflejo de Babinski)
extensor *Referring to the extension of an extremity or part of an extremity.*	extensor
external ear canal, *auditory canal*	meato auditivo externo
external *Outside of the body.*	exterior
extirpate *To totally destroy.*	extirpar
extracapsular *Situated outside a capsule.*	extracapsular
extracellular *Outside the cell.*	extracelular
extract *A substance in a concentrated form.*	extracto
extrapyramidal tract *Motor nerves that are not part of the pyramidal tract.*	tracto extrapiramidal
extrasystole *Either a premature atrial or ventricular contraction.*	extrasístole
extravasation *Referring to a situation in which blood or fluid goes out of a vessel it is normally flowing into.*	extravasación
extremity	extremidad
extrinsic *Coming from outside or external sources.*	extrínseco
exudate *The fluid, cells, and debris found in the tissues or a cavity (like pleural space) during inflammation.*	exudado
eye drops	gotas para los ojos
eyebrow *Supercilium.*	ceja
eyeglasses	espejuelos
eyeground *The fundus that is visualized with an ophthalmoscope.*	fondo del ojo
eyelash	pestaña
eyelid *Palpebra.*	párpado
eyesight	vista
face	rostro, cara
face presentation *Referring to the part of the body coming out of the cervix first during childbirth.*	presentación de cara
facet *A small flat surface of a bone.*	faceta
facial nerve *Cranial nerve VII that supplies the face and tongue.*	nervio facial
facial paralysis *Lack of movement or sensation in the distribution of the facial nerve.*	parálisis facial
facies *A facial expression that is typical for a particular disease.*	facies
faint *Weak and dizzy.*	desmayo
fair	rubio
falciform *Referring to something that is curved. The falciform ligament attaches the liver to the diaphragm.*	falciforme
fallopian tubes *Either of a pair of long narrow ducts located in a female's abdominal cavity that transport the male sperm cells to the egg.*	trompas de Falopio
Fallot, tetrology of *Congenital cardiac defects including ventricular septal defect, pulmonic valve stenosis or infundibular stenosis, and dextroposition of the aorta.*	tetralogía de Fallot
falx cerebri *A fold in the dura that separates the two cerebral hemispheres.*	falx cerebri
familial *Referring to the family*	familiar
family	familia
family history	escrutinio familiar
family planning *Birth control.*	planificación familiar
faradism *The gradual increasing and decreasing of the amplitude of electricity.*	faradismo

English	Spanish
farmer's lung *Coined because farmers are susceptible to this disease by inhaling fungi from hay; also called Aspergillosis.*	pulmón de granjero
fart, to *Slang term for releasing flatus.*	tirarse un pedo
fascia *The fibrous sheath enclosing a muscle or organ.*	fascia
fascicle *A bundle of nerve or muscle fibers.*	fascículo
fasciculation *Involuntary contraction of muscle fibers.*	fasciculación
fasciitis *Inflammation of a fascia.*	fascitis
fasciotomy *Incision into a fascia.*	fascietomía
fasting *Absence of caloric intake for a specified period.*	ayuno
fat	gordo, obeso
fat embolism *A deposit of fat that obstructs a vessel.*	embolia grasosa
fatal	fatal
fatness	gordura
fatty	graso
fatty acid *A carboxylic acid occurring as a an ester in fats and oils.*	ácidos grasos
favus *Tinea capitis caused by Trichopyton schoenleini.*	favo
fear	temor
febrile *Presence of an supraphysiologic temperature.*	febril
fecal impaction *The presence of hard excrement in the rectum that requires manual removal.*	impacción fecal
feces *Excrement.*	heces
fecundity *The capability of producing offspring quickly and frequently.*	fecundidad
feeble-minded *Antiquated term used to describe a person unable to make seemingly simple decisions because of a cognitive impairment.*	zonzo
feeding behavior	conducta de apetencia
feel better, to	sentir mejor
feel, to	sentir
female	hembra
feminine pad *Gauze specially designed to absorb menstrual flow.*	toalla higiénica
femoral artery	arteria femoral
femoral nerve *Supplies the motor function of the quadriceps and the sensation over the anterior and medial thigh.*	nervio femoral
femoral triangle *An area that is bordered by the sartorius muscle, the adductor longus muscle and the inguinal ligament.*	triángulo femoral
femur *The long bone in the thigh.*	fémur
fenestration *Usually referring to a surgical window.*	fenestración
fertility *The ability of a person to contribute to contraception.*	fertilidad
fertilization *The melding of male and female gametes to form a zygote.*	fertilización
fester *To become infected.*	enconarse
festinating gait *Walking with increased speed involuntarily; often seen in Parkinson's disease.*	marcha festinante
fetal alcohol syndrome *A condition caused by acohol use by the mother during pregnancy and exhibited by poor intrauterine growth, decreased muscle tone, delayed development and widened palpebral fissures.*	síndrome alcohólico fetal
fetal distress *Term used to describe an abnormal heart rate or rhythm in a fetus indicating the need for urgent childbirth.*	sufrimiento fetal
fetal heart tone *Refers to the cardiac rate and pattern of the fetus.*	latido cimiento fetal
fetal monitoring	monitorización fetal

English	Spanish
fetal position *Refers to how the fetus lies within the uterus.*	posición fetal
fetal *Referring to the fetus.*	fetal
fetichism *The glorification of an inanimate object.*	fetichismo
fetor *A foul odor.*	fetor
fetus	feto
fever	fiebre
fibrillation *Uncoordinated, ineffective contraction as in atrial fibrillation.*	fibrilación
fibrin *An insoluble protein formed when fibrinogen is acted upon by thrombin.*	fibrina
fibroadenoma *A benign breast mass composed of fibrous and glandular tissue.*	fibroadenoma
fibroblast *A collagen producing cell in connective tissue.*	fibroblast
fibrochondritis *The inflammation of a structure composed of cartilage and fibrous tissue.*	fibrocondritis
fibroelastosis *The abnormal increase in growth of fibrous and elastic tissue.*	fibroelastosis
fibroid *A benign mass, typically uterine, composed of fibrous and muscle tissue.*	fibroide
fibromyoma *A mass containing fibrous and muscle tissue.*	fibromioma
fibrosarcoma *A sarcoma composed primarily of malignant fibroblasts.*	fibroscarcoma
fibrosis *Connective tissue that is scarred and thickened after injury.*	fibrosis cistica
fibrositis *Fibrous connective tissue that is inflammed.*	fibrositis
fibula *The smaller of two bones in the lower leg.*	fíbula,peroné
Fifth disease *Erythema infectiosum is a viral disease caused by parovirus B19.*	quinta enfermedad o eritema infeccioso
filaria *A parasitic nematode worm that is transmitted by flies and mosquitos causing filariasis.*	filaria
file *Patient record or folder.*	lima
filiform *Threadlike.*	filiforme
filum terminale *The thin structure at the end of the conus medullaris which connects the spinal cord with the coccyx.*	filum terminale
fimbria *A slender projection at the end of the fallopian tube near the ovary.*	fimbria
finger	dedo
finger agnosia *The inability to distinguish which finger is being touched.*	agnosia del dedo
finger nose test *A test for dysmetria in which a person reaches out to touch their own nose with an extended finger with their eyes closed.*	prueba de la nariz y el dedo
fingerstick device *A device used to project a lancet into the skin so a drop of blood can be obtained for analysis.*	lanceta
fingertip	punta del dedo
Finkelstein test *Pain elicited with thumb flexion and wrist flexion is indicitive of De Quervain tenosynovitis.*	prueba de Finkelstein.
firm	firme, sólido
first aid	primeros auxilios
fish	pescado
fissure *A general term for a cleft or deep groove. An anal fissure, for example, is a small ulcer adjacent to the anus.*	fisura
fist	puña
fistula *An abnormal communication between two organs or an organ and the skin, as in rectovaginal fistula.*	fístula
fixation *1. An obsessive interest. 2. The securing of a body part.*	fijación
flaccid *Limp. A term applied to an extremity one cannot move actively.*	flácido

English	Spanish
flagellation *1. The protrusion found on flagella. 2. Massage administered by tapping a body part with fingers.*	flagelación
flagellum *A slender appendage that allows protozoa to swim.*	flagelo
flail chest *The term used when one has multiple rib fractures causing a segment of the chest wall to move incongruently with the rest of the chest wall.*	tórax inestable
flame photometer *A device used to measure the intensity of light.*	fotómetro de llama
flap *A term used to describe a piece of tissue partially excised and placed over an adjacent surface.*	colgado
flare *A sudden intensity or dilatation.*	brote
flask	balón
flat	bemol
flat foot *Common term for pes planus.*	pie plano
flatten, to	allanar
flatulence *The gas expulsed from the anus.*	flatunecia
flatus *Term for air that is expelled from the anus.*	flato
flatworm *A class of worms that includes parasitic flukes and tapeworms.*	platelminto
flea	pulga
flesh	carne
flexor *A muscle that bends an extremity or part of an extremity.*	flexor
flexure *The action of bending.*	flexura
floating	flotante
flow	flujo
fluid intake *The amount of oral consumption plus the amount of intravenous fluids administered.*	ingestion fluido
fluke *Parasitic nematode worm; an example is Schistosoma.*	duela
fluoresceine *A fluorane dye used to check for corneal ulcers.*	fluorescina
fluorescent antibody test (FTA test)	técnica del anticuerpo fluorescente
fluorescent screen *A screen used to view x-rays.*	pantalla fluorescente
fluoridation *The addition of fluorine to something.*	fluorización
fluorine *A chemical that causes severe burns if exposed to the skin.*	flúor
fluoroscopy *The continuous viewing of roentgenographic images with a fluorescent screen.*	fluorocopía
flush, to *Term used to describe an irrigation procedure, as in flushing an NG tube.*	irrigar
flushing	bochornos o ruborización
flutter *Used to describe a cardiac rhythm disturbance, as in atrial flutter.*	aleteo
foam	espuma
Foley catheter *A drainage tube placed in the urinary bladder via the urethra.*	catéter de Foley
folic acid *Also called pteroylglutamic acid; a deficiency can cause megaloblastic anemia.*	ácido fólico
follicle stimulating hormone (FSH) *An anterior pituitary gland hormone responsible for production of sperm or ova.*	hormona foliculoestimulante
follicular *Referring to a small secretory gland.*	folicular
fontanelle or fontanel *The space between the bones in the skull that are separate at birth.*	fontanella
food	alimento

English	Spanish
food intake	ingestion alimento
food poisoning	intoxicación alimenticia
foot	pie
foot and mouth disease *A contagious viral disease exhibited by oral and digital vesicles.*	fiebre aftosa
foot drop *Caused by palsy of the nerve controlling foot dorsiflexion.*	pie caído
foramen *An opening in a bone.*	foramen
foramen magnum *The hole in the skull that the spinal cord passes through.*	magnum foramen
foramen ovale *A hole in the atrial septal wall in a fetus.*	foramen oval
forced expiratory flow rate *Amount of air forcibly exhaled in liters per unit of time.*	flujo expiratorio forzado
forced expiratory volume per second (FEV1) *The amount of air exhaled with maximal effort, measured in liters, over one second.*	volumen espiratorio forzado
forceps *A surgical instrument, commonly called tweezers.*	fórceps
forearm	antebrazo
forearm crutch *A long stick with a place for a hand-grip to aid in ambulation when there is lower extremity weakness.*	muleta antebrazo
forebrain *The part of the brain that includes the thalamus, hypothalamus and cerebral hemispheres.*	prosencéfalo
forehead	frente
foreign bodies *Term used to describe objects found in a body orifice that are not part of the body.*	cuerpos extraños
forensic *Referring to the scientific method of studying crime.*	forense
foreskin *Also called prepuce, the skin that naturally covers the glans but can be rolled back.*	prepucio
former	antecedente
formulary *A list of medicines that are permissible to prescribe.*	formulario
fornix *A vaulted structure.*	fornix
forwards	hacia adelante
fossa *A shallow depression.*	fosa
fourchette *The fork shaped fold of skin where the labia minora meet superior to the perineum.*	horquilla
fovea *The area on the retina where the visual acuity is optimal.*	fóvea
fracture	fractura
fracture, avulsion *A broken bone associated with a ligament or tendon pulling a piece of the bone away.*	fractura por avulsión
fracture, closed *A broken bone where there is no break in the skin.*	fractura cerrada
fracture, comminuted *A broken bone where one segment overrides the other.*	fractura communita
fracture, depressed *The presence of concavity associated with a fracture as in a depressed skull fracture.*	fractura con hundimiento
fracture, greenstick *A spiral fracture.*	fractura de tallo verde
fracture, open *A fracture in which there is a break in the skin and bone is exposed.*	fractura expuesta
fracture, pathologic *A fracture due at least in part to another condition, such as a fracture at a location where there is bone cancer.*	fractura patológica
fracture, stress *A fracture associated with overuse.*	fractura de sobrecarga
fragilitas ossium *A condition exhibited by excessively brittle bones. Also called osteogenesis imperfecta.*	fragilitas ossium

English	Spanish
framboesia; yaws *An endemic tropical disease caused by Treponema pertenue.*	frambesía
free	libre
free of	libre de
freedom	libertad
freezing (as in ambient temperature)	helado
fremitus *A vibration that is appreciated with palpation.*	fremitus
frenulum *The tissue that connects the inferior portion of the tongue to the base of the mouth.*	frenulum
frequency	frecuencia
friction	fricción
friction rub *A noise heard during cardiac auscultation in patients with pericarditis, for example.*	roce de fricción
frog	rana
frog in the throat, to have	ronco
frontal *Referring to the anterior aspect, as in frontal lobe.*	frontal
frontal sinuses	senos frontales
frost itch *A pruritis noted when exposed to cold weather.*	prurito de escarcha Dermatitis hiemalis.
frostbite	quemadura por frío
froth	espuma
froth at the mouth, to	echar espuma por la boca
frozen	congelado
frozen shoulder *Common term for adhesive capsulitis.*	hombro congelado
fructosuria *Presence of fructose in the urine.*	fructosuria
FTA test *Fluorescent treponemal antibody test for syphilis.*	prueba de absorción de anticuerpo treponémico fluorescente
full-term *A normal length pregnancy.*	embarazo a término
fulminant *Sudden and severe.*	fulminante
function	función
fundus *Referring to the upper part of the stomach or the part of the globe opposing the pupil.*	fondo
fungicide *An agent that destroys fungus.*	fungicida
fungus *A spore-producing organism that feeds on organic matter.*	fungi, hongo
funiculi of the spinal cord *The white matter of the spinal cord that is further defined by location.*	funículo
funiculitis *Inflammation of the funiculi.*	funiculitis
funnel chest *Anterior thorax funnel shaped depression, also called pectus excavatum.*	tórax en embudo
furuncle *A painful erythematous nodule with a central core.*	furúnculo
furunculosis *The presence of multiple furuncles.*	furunculosis
fusiform *Spindle-shaped.*	fusiforme
gag reflex *Contraction of the pharynx muscles when the back of the pharynx is stimulated by touch.*	reflejo de arcada
gait *The way one walks.*	manera de caminar
galactocele *A milk-filled cyst in the mammary gland.*	galactocele
galactorrhea *Excessive production of milk.*	galactorrea

72

English	Spanish
galactose *A sugar that is a constituent of lactose.*	galactosa
galactosemie *1. Galactose in the blood. 2. A congenital condition exhibited by impaired carbohydrate metabolism.*	galactosemia
gallbladder *The organ adjacent to the liver that stores bile and secretes it into the duodenum.*	vesícula biliar
gallop *An abnormal heart sound.*	galope
gallstones *Calculi produced in the bile duct or gallbladder.*	cálculos en la vesícula
galvanism *The use of electric currents for medical treatment.*	galvanismo
galvanometer *A device used to measure small electric currents.*	galvanómetro
gamete *A germ cell that is able to unite with another germ cell of the opposite gender to form a zygote.*	gameto
gamma globulin *A blood serum protein with little electrophoretic mobility.*	gamma globulina
gamma rays *A type of electromagnetic radiation.*	rayos gamma
ganglionectomy *The removal of a benign swelling on a tendon sheath.*	ganglionectomía
gangrene *Tissue death from either impaired blood flow or an infection.*	gangrena
gaping *Wide open.*	abierto
gargle, to	gargarizar
gargoylism *A congenital anomaly exhibited by mental retardation, bone deformities and an abnormally large head.*	gargolismo
gas gangrene *A life and limb threatening disorder caused associated with tissue death and caused by an anaerobic bacterium in the genus of Clostridium.*	gangrena gaseosa
gastrectomy *Complete or partial surgical resection of the stomach.*	gastrectomía
gastric lavage *Instillation and removal of large quantities of saline into the stomach in order to treat poisoning.*	lavado gástrico
gastric *Referring to the stomach.*	gástrico
gastric secretions	jugo gástrico
gastrin *Hormones that stimulates gastric secretions.*	gastrinas
gastritis *Inflammation of the stomach.*	gastritis
gastrocele *Protrusion of part of the stomach in the form of a hernia.*	gastrocele
gastrocnemius *A large muscle in the lower leg, responsible for ankle plantar flexion, that is attached to the distal femur and achilles tendon.*	gastronemio
gastrocolic reflex *Peristalsis of the colon produced by food entering the stomach.*	reflejo gastrocólico
gastroduodenal ulcer *A lesion in the mucosal lining of the stomach or duodenum.*	úlcera gastroduodenal
gastroenteritis *A bacterial or viral infection that leads to vomiting and diarrhea.*	gastroenteritis
gastroenterostomy *A surgical opening in the stomach or intestine.*	gastroenterotomie
gastrointestinal tract *The alimentary canal from the distal esophagus to the cecum.*	tracto gastrointestina
gastrojejunostomy *A surgical procedure that directly connects the stomach to the jejunum.*	gastroyeyunostomía
gastropexy *Securing the stomach to the abdominal wall.*	gastropexia
gastroscope *A device used to directly visualize the stomach.*	gastroscopio
gastrostomy *A surgical creation of an opening in the stomach.*	gastroscopía
gauge *The size or thickness of something. An 18gauge needle.*	calibre
gauze *A fabric used for dressing changes.*	gasa
gavage syringe	jeringa gastrogavaje

English	Spanish
gavage *The instillation of food into the stomach with use of a tube.*	gavaje
gavage tube *A tube used for instillation of liquids into the stomach.*	sonda gastrogavaje
gaze	mirada
gel	gel
gene *A unit of heredity that is passed on from parent to child.*	gen
general	general
general appearance	aspecto general
genetic counseling	asesoramiento genético
genetic *Referring to genes or heredity.*	genético
geniculate *Bent at a sharp angle.*	geniculado
geniculate body *Protrusions on the thalamus that relay visual and auditory signals to the brain.*	cuerpo geniculado
geniculate ganglion *The sensory ganglion of the facial nerve.*	ganglio geniculado
geniculate neuralgia *Severe intermittent pain in the external ear and deep in the ear.*	otalgia geniculada
genital ambiguity *A disorder of sexual development in which the genitalia are not sufficiently developed to tell clearly if the person is male or female.*	ambigüedad genital
genital herpes *A sexually transmitted infection caused by herpes simplex.*	herpes genital
genital wart *The common term for Condylomata acuminata.*	verruga genital
genitalia *Genitals.*	genitales
genitourinary	genitourinario
genome *A full set of genetic information for an organism.*	genoma
gentian violet *An antiseptic derived from rosaniline.*	violeta de genciana
genu valgum *A condition exhibited by the knees turning inward, commonly referred to as knock-knee.*	genu valgum
genu varum *A condition exhibited by the knees turning outward, commonly referred to as bowleg.*	genu varum
GERD gastroesophageal reflux disease *A condition characterized by gastric contents being regurgitated into the esophagus or mouth.*	ERGE enfermedad del reflujo gastroesofágico
geriatrics *The study of the health of old people.*	geriatría
germ	germen
German measles *(rubella) A contagious viral infection.*	rubeola
gerontology *The study of old persons.*	gerontología
gestation *The development of a fetus from conception until birth.*	gestación
gestation; *pregnancy*	embarazo
giant	gigante
giardiasis *A flagellate protozoa, Giardia lamblia, that causes diarrhea.*	giardiasis
gigantism *Abnormally large size.*	gigantismo
gingival *Referring to the gums.*	gingival
gingivitis *Inflammation of the gums.*	gingivitis
ginglymus *A joint that allows movement in one direction only.*	gínglimo
glabella *The area of the forehead above and between the eyebrows.*	glabela
glance	mirada
glans *The distal aspect of the penis or clitoris.*	glande
glare	resplandor
Glasgow coma scale *A scale used to grade one's level of consciousness with a score of 3 being totally unresponsive and a score of 15 being normal.*	escala de coma de Glasgow

glaucoma *A condition characterized by increased intraocular pressure.* — glaucoma

glenoid *Referring to the fossa that is a shallow depression, such as the hollow of the scapula where the humeral head sets.* — glenoideo

glioma *A neural malignant tumor of glial cells.* — glioma

gliomyoma *A mass with gliomatous and myomatous characteristics.* — gliomioma

globus pallidus *A portion of the lentiform nucleus in the brain.* — globo pálido

glomerulonephritis *Inflammation of the renal glomeruli, usually from hemolytic streptococcus.* — glomerulonefritis

glomerulus *A grouping of capillaries where waste is filtered from the blood.* — glomérulo

glomus tumor *A reddish-blue painful papule that occurs on the distal aspects of the digits.* — globo

glossal *Referring to the tongue.* — glosa, lengua

glossectomy *Surgical resection of the whole or part of the tongue.* — glosectomía

glossitis *Inflammation of the tongue.* — glositis

glossodynia *Tongue pain.* — glosodinia

glossopharyngeal *The name for cranial nerve IX that supplies the tongue and pharynx.* — glosofaríngeo

glottis *Essentially the vocal structure, including the true vocal cords and the opening between them.* — glotis

glove — guante

glove anesthesia *Absence of sensation of the hand and wrist.* — anestesia en guante

glucagon *A pancreatic enzyme responsible for breakdown of glycogen to glucose.* — glucagón

glucose tolerance test *The oral administration of a carbohydrate load and then evaluation of the blood sugar at timed intervals.* — prueba de tolerancia a la glucosa

glue — pegamento

glue sniffing addiction — adicción inhalación de cemento

gluteal *Referring to the gluteus.* — glúteo

gluteal fold *The horizontal crease between the buttock and upper thigh.* — pliegue glúteo

gluteal or gluteus muscle *A paired set of three muscles, the gluteus maximus, medius and minimus, that all have origins in the ilium and insertions in the femur. (buttocks)* — músculo glúteo

glycemia *The amount of glucose in the blood.* — glucemia

glycerin *A byproduct in the manufacture of soap that is used as a laxative.* — glicerina

glycogen *A compound that stores glucose and when it undergoes hydrolysis forms glucose.* — glucógeno

glycogenesis *The production of glycogen from glucose.* — glucogénesis

glycolysis *The production of energy and pyruvic acid when glucose is broken down by enzymes.* — glicólisis

glycoprotein *A protein that has a carbohydrate attached to its polypeptide chain.* — glicoproteína

glycosuria *Presence of glucose in the urine.* — glucosuria

gnathic *Referring to the jaws.* — gnático

gnosia *Ability to recognize things and people.* — gnosia

goblet cells *They aid in the secretion of respiratory and intestinal mucous.* — célula calciforme

goggles — las gafas de buceo

goiter *Swelling of the thyroid gland.* — bocio

English	Spanish
gold	oro
gonad *A testis or an ovary.*	gónada
gonadal dysgenesis *The lack of complete development of the gonads.*	disgenesia gónada
gonadotrophin *Pituitary hormone that promotes gonadal activity.*	gonadotropina
gonococcus *A diploccocal bacteria that is the causative agent in gonorrhea, formally Neisseria gonorrhoeae.*	gonococo
gonorrhea *A sexually transmitted disease that is exhibited by purulent discharge from the vagina or penis.*	gonorrea
gonorrheal arthritis *A type of arthritis caused by the gram negative diplococcus Neisseria gonorrhoeae.*	artritis gonorreico
gonorrheal ophthalmia *An acute purulent conjunctivitis that can occur in neonates within 2-5 days of birth.*	oftalmía gonorreica
goose bumps	carne de gallina
gouge *A chisel with a concave blade used in surgery.*	gubia
gout *Monosodium urate crystal deposition disease.*	gota
gown	vestido de camisa
grade	grado
Graefe's sign *Also called lid lag, a sign characterized by the upper eyelid not closing over the globe. This is seen commonly in exophthalmic goiter.*	Graefe, signo de
graft	injerto
gram	gramo
granular layer *A deep layer of the cerebellum.*	capa granular
granulation tissue	tejido de granulación
granulocyte *A white blood cell with cytoplasmic secretory granules.*	granulocito
granuloma *A mass of granulation tissue.*	granuloma
grasp reflex *Flexion of the fingers or toes when stimulated.*	reflejo de prensión
Graves' disease *A form of hyperthyroidism exhibited by a goiter and exophthalmos.*	exophthalmic goiter
gravida *Pregnant.*	mujer embarazada
gray matter *The section of the brain and spinal cord composed of branching dendrites and nerve cell bodies.*	sustancia gris
greater than normal	supranormal
grief	pesar
grip strength *Quantitative measurement of the force of a hand grip.*	fuerza compresiva
groan	gemir
groggy	atontado
groin pull *A muscle strain in the inguinal region.*	tirón de la ingle
groin *The genital region.*	ingle
gross	grueso
ground itch *Marked pruritis caused by a hookworm larvae, known otherwise as cutaneous larva migrans.*	prurito del suelo
growth	desarrollo
growth hormone-releasing factor	factor de liberación de la hormona de crecimiento
grunting *A low guttural sound used to describe a person with profound respiratory difficulty.*	gruñido

English	Spanish
guaiac *A substance derived from guaiacum trees used to test for trace amounts of blood, in stool for instance.*	guayaco
guarding *A symptom used to describe a patient resisting an examination because of severe pain; often seen in patients with peritonitis.*	defensa
Guillain-Barré syndrome *An acute autoimmune disorder that causes nerve inflammation subsequently muscle weakness.*	Guillan-Barré, síndrome de
guinea worm *A parasitic nematode worm that lives under the skin, formally called Dracunculus medinensis.*	dracunculiasis
gum	encía
gum (chewing gum)	chicle
gumboil *Swelling noted on the gingiva over a dental abscess.*	postemilla
gumma *A soft granulomatous tumor of the skin or cardiovascular system seen in tertiary syphilis.*	goma
gunshot wound	herida de bala
gustatory agnosia *The loss of the sense of taste.*	agnosia gustativo
gustatory *Referring to sense of taste.*	gustativo
guttural	gutural
gynecology *The branch of medicine associated with the reproductive system of women.*	ginecología
gynecomastia *Enlargement of the breasts.*	ginecomastia
gyrus *Convolutions of the brain where there is infolding.*	circonvolución
habit	hábito
hair (of body)	vello
hair (of head)	cabello
hair cell *Epithelial cells with hairlike projections.*	célula pilosas
hair follicle	folículo piloso
hairy	peludo
hairy tongue *Lingua villosa, a benign condition associated with antibiotic used caused by candida albicans infection.*	lengua vellosa
half	mitad
half-life *The time a drug decreases its effect in half over time.*	vida media
halitosis *Foul odor eminating from the mouth.*	halitosis
hallucination *A perception that is not based on reality.*	aluncinación
hallucinogen *A substance that elicits hallucinations.*	alucinógeno
hallux *Referring to the first toe.*	dedo gordo del pie
hallux valgus *Also called bunion, it is the lateral deviation of the great toe.*	hallux valgus
hallux varus *Medial deviation of the great toe.*	hallus varus
hamartoma *A nodule of superfluous tissue.*	hamartoma
hamate bone; uncinate bone *The medial bone in the distal row of carpal bones adjacent to the fifth metacarpal.*	hueso ganchoso
hammer toe *A condition characterized by extension of the proximal phalanx and flexion of the second and distal phalanges.*	dedo en garra
Hampton maneuver *Rolling a patient during gastrointestinal fluoroscopy in order to obtain an air contrast of the antrum and duodenum.*	maniobra de Hampton
hamstrings *Tendons of the posterior thigh.*	tendones de la corva
hand	mano
hangnail	padrastro
Hansen's disease *Leprosy*	enfermedad de Hansen

English	Spanish
haploid *Either a single set of chromosomes or a set of nonhomologous chromosomes.*	haploide
hapten *The molecular component that determines immunologic specificity.*	hapteno
hard	duro
hard of hearing	medio sordo
harmless	inofensivo
hay fever *An allergy exhibited by pruritis of the eyes and nose, rhinorrhea and excessive lacrimal secretion.*	fiebre del heno
hazy	anieblado
head	cabeza
head trauma *Any injury to the brain.*	traumatismo del cráneo
headache	cefalagia
healing	curación
health	salud
health center	salud de centro
healthy	sano
hearing	audición
hearing aid	audífono
heart	corazón
heart beat	latido, pulsación
heart block *An alteration in the cardiac electrical conduction system.*	bloqueo del corazón
heart burn *Synonym of pyrosis.*	acedía
heart lung machine *Device used during cardiac surgery to replace the function of the heart and lungs while surgery is performed.*	máquina corazón-pulmón
heart murmur	soplo cardíaco
heart rate	frecuencia cardíaca
heat	calor
heat exhaustion *A condition that occurs secondary to prolonged exposure to high ambient temperature; it is exhibited by subnormal temperature, dizziness and nausea.*	colapso por calor
heat stroke *A condition caused by excessive exposure to high ambient temperature; it is exhibited by dry skin, thirst, vertigo, muscle cramps and nausea. The three forms are heat exhaustion, heat cramps and sunstroke.*	insolación calor
heavy	pesado
hebephrenia *A type of schizophrenia exhibited by hallucinations and inappropriate laughter.*	hebefrenia
Heberden's node *Hard nodules formed at the distal interphalangeal joints in osteoarthritis.*	nódulos de Heberden
hedonism *Devoting oneself to being happy.*	hedonismo
heel	talón
height	altura
Heimlich maneuver *A forceful upward thrust to the diaphragm to dislodge an airway obstruction.*	maniobra de Heimlich
heliotherapy *Treatment of disease with sunlight.*	helioterapia
helium *An inert gas that is the lightest of the noble gases.*	helio
helminth *A fluke, tapeworm or nematode.*	helminto
helminthiasis *Being infected by a helminth.*	helmintiasis
hemagglutinin *An antibody that facilitates the agglutination of blood.*	hemoaglutinación

English	Spanish
hemangioma *A benign tumor composed of blood vessels.*	hemangioma
hemarthrosis *Presence of intra-articular blood.*	hemartrosis
hematemesis *Vomiting blood.*	hematemesis
hematin *The insoluble iron protoporphyrin component of hemoglobin.*	hematina
hematinic *A substance that increases hemoglobin in the blood.*	hemático
hematocele *A mass or area of swelling caused by the accumulation of blood.*	hematocele
hematochezia *Presence of blood in the excrement.*	hematoquesia
hematocrit *The measurement of the volume of red blood cells compared to the total volume of blood; recorded in percent.*	hematócrito
hematoma *A mass containing blood.*	hematoma
hematometra *The accretion of blood in the uterus.*	hematómetra
hematomyelia *Accumulation of blood in the spinal cord.*	hematomielia
hematoporphyrin *A derivative of heme that does not contain iron.*	hematoporfirina
hematosalpinx *Presence of blood in the fallopian tube.*	hematosálpinx
hematuria *The presence of blood in the urine.*	hematuria
heme *A constituent of hemoglobin that is an insoluble iron protoporphyrin.*	hem
hemeralopia *Night blindness.*	hemeralopía
hemianopsia *Blindness over half the field of vision.*	hemianopia
hemiballismus *Severe motor restlessness unilaterally, usually from a subthalamic lesion.*	hemibalismo
hemicolectomy *Surgical removal of part of the colon.*	hemicolectomía
hemicrania *1. Pain on one side of the head. 2. Incomplete anencephaly.*	hemicrania
hemiparesis *Unilateral muscle weakness (half the body).*	hemiparesis
hemiplegia *Paralysis of one side of the body.*	hemiplejía
hemisphere *Referring to either the right or left portion of the cerebrum.*	hemisferio
hemizygote *A cell with only one set of genes.*	hemicigoto
hemochromatosis *A hereditary condition exhibited by iron deposition in the tissue and leading to liver disease, bronze discoloration of the skin and diabetes.*	hemocromatosis
hemoconcentration *Decrease in the total fluid content of the blood, leading at times to a falsely elevated hematocrit.*	hemoconcentración
hemocytometer *A device used for counting cells from a blood sample.*	hemocitómetro
hemodialysis *The process of filtering blood outside the body to remove toxins normally excreted by functioning kidneys.*	hemodiálisis
hemoglobin *An iron containing protein used for the transport of oxygen in blood.*	hemoglobina
hemoglobinuria *Presence of free hemoglobin in the urine.*	hemoglobinuria
hemolysis *Breakdown of hemoglobin.*	hemólisis
hemolytic *Something that causes hemolysis.*	hemolítico
hemolytic anemia *Reduced number of erythrocytes due to shortened survival and inability of the bone marrow to compensate.*	anemia hemolítica
hemopericardium *Abnormal presence of blood in the pericardium.*	hemopericardio
hemoperitoneum *Abnormal presence of blood in the peritoneum.*	hemoperitoneo
hemophilia *A hereditary bleeding disorder characterized by hemarthroses and deep tissue bleeding as a result of absence of a coagulation factor such as factor VIII.*	hemofilia
hemophiliac *A person with hemophilia.*	hemofílico
hemophilic arthropathy	artropatía hemofílico
hemophthalmia *Bleeding within the eye.*	hemoftalmía

English	Spanish
hemopneumothorax *Accumulation of blood and air in the pleural space.*	hemoneumotórax
hemopoiesis *The production of blood cells from stem cells.*	hemopoyesis, hematopoyesis
hemopoietin *A hormone secreted by the kidneys that stimulates the bone marrow to produce erythrocytes.*	hemopoyetina
hemoptysis *Expectoration of blood.*	hemoptisis
hemorrhage *Bleeding from a damaged blood vessel.*	hemorragia
hemorrhoidectomy *Surgical excision of a hemorrhoid.*	hemorroidectomía
hemorrhoids *Engorgement of the veins in the anus or rectum.*	hemorroide
hemostasis *The control of bleeding.*	hemostasis
hemothrorax *The abnormal presence of blood in the pleural cavity.*	hemotórax
hence	de aquí
Henoch purpura *Exhibited by vomiting, diarrhea, abdominal pain and hematuria; a non-thrombocytopenic purpura.*	púrpura de Henoch-Schönlein
Henri, syndrome of *Congenital anomaly exhibited by different sized external orifices of the nostrils.*	síndrome de Henri
heparin *A polysaccharide that occurs naturally in the liver and is used as a medication to induce a hypocoagulable state.*	heparina
hepatectomy *Partial or complete surgical resection of the liver.*	hepatectomía
hepatic duct *The right and left hepatic ducts join the cystic duct to form the common bile duct.*	ducto hepático
hepatic flexure of the colon *The junction of the ascending and transverse portion of the colon.*	flexura hepática
hepatic *Referring to the liver.*	hepático
hepatitis *Inflammation of the liver.*	hepatitis
hepatocyte *A liver cell.*	hepatocito
hepatojugular reflex *The presence of jugular venous distension with compression of the abdomen for at least 10 seconds.*	reflejo hepatoyugular
hepatoma *A tumor of the liver.*	hepatoma
hepatomegaly *Enlargement of the liver.*	hepatomegalia
hepatosplenomegaly *Enlargement of the spleen and the liver.*	hepatosplenomegalia
hereditary spherocytosis *A familial hemolytic disease exhibited by abnormally thick erythrocytes.*	esferocitosis hereditario
hereditary *That which is transmitted genetically*	hereditario
hermaphrodite *A person possessing gonadal characteristics of both sexes.*	hermafrodita
hernia, femoral *A bulge in the upper thigh/groin region because of bowel protruding through the muscle.*	hernia femoral
hernia, incarcerated *An irreducible hernia.*	hernia incarcerada
hernia, inguinal *Protrusion of abdominal-cavity contents through the inguinal canal.*	hernia inguinal
hernia, lumbar *Defect in the lumbar muscles or the posterior fascia, below the 12th rib and above the iliac crest.*	hernia lumba
hernia, umbilical *Protrusion of abdominal contents at the umbilicus.*	hernia umbilical
herniated disc *Prolapse of the nucleus pulposus into the spinal cord.*	disco herniado
herniorrhaphy *The surgical repair of a hernia.*	herniorrafía
heroin *A morphine derivative that is highly addictive.*	heroína
herpangina *An infectious disease caused by Coxsackie virus exhibited by vesicular lesion on the soft palate.*	herpangina

English	Spanish
herpes *A skin condition exhibited by formation of clustered vesicular lesions; herpes simplex is at times referred to, albeit incompletely, as herpes.*	herpes
herpes zoster; shingles *A unilateral vesicular rash along one dermatome and caused by inflammation of a posterior nerve root by "the chicken pox virus".*	herpes zóster
herpetic *Referring to herpes.*	herpético
herpetiform *Something that is characteristic of herpes.*	herpetiforme
heterochromia iridis or syndrome of Eric *Congenital anomaly in which the iris of each eye is of a different color.*	heterocromía del iris
heterogenous *That which originates outside the organism.*	heterogéneo
heterotropia *Synonym of strabismus.*	heterotopía
heterozygous *Having different alleles concerning a certain trait.*	heterocigótico
hiatus hernia *Protrusion of part of the stomach through the esophageal hiatus of the diaphragm.*	hernia hiatal
hiccup	hipo
hidradenitis *Inflammation of a sweat gland. When there is purulent discharge it is called hidradenitis suppurativa.*	hidradenitis
hidrosis *The production and secretion of sweat.*	hidrosis
high	alto
high blood pressure	presión alta
high cholesterol	alto nivel de colesterol
hilar *Referring to a hilus.*	hiliar
Hillis-Müller maneuver *A procedure to determine the descent of the head during active labor.*	maniobra de Hillis-Müller
hilum or hilus *A depression where blood vessels and nerve fibers enter an organ.*	hilio
hindbrain *The brainstem which includes the pons, medulla oblongata and cerebellum.*	cerebro posterior
hip	cadera
hip girdle *The bony supporting structure for the legs.*	cintura pelviana Cíngulo de las extremidades inferiores
hip joint	articulación de la cadera
hip replacement	restitución de la cadera
hippocampus *The area at the base of the cerebral ventricles thought to be the center of memory and emotion.*	hipocampo
Hippocratic oath *An vow taken by doctors, indicating they will treat people properly.*	juramento hipocrático
hirsutism *Abnormal growth on hair on a person's face and body.*	hirsutismo
histamine *A chemical responsible for the reaction exhibited when a person has an allergic reaction.*	histamina
histidine *An amino acid precursor to histamine.*	histidina
histiocyte *A phagocytic cell found in connective tissue.*	histiocito
histochemistry	histoquímica
histology *The study of the structure and composition of minute structures.*	histología
histoplasmosis *A fungal pulmonary infection from bat and bird excrement.*	histoplasmosis
hit	dar
HIV *Abbreviation for human immunodeficiency virus.*	VIH virus de inmunodeficiencia humano

English	Spanish
hoarse *A rough, harsh sounding voice.*	ronco
Hodgkin's disease *Also called Hodgkin's lymphoma, it is a cancer that begins in the lymphocytes.*	enfermedad de Hodgkin
hollow	hueco
homeless	sin hogar
homeopathy *A treatment of disease by use of minute doses of toxic substances that would normally be harmful.*	homeopatía
homeostasis *The tendency of an organism to maintain a stable and uniform state.*	hemeostasis
homicide *When one person kills another.*	homicidio
homograft *A graft of tissue from the same species as the recipient.*	homoinjerto
homolateral *Ipsilateral.*	homolateral
homologous *Referring to something derived from the same species but different genotype.*	homólogo
homosexual *A person sexually attracted to someone of the same gender.*	homosexual
homozygous *Having identical alleles for a particular trait.*	homocigótico
hookworm *A parasitic infection of the family Strongylidae that can cause anemia.*	uncinaria
hordeolum *Inflammation of the sebaceous gland of the eye.*	orzuelo
hormone *A substance produced in the body that effects a specific organ.*	hormona
horn *A keratinized outgrowth.*	asta, cuerno
horseshoe kidney *Anomalous renal development.*	riñón en herradura
hospital	hospital
hospital discharge	dar de alta
hot	caliente
hot flash *A symptom of menopause manifested as a sudden sensation of fever.*	fogaje
housemaid's knee *Also referred to as prepatellar bursitis.*	rodilla de mucama
HPV human papillomavirus *The virus that causes genital warts.*	VPH virus del papiloma humano
Hueter's maneuver *The application of downward and forward pressure on the tongue while passing an gastric tube.*	maniobra de Hueter
human	humano
humerus *The long bone in the upper arm.*	húmero
humor, aqueous *The gelatinous fluid circulating between the cornea and lens.*	humor acuoso (a)
humor, vitreus *The fluid circulating between the lens and retina.*	humor vítreo
hunchback *Synonym of kyphosis.*	corcova
hunger	hambre
Huntington's chorea *A neurodegenerative disease characterized initially by behavioral changes and later by a movement disorder. Called Huntington's disease now.*	corea de Huntington
Hutchington's mask *The sensation the face is covered in cobwebs, associated with tabes dorsalis.*	máscara de Hutchinson
Hutchinson's pupil *Dilation of a pupil related to third nerve palsy on the side of the lesion as seen in herniation.*	pupilo de Hutchinson
hyaline *Having a glassy, transparent appearance.*	hialino
hyaloid *Transparent.*	hialoide
hybrid *An animal or plant produced from two different species.*	híbrido
hydatid cyst *A cyst produced by and containing tapeworm larvae.*	quiste hidatídico

English	Spanish
hydatiform *Referring to a hydatid cyst.*	hidatidiforme
hydrarthrosis *An accumulation of water-like fluid in a joint cavity.*	hidrartrosis
hydration *Used to describe fluid balance.*	hidratación
hydrocele *The accumulation of fluid in a body sac.*	hidrocele
hydrocephalus *The excessive accumulation of cerebral spinal fluid in the brain causing enlargement of the head.*	hidrocéfalo
hydrochloric acid *A solution with a low pH formed by dissolving hydrogen chloride in water.*	ácido clorhídrico
hydrochloride	clorhidrato
hydrocortisone *A natural steroid hormone secreted by the adrenal cortex and used in a synthetic formulation for treatment of various medical conditions.*	hidrocortisona
hydrolysis *A reaction with water causing a compound to breakdown.*	hidrólisis
hydronephrosis *Enlargement of a kidney due to interruption of outflow of urine from that kidney.*	hidronefrosis
hydrophobia *Abnormal fear of water.*	hidrofobia
hydropneumothorax *Abnormal accumulation of fluid and air in the pleural space.*	hidroneumotórax
hydrops *The abnormal collection of fluid in a cavity.*	hidropesía
hydrops fetalis *The total body accumulation of fluid in a fetus; the result of a hemolytic reaction in a Rh neg mother.*	hidropesía fetal
hydrosalpinx *Collection of fluid in a fallopian tube.*	hidrosálpinx
hydrothorax *Accumulation of fluid within the thoracic cavity.*	hidrotórax
hygroma *A cyst or bursa filled with fluid.*	hidroma
hygroscopic *The tendancy to absorb moisture from the air.*	higroscópico
hymen *A membrane in the vagina.*	himen
hymenotomy *Surgically creating an opening in the hymen.*	himenotomía
hyoid bone *A horseshoe shaped bone located between the chin and thyroid cartilage.*	hioides
hyperacidity *An abnormally high acid level.*	hiperacidez
hyperactivity *Abnormal increase in activity.*	hiperactividad
hyperalgesia *Greater than normal sensitivity to pain.*	hiperalgesia
hyperbaric *Use of gas at a higher than normal pressure.*	hiperbárico
hyperbaric chamber *A device used to treat decompression illness.*	cámara hiperbárica
hyperbilirubinemia *Higher than normal level of bilirubin in the blood.*	hiperbilirrubinemia
hypercalcemia *Higher than normal level of calcium in the blood.*	hipercalcemia
hypercapnia *Higher than normal level of carbon dioxide in the blood stream.*	hipercapnia
hypercholesterolemia *Higher than normal level of cholesterol in the blood.*	colesterol alto
hyperchromia *An excessive level of hemoglobin in erythrocytes.*	hipercromía
hyperemia *An increase in blood for the area of concern.*	hiperemia
hyperesthesia *Higher than normal skin sensitivity.*	hiperestesia
hyperextension *Extension of an articulation beyond the normal range.*	hiperextensión
hyperflexion *Flexion of an articulation beyond the normal range.*	hiperflexión
hyperglycemia *Higher than normal level of glucose in the blood.*	hiperglucemia
hypergonadism *A condition of excessive gonadal activity and subsequently precocious sexual development.*	hipergonadismo
hyperhidrosis *Excessive perspiration.*	hiperhidrosis
hyperkalemia *Higher than normal level of potassium in the blood stream.*	hipercalemia

English	Spanish
hyperkeratosis *Excessive thickening of the outer layer of skin.*	hiperqueratosis
hyperkinesis *Excessive activity and inability to concentrate.*	hipercinesia
hyperlipidemia *Higher than normal level of lipids in the blood stream.*	hiperlipidemia
hypermetropia *Farsightedness.*	hipermetropía
hypermnesia *Unusually good memory.*	hipermnesia
hypermyotonia *Excessive muscle tone.*	hipermiotonía
hypernatremia *Elevated level of sodium in the blood.*	hipernatremia
hypernephroma *A renal tumor that mimic adrenal cortical tissue.*	hipernefroma
hyperonychia *Hypertrophic nails.*	hiperoniquia
hyperopia *Farsightedness.*	hiperopia
hyperosmia *Increased sense of smell.*	hiperosmia
hyperparathyroidism *Excessive level of parathyroid hormones in the blood stream causing weak bones and hypocalcemia.*	hiperparatiroidismo
hyperphagia *Excessive food ingestion.*	hiperfagia
hyperphoria *Upward deviation of the visual axis of the eye.*	hiperforia
hyperpituitarism *Excessive eosinophilic hormone resulting in acromegaly or excessive basophilic hormone resulting in pituitary compression and ultimately hypopituitarism.*	hipertituitarismo
hyperplasia *Excessive growth of normal cells.*	hiperplasia
hyperpnea *Abnormal increase in rate and depth of respiration.*	hiperpnea
hyperpyrexia *Fever.*	hiperpirexia
hyperreflexia *Abnormally brisk and vigorous reflex.*	hiperreflxia
hypersensitivity *Abnormal increase in sensitivity.*	hipersensibilidad
hypersplenism *Excessive splenic activity resulting in decreased peripheral blood elements and sometimes splenomegaly.*	hiperesplenismo
hypertension *Higher than normal blood pressure.*	hipertensión
hyperthermia *Fever.*	hipertermia
hyperthyroidism *Increased thyroid activity resulting in exophthalmos and increased metabolic rate.*	hipertiroidismo
hypertonia *Excessive tone or tension.*	hipertonía
hypertonic *Increased osmotic pressure.*	hipertónica
hypertrichosis *Excessive hair growth.*	hipertricosis
hypertrophy *Pathologic organ enlargement.*	hipertropia
hyperuricemia *Elevated level of uric acid in the blood.*	hiperuricemia
hyperventilation *Rapid and deep respirations.*	hiperventilación
hypervolemia *Abnormally large amount of fluid in the blood stream.*	hipervolimia
hyphema *A blood collection in the front of the eye.*	hifema
hypnotic *Sleep inducing agent.*	hipnótico
hypocalcemia *Lower than normal level of calcium in the blood.*	hipocalcemia
hypocapnia *A decreased level of carbon dioxide in the blood.*	hipocapnia
hypochlorhydria *A state of decreased secretion of hydrochloric acid in the stomach.*	hipocloridria
hypochondriac *A person suffering from hypochondriasis.*	hipocondríaco
hypochondriasis *Abnormal increase in concern about one's own health.*	hipocondriasis
hypochondrium *The upper abdomen lateral to the epigastrium.*	hipocondrio
hypochromic *Referring to the abnormal decrease in hemoglobin content of erythrocytes.*	hipocromía

84

English	Spanish
hypodermic needle	jeringa hipodérmico
hypoesthesia *Abnormally decreased skin sensitivity.*	hipoestesia
hypofibrinogenemia *Diminished blood fibrinogen level.*	hipofibrinogenemia
hypogastric *Referring to the hypogastrium.*	hipogástrico
hypogastrium *The area of the central abdomen located below the stomach.*	hipogastrio
hypoglossal nerve *Twelfth cranial nerve pair.*	nervio hipogloso
hypoglycemia *Abnormally low blood sugar.*	hipoglicémico
hypogonadism *Abnormal decrease in gonadal function with associated diminished growth and sexual development.*	hipogonadismo
hypokalemia *Diminished level of potassium in the blood stream.*	hipocalemia
hypokalemic periodic paralysis *An inherited disorder that leads to muscle weakness related to a low serum potassium level.*	parálisis periódica hipocaliémica
hypomania *A moderate form of mania.*	hipomanía
hyponatremia *Diminished level of sodium in the blood stream.*	hiponatremia
hypoparathyroidism *Abnormal decrease in parathyroid function.*	hipoparatiroidismo
hypophoria *Downward deviation of the visual axis of the eye.*	hipoforia
hypophosphatasia *A genetic defect of diminished alkaline phosphatase in the cells leading to bone demineralization.*	hipofosfatasia
hypophysectomy *Surgical removal of the pituitary gland.*	hipofisectomía
hypophysis *Pituitary gland.*	hipófisis
hypopituitarism *Diminished pituitary activity exhibited by obesity and persistence of adolescent characteristics.*	hipopituitarismo
hypoplasia *Incomplete development.*	hipoplasia
hypopyon *The presence of purulent fluid in the anterior chamber of the eye.*	hipopión
hyposalivation *Secretion of saliva below the normal rate.*	hiposalivación
hypospadias *Congenital condition exhibited by development of the urethral meatus on the inferior aspect of the penis.*	hipospadias
hypostasis *The formation of a deposit.*	hipostasis
hypotension *Abnormally low blood pressure.*	hipotensión
hypothalamus *Located inferior to the thalamus it controls visceral activities, water balance, temperature and sleep.*	hipotálamo
hypothenar eminence *The prominence on the palm at the base of the fingers adjacent to the ulna.*	eminencia hipotenar
hypothermia *Lower than normal temperature.*	hipotermia
hypothyroidism *Reduced functioning of the thyroid.*	hipotiroidismo
hypotonia *Reduced tone or activity.*	hipotonía
hypoxia *Diminished oxygen content.*	hipoxia
hysterectomy *Surgical removal of the uterus.*	histerectomía
hysteria *A psychological condition exhibited by uncontrolled emotion or exaggerated manifestations.*	histeria
hysterography *1. Recording of uterine contractions. 2. Roentgenography of the uterus after administration of contrast media.*	histerografía
hysteromyomectomy *Surgical removal of a uterine myoma.*	histeromiomectomía
hysteropexy *Surgical fixation of the uterus by shortening of the round ligaments or by other means.*	histeropexia
hysterosalpingography *Roentgenography of the uterus and fallopian tubes after instillation of contrast media.*	histerosalpingografie
hysterotomy *Surgical opening of the uterus.*	histerotomía

English	Spanish
i.e. *A latin derived abbreviation for "that is to say"(In latin: id est)*	es decir
iatrogenic *A problem caused by medical treatment.*	iatrogénico
ichthyosis *A congenital anomaly exhibited by excessively dry, thick skin.*	ictiosis
icterus *Yellowing of the skin and sclerae because of excess bilirubin.*	icterus
identical twins *Twins from the same zygote.*	gemelo monocigóticos
idiopathic *Relating to a disease with an unknown cause.*	idiopático
ileitis *Inflammation of the ileum.*	ileítis
ileocecal valve *The membranous folds between the ileum and cecum.*	válvula ileocecal
ileocolitis *Inflammation of the ileum and cecum.*	ileocolitis
ileocolostomy *Creating a surgical opening between the ileum and colon.*	ileocolostomía
ileoproctostomy *Creating a surgical opening between the ileum and the rectum.*	ileoproctostomía
ileostomy *Surgical creation of an opening in the ileum that is placed at the skin surface.*	ileostomía
ileum *The portion of the small bowel from the jejunum to the cecum.*	íleon
ileus *A temporary obstruction in the intestine.*	íleo
iliac crest *The upper border of the ilium.*	cresta ilíaca
iliococcygeal *Referring to the ilium and coccyx.*	iliococcígeo
ilium *The large bone at the superior aspect of the pelvis which is present bilaterally.*	ilium
illiterate	analfabeto, analfabeta
immune *Being resistant to an infection.*	inmune
immune response *The body's reaction to what is perceived as a foreign substance.*	repuesta inmune
immunization *A medication given to provide immunity.*	inmunización
immunochemistry *The study of immune response and biochemistry.*	inmunoquímica
immunodeficiency *An inadequate immune response.*	inmunodeficiencia
immunoelectrophoresis *A means of differentiating proteins and other compounds by comparing their mobility and antigenic specificities.*	inmunoelectroforesis
immunoglobulin *Serum and cellular proteins of the immune system.*	inmunoglobulina
immunosuppression *The inhibition of the immune response.*	inmunosupresión
impacted tooth *A tooth that does not erupt because adjacent teeth prevent it.*	impacción dental
impaired	defectuoso
impairment	deterioro
imperforate *Lack of an opening. An infant with an imperforate anus has a congenital defect with no anal opening.*	imperforado
impervious *Not affected by.*	impenetrable
implant	implante
implementation	ejecución
impotence *Absence of power. A term used to describe erectile dysfunction.*	impotencia
inanition *Generalized weakness from lack of nutrition.*	inanición
inarticulate *Indistinct speech.*	inarticulado
incest *Sexual relations between related people.*	incesto
incipient *Starting to happen.*	incipiente
incision	incisión
incisor *Sharp-edged tooth; humans have four incisors.*	incisivo
incisura *A notch or indentation usually on the edge of a bone.*	incisura
incisure *A notch or incision.*	incisura

English	Spanish
inclusion body *Variably shaped bodies in the nuclei of cells found in infections such as rabies and herpes.*	inclusión celulares
incoherent *Absence of intelligible speech.*	incoherente
incontinence *Inability to control urination.*	incontinencia
incoordination *Absence of smooth, efficient body movement.*	incoordinación
increment	incremento
incubator *A warming device for infants.*	incubadora
incus *The middle ear bone between the stapes and malleus.*	incus
indeed	ciertemente
indigenous *Naturally occurring.*	indígena
indigestion *Inadequate digestion for various reasons.*	indigestión
indolent *1. Causing little pain. 2. Slow healing ulcer.*	indolente
induce, to *Facilitated. When referring to labor, it means medication was given to assist in delivery of the fetus.*	inducir
induced abortion *Surgical or medical evacuation of the fetus.*	aborto inducido
induration *An area that is abnormally hard.*	induración
indwelling catheter *Continuous use tube usually referring to a tube in the urinary bladder.*	catéter permanente
indwelling foley *A catheter inserted into the urinary bladder with an inflatable ballon on the tip.*	catéter de Foley
inebriation *Intoxication with drugs or alcohol.*	inebriación
ineffective	ineficaz
inertia *The tendency to remain unchanged.*	inercia
inevitable *Not preventable.*	inevitable
infancy	infancia
infant	lactante
infant, post-term	lactante postérmino
infant, pre-term	lactante pretérmino
infant, term	lactante de término
infantile *Referring to babies or young children.*	infantil
infarct *Referring to dead tissue.*	infarto
infarction *Dead tissue, for example, myocardial infarction.*	infarto
infectious	infeccioso
inferior	inferior
inferior pelvis strait *The pelvic outlet.*	salida pélvica
infestation *The presence of large numbers, as in lice infestation.*	infestación
inflammation *Localized redness, excessive warmth and swelling.*	inflamación
influenza *Viral infection causing fever, muscle aches and catarrh.*	gripe, influenza
infraspinous *Below the scapular spine.*	infraespinoso
infundibulum *The connection between the hypothalamus and the posterior pituitary gland.*	infundíbulo
infusion *The injection of fluid into tissue or a vein.*	infusión
ingestion *The intake of food or liquid orally.*	ingestión
ingrown nail *Also referred to as onychocryptosis.*	uña encarnada
inguinal *Referring to the groin.*	inguinal
inhalation *The act of breathing in.*	inhalación
injection *The act of a needle being inserted into a body.*	inyección

English	Spanish
injure, to	lesionar
injury	lesión
injury, closed head *Brain trauma not associated with damage to the dura or skull.*	lesión céfalica cerrada
injury, contrecoup of brain *An injury to the brain on the side opposite of that which was struck.*	lesión encontragolpe del cerebro
injury, degloving *Trauma that involves the ripping of skin and subcutaneous tissue from the underlying tissue.*	lesión por desguantamiento o desguante
injury, hyperextension-hyperflexion *An injury, usually to the cervical spine, that involves rapid deceleration, causing pronounced extension and flexion.*	lesión de hiperextensión-hiperflexión
inner ear *Made up of the cochlea and semicircular canals.*	oreja interno
innervation *The presence of a nerve supply.*	inervación
innominate artery *The first branch off the aortic arch that branches into the right common carotid and right subclavian arteries.*	arteria innominada
innominate *Referring to the innominate artery.*	innominado
inoculation *Injection with a vaccine to provide immunity.*	inoculación
inorganic *Not coming from natural growth.*	inorgánico
insane *A term not used in formal medical evaluations that when used by a layperson means a serious mental illness.*	insano
insanity *Referring to a serious mental illness.*	insania
insensible *Unable to perceive a stimulus.*	insensible
insertion	inserción
inside	dentro de
insidious *A slow, gradual and harmful advancement.*	insidioso
insomnia *Sleeplessness.*	insomnio
inspiration *Drawing in a breath.*	inspiración
inspiratory reserve volume *The amount of air that can be inhaled after a normal inhalation.*	volumen de reserva inspiratoria
inspissate, to *To thicken or congeal.*	espesar
instep *The medial aspect of the foot between the ankle and the ball of the foot.*	empeine
insulin *A hormone produced by the pancreas and synthetically to control blood glucose levels.*	insulina
insulinoma *An islet cell tumor that causes abnormally high insulin secretion and thus hypoglycemia.*	insulinoma
intake	consumo
integument *Outer protective layer.*	integumento
intelligence quotient (IQ) *A number representing a person's ability to problem solve compared to a matched-control.*	cociente de inteligencia (CI)
intensive	intensivo
intensive care	cuidado intensivo
intention tremor *The tremulous movement noted when a person is beginning to perform a task but not seen at rest.*	temblor intencional
interarticular *Between the articular surfaces of a joint.*	interarticular
intercellular *Between cells.*	intercelular
intermittent	intermitente
internal	interno

English	Spanish
interosseous *Referring to something between bones, like the interosseous muscles of the hand.*	interóseo
interstitial *Referring to the interstices of tissue.*	intersticial
intertrigo *Irritation present because adjacent surfaces rub together.*	intertrigo
intertrochanteric *Referring to the space within the trochanter.*	intertrocantéreo
interval	intervalo
interventricular *Between the ventricles.*	interventricular
intestinal obstruction *Blockage of the intestine by mass or volvulus.*	obstrucción intestinal
intestinal *Referring to the intestines.*	intestinal
intestine *A general term used for the section of bowel from the stomach to the anus.*	intestino
intraabdominal abscess	abasceo intraabdominal
intraabdominal *Within the abdominal cavity.*	intraabdominal
intraarticular *Within a joint space.*	intraarticular
intracellular *Within a cell.*	intracelular
intracerebral *Within the cerebrum.*	intracerebral
intracranial *Within the cranial vault.*	intracraneal
intradermal *Within the dermis.*	intradérmico
intradural *Within the dural space.*	intradural
intramedullary *1. Within the medulla oblongata. 2. Within the bone marrow.*	intramedular
intramuscular *Within a muscle.*	intramuscular
intraocular fluid *Fluid within the globe.*	fluido intraocular
intraosseous *Within a bone.*	intraóseo
intraperitoneal *Within the peritoneal cavity.*	intraperitoneal
intrathecal *Technically means within a sheath but this term is used when medication is instilled in the dura mater spinalis.*	intratecal
intrauterine contraceptive device (IUD) *A device used to physically prevent the implantation of a fertilized ovum.*	dispotivo intrauterino anticonceptivo (DIUA)
intrauterine *Within the uterus.*	intrauterino
intravenous infusion *Administration of fluid into a vein.*	infusión intravenoso
intravenous tubing	tubo intravenoso
intravenous *Within a vein.*	intravenoso
intubation *Placement of a tube; commonly used to refer to endotracheal intubation.*	intubación (intubación endotraqueal)
intussusception *The inversion of one portion of the bowel into another.*	intususcepción
inulin *A polysaccharide used in the testing of renal function.*	inulina
inunction *The application of lotion with friction.*	inunción
involucrum *A wrap or covering (referring to a sequestrum).*	involucrum
involutional *The shrinkage of an organ when it is not in use, as in the uterus after childbirth.*	involutivo
involved	enredado
iodine *A chemical used as an antiseptic and a deficiency of it can lead to goiter.*	yodo
iodism *A condition caused by excessive iodine intake resulting in diarrhea , weakness, and convulsions.*	yodismo
ion channel *A selectively permeable cell membrane to certain ions.*	canal iónico
ionizing radiation *High energy radiation that produces ion pairs in matter.*	radiación ionizante
ipsilateral *On the same side.*	ipsilateral

English	Spanish
iridectomy *Surgical removal of part of the iris.*	iridectomía
iridocyclitis *Inflammation of the ciliary body and the iris.*	iridocilitis
iridoplegia *Paralysis of part of the iris with subsequent lack of contraction or dilation of the pupil.*	iridoplejía
iridotomy *A surgical opening of the iris.*	iridotomía
iris *The colored membrane posterior to the cornea.*	iris
iron *An element found in hemoglobin.*	hierro
iron-deficiency anemia *A microcytic anemia.*	anemia ferropénica
irradiation *The process of being irradiated.*	irradiación
irrelevant *Not pertinent.*	irrelevante
irritable bowel syndrome *A condition exhibited by chronic diarrhea or constipation and abdominal pain; it is sometimes associated with a labile emotional state.*	síndrome del intestino irritable
ischemia *Inadequate blood supply to a part of the body.*	isquemia
ischemic contracture *A muscle's resistance to passive stretch that is related to a decrease in arterial flow from any reason.*	contractura isquémica
ischemic heart disease *Inadequate blood supply to the heart.*	insuficiencia coronaria
ischemic optic neuropathy *A general category of a cause of blindness with several subcategories.*	neuropatía óptica isquémica
ischium *The inferoposterior portion of the pelvis.*	isquión
islet *Tissue that is structurally separate from adjacent tissues.*	islote
isoantibody *A situation in which an antibody of person A reacts with an antigen of person B.*	isoanticuerpo
isolation *A ward where patients with infectious disease are housed.*	aislamiento
isthmus *A narrow piece of tissue connecting two larger body parts.*	istmo
itch	prurito
jaundice *Yellowing of the sclerae and skin because of excessive bilirubin in the blood.*	ictericia
jaw *Mandible.*	mandíbula
jejunectomy *Surgical removal of the jejunum.*	yeyunectomía
jejunostomy *Surgical creation of an opening in the jejunum.*	yeyunostomía
Jendrassik's maneuver *A method of distracting a patient while checking the patellar reflex.*	maniobra de Jendrassik
jock itch *Pruritis caused by tinea cruris.*	prurito inguinal
jugular notch *The notch on the upper border of the sternum.*	incisura supraesternal
jugular *Referring to the neck, as in jugular vein.*	yugular
juvenile angiofibroma *A noncancerous growth in the nose or pharyngeal region.*	angiofibroma juvenil
juxta-articular *Positioned near a joint.*	yuxtaarticulación
juxtaglomerular apparatus *Cells located in the tunica media of the afferent glomerular arterioles.*	aparato yuxtaglomerular
kala-azar *A disease caused by Leishmania donovani that is exhibited by weight loss, fever, anemia and hepatosplenomegaly.*	kala azar Leishmaniasis visceral.
karyokinesis *A part of mitosis involving the cell nucleus division.*	cariocinesis
karyotype *The arrangement of chromosomes in a single cell.*	cariotipo
keloid *Hypertrophic scar tissue that forms after a minor cut or surgical procedure.*	queloide
keratectasia *Obtrusion of the cornea.*	queratectasia

90

English	Spanish
keratectomy *Excision of a portion of the cornea.*	queratectomía
keratic *Referring to the cornea.*	querático
keratin *A protein found in the skin, hair, nails and enamel of the teeth.*	queratina
keratoma *A protuberance of horny tissue.*	queratoma
keratomalacia *Softening of the cornea.*	queratomalacia
keratosis *A growth of keratin such as a wart or callosity.*	queratosis
kernicterus *A condition associated with high bilirubin levels that causes yellow staining of cerebral tissues and subsequent neurologic dysfunction.*	kernicterus
ketoacidosis *Usually referring to diabetic ketoacidosis in which ketones are broken down, causing a decrease in blood pH.*	cetoacidosis
ketone	cetone
ketonemia *Presence of ketone in the blood.*	cetonemia
ketonuria *Presence of ketone in the urine.*	cetonuria
ketosis *The presence of an abnormally high level of ketones in the blood and body tissues.*	cetosis
kick, to	acocear
kidney *One of two glandular organs that form urine.*	riñón
kinase *An enzyme that facilitates movement of phosphate from ATP to another molecule.*	cinasa
kineplasty *An amputation done in a fashion to facilitate ambulation.*	cineplastia
kinesis *Movement of a part in response to a stimulus.*	cinesia
knee	rodilla
knee elbow position *Knees and elbows are on the table and the chest is in the air.*	posición rodilla-codo
knee jerk reflex *Contraction of the quadriceps, yielding leg extension when the quadriceps tendon is tapped.*	reflejo de sacudida de la rodilla
kneecap *Common term for patella.*	rótula
kneeling	arodillarse
knock knees *Common term for genu valgum.*	patizambo Genu valgum.
knot	nudo
known	conocido
knuckle	nudillo
koilonychia *Thin and concave fingernails.*	coiloniquia
Koplik's spots *Red buccal macules with a blue center; seen in measles.*	mancha de Koplik
kopophobia *A morbid fear of fatigue.*	copofobia
Köhler's disease *Malformation of the navicular bone.*	enfermedad de Köhler
kraurosis vulvae *Dryness and shrinkage of the vulva.*	craurosis vulvar Leucocraurosis.
Krebs cycle *The process of aerobic respiration by which living cells generate energy.*	ciclo del ácido tricarboxílico
kubisagari *Vestibular neuronitis.*	kubisagari Vértigo epidémico.
Kussmaul respiration *The slow, deep breathing noted in patients with acidosis.*	respiración de Kussmaul
kwashiorkor *A form of malnutrition from inadequate protein intake.*	kwashiorkor
kyphoscoliosis *An abnormal outward and lateral curvature of the spine.*	cifoescoliosis
kyphosis *Abnormal outward curvature of the spine.*	cifosis

91

English	Spanish
lab result	resultado labatororio
labial *Referring to the lip.*	labial
labile *Easily altered; emotionally unstable.*	lábil
labium majus (plural= labia majora) *The folds of skin forming the lateral borders of the pudendal cleft.*	labio pudendo mayor
labium minus (plural=labia minora) *The folds of skin posterior to the labia majora.*	labio pudendo menor
labium *Referring to any lip shaped structure.*	labium
laboratory	laboratorio
labyrinthitis *Inflammation of the labyrinth.*	laberintitis
labrum *An edge or lip. The labrum acetabular is the fibrocartilagous rim attached to the acetabulum.*	labrum
labyrinth *Inner ear structure concerned with balance.*	laberinto
laceration *An injury that produced a cut in the skin or tissue such as a tear during childbirth.*	laceración
lacrimal *Referring to the secretion of tears.*	lagrimal
lacrimation *The secretion of tears.*	lagrimeo
lactalbumin *Proteins found in milk.*	lactalbúmina
lactase *An enzyme that facilitates the breakdown of lactose to glucose and galactose.*	lactasa
lactation *The secretion of milk from mammary glands.*	lactación
lactic *Referring to milk.*	láctico
lactiferous duct *A canal that carries milk.*	conducto lactíferos
lactose *A disaccharide present in milk.*	lactosa
lactose intolerance *The inability of the small bowel to digest lactose.*	intolerencia a la lactosa
lacuna *A small cavity or depression.*	laguna
lagophthalmos *Characterized by the inability to close the eyelid completely over the eye.*	lagoftalmos
laliophobia *Abnormal fear of speaking or stuttering.*	lalofobia
lalochezia *Relief of stress by uttering obsenities.*	laloquecia
lambdoid *The suture connecting the parietal bones with the occipital bone.*	sutura lambdoidea
lamella *A thin layer of bone.*	laminilla
laminectomy *The surgical removal of part of a vertebrae.*	laminectomía
lancet *A small sharp instrument used to obtain a drop of blood for testing.*	lanceta
laparoscope *A fiber-optic instrument used to visualize the peritoneal contents.*	laparoscopio
laparoscopy *A procedure utilizing a laparoscope.*	laparoscopia
laparotomy *A surgical incision of the abdomen.*	laparotomía
laryngeal *Referring to the larynx.*	laríngeo
laryngectomy *Surgical removal of the larynx.*	laringectomía
laryngismus stridulus *Sudden, severe laryngeal spasm.*	laringismo
laryngitis *Inflammation of the larynx.*	laringitis
laryngology *The study of the larynx and related diseases.*	laringología
laryngopharynx *The pharyngeal space between the superior aspect of the glottis and the opening of the larynx.*	laringofaringe
laryngospasm *Sudden, involuntary muscle contraction of the larynx.*	laringoespasmo
laryngostenosis *Abnormal narrowing of the larynx.*	laringoestenosis
laryngotomy *Surgical creation of an opening in the larynx.*	laringotomía

English	Spanish
larynx *A hollow muscular structure that contains the vocal cords.*	laringe
last	pasado
late	tarde
lateral *Referring to the side of the body.*	lateral
laterodeviation	laterodesviación
lathyrism *A disease characterized by tremors, spastic paralysis and paresthesias caused by Lathyrus sativus.*	latirismo Lupinosis.
laugh, to	reír
laxity *A description of a joint that is loose.*	flojedad
layer	capa
lead *An element with an atomic number of 82.*	plomo
lead poisoning *The ingestion of lead, exhibited in severe cases by paralysis, encephalopathy, purple gingiva, and colic.*	envenenamiento por plomo
leaflet *Cusp.*	valva, cúspide
leakage	fuga
learning	aprendizaje
lecithin *A compound widely used by tissues, derived from egg yolks and it consists of phospholipids linked to choline.*	lecitina
leech *An annelid used in some tropical regions for drawing out blood; they have an anticoagulant effect locally and have been attached to digits of persons with acute peripheral ischemia.*	sanguijuela
left	izquierda
left handed	sinistrómano Zurdo
leg	pierna
legionnaires' disease *The name was derived after an outbreak at a convention of the American Legion; it is manifested by fever, chills, dyspnea, and cough.*	enfermedad de los legionarios
leishmaniasis *A condition caused by a flagellate protozoan parasite that is exhibited by visceral or dermatologic manifestations.*	leishmaniasis
length	longitud
lengthening	alargamiento
lens *The transparent chamber between the posterior chamber and the vitreous body.*	lens
lenticular *Referring to the lens of the eye.*	lenticular
lentigo *A benign condition exhibited by flat brown patches on the skin.*	léntigo
leontiasis ossea *Bilateral hypertrophy of the bones of the face and cranium.*	leontiasis ósea Enfermedad de Virchow.
Leopold's maneuver *Used to determine fetal position.*	maniobra de Leopold
leproma *A superficial granulatomous papule that is seen in leprosy.*	leproma
leprosy *A contagious disease caused by Mycobacterium leprae that causes insensate papules and disfiguration.*	lepra
leptomeningitis *A general term used to describe meningitis of the pia and arachnoid of the brain.*	leptomeningitis
leptospirosis *A zoonosis caused by the spirochete Leptospira interrogans transmitted by rats and contaminated water.*	leptospirosis
lesbian	lesbiana
less	menos
lethal	letal

English	Spanish
lethal dose *The amount of a drug required to cause death.*	dosis letal
lethargy *Absence of energy.*	letargia
leucinosis; maple syrup urine disease *A condition characterized by an enzyme defect causing an increase in leucine in the urine.*	leucinosis
leukemia *A malignant disease causing an increase in the number of abnormal and immature leukocytes.*	leucemia
leukine (or leucine) *An amino acid obtained from hydrolysis of some proteins.*	leucina
leukocyte *A white blood cell.*	leucocito
leukocythemia *Synonym of leukemia.*	leucocitemia
leukocytolysis *Destruction of white blood cells.*	leucocitólisis
leukocytosis *An increase in the number of leukocytes.*	leucocitosis
leukodermia *A localized loss of skin pigment.*	leucodermia
leukonychia *A whitish discoloration of the fingernails and toenails.*	leuconiquia
leukopenia *A decreased number of leukocytes in the blood.*	leucopenia
leukopoiesis *Production of white blood cells.*	leucopoyesis
leukorrhea *Thick white vaginal discharge.*	leucorrea
levator *A muscle that raises part of the body; the levator labii superioris raised the upper lip.*	levator
levulose *Synonym for fructose.*	levulosa Fructosa
libido *Sexual desire.*	libido
library	biblioteca
lice *Plural for louse, a small parasite that lives on the skin. Pediculus humanus capitis is a head louse.*	piojo
lichen *A term used to describe a variety of papular skin diseases. Lichen planus is a shiny, flat, violaceous eruption of the mucous membranes, skin and genitalia.*	liquen
life expectancy	expectativa de vida
life-threatening	enfermedad mortífera
lifetime	curso de la vida
lift, to	levantar
ligament	ligamento
ligature *A thread used to tie a vessel.*	ligadura
light	luz
light adaptation *The pupillary adjustment after going from a dark environment to one of bright light.*	adaptación a la luz
likelihood	probabilidad
limb	segmento
limbus *The margin of a structure, for example, of the cornea and sclera.*	límbico
liminal *Referring to a threshold.*	liminal
lincture *A medicine mixed with a sweet substance.*	linctura
linea alba *The tendinous portion of the anterior abdomen between the two rectus muscles.*	línea de Hunter
lingua nigra *A condition characterized by a dark fur-like covering on the dorsum of the tongue.*	lengua nigra
lip, lower *Labium inferius oris.*	labio inferior
lip, upper *Labium superius oris.*	labio superior de la boca
lipase *A pancreatic enzyme that facilitates the breakdown of fats.*	lipasa

English	Spanish
lipemia *Abnormally high fat content in the blood.*	lipemia
lipid *A compound that is a fatty acid which is insoluble in water but soluble in organic solvents.*	lípido
lipid-lowering agent *A medication used to treat hyperlipidemia.*	reductor de colesterol
lipoatrophy *Fatty tissue atrophy.*	lipoatrofia
lipochondrodystrophy *A congenital condition exhibited by short stature, kyphosis, mental deficiency and short fingers.*	lipocondrodistrofia
lipocyte *A fat cell.*	lipocito
lipodystrophy *Abnormal fat metabolism.*	lipodistrofia
lipoid *Referring to fat.*	lipoide
lipoidosis *Abnormal lipid metabolism.*	lipoidosis
lipoma *A benign tumor consisting of fat cells.*	lipoma
lipoprotein *A soluble protein used to transport fat or lipids.*	lipoproteína
lipotrophic substance *A compound which causes an increase in body fat.*	sustancia lipotrófico
lisping *A speech problem in which "s" and "z" are pronounced "th".*	ceceo
liter	litro
lithagogue *A treatment of a calculus.*	litagogo
litholapaxy *The crushing and then removal of a calculus.*	litolapaxia
lithotomy *Surgical removal of a calculus.*	litotomía
lithotritor *An instrument used to crush a calculus.*	litotrito
litmus *A dye that turns red with low pH and blue with high pH.*	tornasol
liver *A large glandular organ in the right upper quadrant that functions in digestive processes, as well as, neutralizing toxins.*	hígado
liver abscess	absceso hígado
lobar *Referring to a lobe.*	lobar
lobe *A body part divided by a fissure.*	lóbulo
lobectomy *Surgical removal of a lobe (generally lung or liver).*	lobectomía
lobotomy *Surgical incision into the prefrontal lobe; historically a treatment of mental illness.*	lobotomía
Lobo's disease *A condition exhibited by small, red, hard papules in the sacral region caused by Lacazia loboi.*	enfermedad de Lobo, Lobomicosis
lobule *A small lobe.*	lobulillo
localization *Establishment of a site of a disease process.*	localización
localized *Toward one point or area.*	localizado
lochia *Vaginal secretions noted within two weeks of childbirth.*	loquios
locked-in syndrome *A neurologic condition characterized by a person being conscious of their surroundings but being unable to verbally communicate that understanding.*	síndrome de encierro
loculated *Divided into small cavities.*	loculado
loiasis *A disease caused by the filarial nematode Loa loa.*	loasis
long acting	de larga acción
long time	mucho tiempo
long-standing	de larga duración
longevitiy	longevidad
longsighted *Synonym of hyperopia.*	hiperopía. Presbicia.
loose	suelto
looseness	soltura

95

English	Spanish
lordosis *An abnormal depth of the inward curvature of the spine.*	lordosis
loss of consciousness *Unresponsive to verbal and tactile stimuli.*	pérdido el conocimiento
loss of function	pérdida de función
loss of motion	pérdida de movimiento
lost to follow-up *This describes a situation in which a patient has a chronic medical problem but has not been seen regularly.*	pérdido el seguimiento
lots of	mucho
low back pain	lumbago
low nasal bridge *A flattening of the top part of the nose.*	puente nasal bajo
low-fat foods	alimentos bajos en grasas
lower extremity edema	edema por declive
lubricant	lubricante
lumbago *Pain in the region of the lumbar spine.*	lumbago
lumbar puncture *Insertion of a needle into the spinal canal in the region of L3-4 to obtain a sample of CSF.*	punción lumbar
lumbar *Referring to the spinal region inferior to the thoracic spine.*	lumbar
lumen *A hollow cavity.*	lumen
lump	protuberancia
lunate bone *A carpal bone that articulates with the wrist.*	hueso lunar
lung	pulmón
lung capacity *The amount of air in the lungs after a maximal inhalation.*	capacidad vital
lunula *The pale area at the base of a fingernail.*	lúnula
lupus erythematosous *An autoimmune inflammatory disease exhibited by a butterfly shaped rash on the face along with visceral and connective tissue abnormalities.*	lupus eritematoso
luteinizing hormone (LH) *A pituitary hormone that stimulates ovulation in females and androgen in males.*	hormona luteinizante
luteotropic *Synonym of prolactin.*	luteotrófico
lymph *A transparent and sometimes opalescent fluid that flows in the lymph channels.*	linfa
lymph node *An area of organized lymphatic tissue.*	ganglio linfático
lymphadenitis *Inflammation of a lymph node.*	linfadenitis
lymphangiectasis *Distention of the lymph channels.*	linfangiectasia
lymphangioma *A mass composed of newly formed lymph tissue.*	linfangioma
lymphangitis *Inflammation of the lymph vessels.*	linfangitis
lymphatic *Referring to the lymph system.*	linfático
lymphocyte *A white blood cell produced by the lymph tissue.*	linfocito
lymphocythemia *Abnormally high number of lymphocytes in the blood.*	linfocitemia
lymphocytic leukemia *Chronic accumulation of functionally incompetent lymphocytes.*	leucemia linfocítica
lymphocytopenia *Decrease in the usual number of lymphocytes in the blood.*	linfocitopenia
lymphocytosis *The organization of cysts containing lymph.*	linfocitosis
lymphoid *Similar to lymph.*	linfoide
lymphoma *A malignant disease of the lymph system, Hodgkin's lymphoma for example.*	linfoma
lymphosarcoma *A malignant disease of the lymph system that does not include Hodgkin's lymphoma.*	linfosarcoma

English	Spanish
lysine *An amino acid found in most proteins.*	lisina
lysis *The rupture of a cell wall or membrane.*	lisis
lysosome *An organelle contained in the cytoplasm of eukaryotic cells.*	lisosoma
lysozyme *An enzyme in tears that facilitates destruction of certain bacterial cell walls.*	lisozima
lytic *Referring to lysis.*	lítico
macrocheilia *Abnormally large lips.*	macroqueilia
macrocyte *A large red blood cell.*	macrocito
macrocytosis *Referring to the status of an increased number of large erythrocytes as seen in Vitamin B12 deficiency.*	macrocitosis
macrodactyly *Abnormally large digits.*	macrodactilia
macroencephaly *Having an abnormally large head.*	macroencefalia
macroglobulinemia *A condition exhibited by an increase number of macroglobulins in the blood.*	macroglobulinemia
macroglossia *Abnormally large tongue.*	macroglosia
macromastia *Abnormally large breasts.*	macromastia
macromelia *Abnormally large head or extremity.*	macromelia
macrophage *A phagocytic cell that originates in the tissues.*	macrófago
macrostomia *Abnormal increase in the width of the mouth.*	macrostomía
macula *1. The area of the eye of greatest visual acuity that surrounds the fovea. 2. A small flat discoloration of the skin (synonym for macule).*	macula
macula solaris *Formal medical term describing a freckle.*	peca
maculopapule *A skin lesion that is similar to both a macule and a papule.*	maculopápula
mad cow disease *Bovine spongiform encephalopathy, a disease that cause cerebral degeneration exhibited by ataxia.*	encefalopatía espongiforme bovina
madness	locura
magnet	imán
magnetic	magnético
magnetic resonance imaging (MRI) *Images are produced by evaluating the response of body tissue. nuclei to radio waves in a magnetic field.*	imágenes por resonancia magnética
maiden name	apellido de soltera
maintenance	mantenimiento
Malabar itch. *Pruritis associated with tinea imbricata which is characterized by overlapping rings of papulosquamous patches. It is also known as oriental ringworm.*	prurito de Malabar. Tiña imbricata.
malacia *The abnormal softening of a body part or tissue.*	malacia
maladjustment	inadaptación
malaise	malestar
malalignment (dental) *Displacement of the teeth from their normal position.*	malalineación
malaria *A condition caused by a protozoan of the genus Plasmodium. It is transmitted by mosquitos and is exhibited by fever, chills, headache. In the severe form it can lead to convulsions, increased ICP and death.*	paludismo
malignant	maligno
malignant hypertension *Sudden, severe hypertension associated with neuroretinitis.*	hipertensión maligno
malingering *Feigning illness.*	simulación
malleolus *A bony protrusion on medial and lateral aspect of each ankle.*	maléolo
malleolus, lateral *The lateral aspect of the distal fibula.*	maléolo lateral

English	Spanish
malleolus, medial *The medial aspect of the distal portion of the tibia.*	maléolo interno
mallet finger *Flexion contracture of the distal phalanx.*	dedo en maza
malleus *Small bone in the inner ear that articulates with the incus.*	malleus
malnutrition *Lack of appropriate nutrition.*	desnutrición
malpractice *Negligent professional activity.*	malpraxis
maltose *A disaccharide hydrolyzed by amylase.*	maltosa
malunion *The union of a fracture in a faulty position.*	malaunión
mammaplasty *Plastic surgery of the breast.*	mamoplastia
mammary *Referring to the breast.*	mamario
mammary gland *The mass of tissue posterior to the nipples which has the essential task of milk production.*	glándula mamaria
mammillary *Referring to a nipple.*	mamilar
mammography *Roentgenography of the breasts, used as a screening test for cancer.*	mamografía
man	hombre
management	gestión
mandatory	obilgatorio
mandible *The lower jaw.*	mandíbula
mania *A mental disorder exhibited by hyperexcitability, delusions and euphoria.*	manía
manic-depressive psychosis *A mental disorder exhibited by alternating periods of depression and mania.*	psicosis maniacodepresiva
manometer *Device used for pressure monitoring.*	manómetro
manubrium sterni *The superior segment of the sternum which articulates with the clavicle and first rib.*	manubrio del esternón
maple syrup urine disease *A condition characterized by an enzyme defect causing an increase in leucine in the urine.*	enfermedad de la orina en jarabe de arce
mapping	mapeo
marasmus *Progressive weight loss and emaciation.*	marasmo
Marfan syndrome *A connective tissue disease exhibited by long limbs, joint laxity and cardiovascular defects.*	síndrome de Marfan
marijuana *Cannabis.*	marijuana o marihuana
marital counseling	asesoramiento matrimonial
marital status	status matrimonial
marsupialization *Creation of a surgical pouch.*	marsupialización
mass *Tumor.*	masa
mast cell *A cell containing basophilic granules that releases histamine and other substances during allergic reactions.*	célula mastocito
mastectomy *Surgical resection of one or both breasts.*	mastectomía
mastication *Chewing.*	masticación
mastitis *Inflammation of the breast.*	mastitis
mastodynia *Breast pain.*	mastodinia
mastoid *Referring to the mastoid process.*	mastoideo
mastoid process *The posterior part of the temporal bone bordered by the parietal bone superiorly and the occipital bone posteriorly.*	apófisis mastoides
mastoidectomy *Surgical removal of the mastoid.*	mastoidectomía
mastoiditis *Inflammation of the mastoid process.*	mastoiditis
matching	compatibilización

98

English	Spanish
mattress	colchón
mattress suture *A double stitch that forms a loop and there is eversion of the edges when tied.*	sutura de colchonero
maxilla *The upper jaw that also forms the inferior portion of the orbit and part of the nose.*	maxilar
maxillofacial	maxilofacial
mazamorra *Dermatitis caused by hookworm larvae indigenous to Peurto Rico.*	mazamorra
Mcdonald's maneuver *A measurement of the uterus in centimeters that corresponds to gestational age in weeks.*	maniobra de Mcdonald
meaningless	sin sentido
measles *A childhood viral, infectious disease exhibited by rash and fever.*	sarampión
meatus *Opening to the body, such as urethral meatus.*	meato
meconium *The first newborn feces which are green. Presence of meconium on the newborn is a sign there was fetal distress in utero.*	meconio
medial *Situated toward the midline.*	medial
medianoscopy *Visual inspection of the mediastinum with a scope.*	mediastinoscopia
mediastinum *The thoracic area between the lungs.*	mediastino
medical record	registro médico
medication	medicación
medicine	medicina
medicosurgical *Referring to medicine and surgery.*	medicoquirúrgico
medulla oblongata *The inferior portion of the brainstem.*	médula oblongata
medullary *1. The inner part of an organ. 2. Referring to the medulla oblongata.*	medular
medulloblastoma *A malignant tumor of the cerebellum found mostly in children.*	meduloblastoma
megacephaly *Having a larger than normal cranial capacity.*	megacefalia
megacolon	megacolon
megakaryocyte *A cell found in the bone marrow that is a source of platelet production.*	megacariocito
megaloblast *A large red blood cell noted primarily in pernicious anemia.*	megaloblasto
megalomania *A mental disorder characterized by abnormal feelings of self-importance.*	megalomanía
meibomian cyst *An enclosed fluid collection along a sebaceous gland of the eyelid.*	quiste de Meibomio. Chalazión.
meiosis *Cell division creating two daughter cells each with half the number of cells as the parent cell.*	meiosis
melancholia *Profound sadness.*	melancolía
melanin *A dark pigment found on the skin, hair or iris.*	melanina
melanoma *Malignant cancer, typically found in the skin.*	melanoma
melanotic whitlow	panadizo melanótico Melanoma subungular.
melena *The passage of black, tarry stools indicative of upper gastrointestinal bleeding.*	melena
melissophobia *Also called apiphobia, a fear of bees.*	melisofobia
melitis *Inflammation of the cheek.*	melitis Inflamación de la mejilla.
member *Referring to an extremity (arm or leg).*	miembro
memory	memoria

English	Spanish
menarche *The time of the initial menstrual period.*	menarca
meningeal *Referring to the dura mater, arachnoid and the pia mater.*	meníngeo
meningioma *A tumor of the meningeal tissue; generally benign.*	meningioma
meningism *Signs and symptoms of meningitis without infection of the meninges.*	meningismo
meningitis *Inflammation of the meninges exhibited by fever, photophobia, nuchal rigidity and in severe cases coma and convulsions.*	meningitis
meningocele *A congenital defect exhibited by protrusion of the meninges through a defect in the spinal column.*	meningocele
meningococcemia *Presence of N. meningitidis in the blood.*	meningococemia
meniscectomy *Surgical excision of a meniscus.*	meniscectomía
meniscus *A thin cartilage between joint surfaces.*	menisco
menopause *The time when menstruation ceases.*	menopausia
menorrhagia *Abnormally large amount of menstrual blood.*	hipermenorrea
menses *The blood and other material expelled from the uterus during menstruation.*	menstruo
menstruation	menstruación
mental	mental
mention, to	mencionar
mesarteritis *Inflammation of the middle layer of an artery.*	mesarteritis
mesencephalon *Midbrain.*	mesencéfalo
mesenchyme *Organized mesodermal cells that produce connective tissue, lymphatics and bone.*	mesénquima
mesentery *The fold of peritoneum that connects the small bowel, pancrease and spleen to the posterior portion of the abdominal wall.*	mesenterio
mesoappendix *The portion of the mesentery vermiform appendix.*	mesentario del apéndice
mesocolon *The mesentery connecting the colon to the posterior abdominal wall.*	mesocolon
mesoderm *The middle germ layer in an embryo that is the source of bone, muscle and skin.*	mesodermo
mesonephroma *Usually a tumor of the female genital tract that is thought to stem from the mesonephros.*	mesonefroma
mesosalpinx *A portion of the broad ligament supporting the fallopian tubes.*	mesosálpinx
mesothelioma *A tumor that stems from mesothelial tissue; a known cause is asbestos exposure.*	mesotelioma
mesovarium *The portion of the mesentery connecting the ovary with the abdominal wall.*	mesoovario
metabolic *Referring to the physical and chemical reactions involved with keeping an organism functioning.*	metabólico
metacarpal *The name for any of the five hand bones.*	metacarpiano
metacarpophalangeal *Referring to the metacarpus and the phalanges.*	metacarpofalángico
metaphysis *The region between the diaphysis and the epiphysis.*	metáfisis
metaplasia *Abnormal change in the nature or character of tissue.*	metaplasia
metatarsal *Any of the bones of the foot.*	metatarsiano
metatarsalgia *Foot pain.*	metatarsalgia
meter	metro
methemoglobin *A substance formed with the oxidation of hemoglobin.*	metahemoglobina
methionine *A sulfur-containing amino acid used in the biosynthesis of cysteine.*	metionina
metric system	sistema métrico
metrorrhagia *Uterine bleeding in normal amounts but at irregular intervals.*	metrorragia

English	Spanish
microbe *A microorganism.*	microbio
microbiology *The study of microorganisms.*	microbiología
microcephalic *A congenital deformity exhibited by an abnormally small head.*	microcefálico
microcyte *An unusually small erythrocyte associated with anemias, such as iron deficiency anemia.*	microcito
micrognathia *Abnormally small maxilla or mandible.*	micrognatia
microgram *One millionth of one gram.*	microgramo
micrometer *One millionth of one meter.*	micrómetro
microorganism *An organism only seen with a microscope.*	microorganismo
microphthalmos *A congenital condition characterized by smallness of the eyes.*	microftalmo
microscope	microscopio
micturition *Synonym of urination.*	micturición
midbrain *The portion of the brainstem superior to the pons.*	cerebro medio Mesencéfalo.
middle ear *The portion of the ear containing the stapes, incus and malleus.*	auris media
midline	línea media del cuerpo
midstream urine *A specimen of urine that is collected after the initial stream of urine is initiated and before one finishes urinating.*	muestra de orina limpia
midwife *A person trained to assist in childbirth.*	partera
midwifery *The occupation of assisting in childbirth.*	partería
migraine *An episodic, unilateral headache accompanied by nausea.*	migraña
mild	moderado
milestone *An event indicative of a certain stage of development.*	hito
miliary *Referring to a disease that is exhibited by small seed-like lesions (millet), such as miliary tuberculosis.*	miliar
milligram	miligramo
milliliter	mililitro
millimeter	milímetro
Milroy's disease *Hereditary disease exhibited by leg edema.*	enfermedad de Milroy
minute *A unit of time.*	minuto
minute *Something very small.*	diminuto
mirror	espejo
miryachit *A disease of Siberia characterized by an exaggerated startle response.*	miriaquita
misanthropy *A severe dislike of homo sapiens.*	misantropía
miscarriage *Spontaneous abortion.*	aborto espontáneo
misspelling	flata de ortografía
mite fever *Synonym of typhus fever.*	fiebre ácaro
mitochondria *Organelle found in cells responsible for energy production.*	mitocondria
mitosis *Cell division in which two daughter cells are formed that have the same number of chromosomes as the parent cell.*	mitosis
mitral *Referring to the mitral valve.*	mitral
mitral regurgitation *Backflow of blood from the left ventricle to the left atrium because of dysfunctional valve.*	regurgitación mitral
mitral stenosis *Narrowing of the left atrioventricular orifice.*	estenosis mitral
mitral valve *The valve with two cusps between the left atrium and ventricle.*	válvula mitral
modiolus *A column located in the cochlea.*	columela

English	Spanish
moist	húmedo
molality *The number of moles of a solution per kilogram of pure solvent.*	molalidad
molar teeth *The most posterior teeth bilaterally which includes 8 deciduous and usually 12 permanent teeth.*	diente molar
molecule *A combination of at least two atoms.*	molécula
monitoring	monitoreo
monkey-paw *An appearance due to median nerve palsy causing atrophy of the thenar eminence with adduction and elevation of the thumb, resembling that of a simian.*	pato o garra de mono
monkeypox *A viral disease that is similar to smallpox which occurs primarily in monkeys and rarely in humans.*	viruela de los monos
monoamine oxidase inhibitor (MAOI) *A drug used to treat depression that allows accumulation of serotonin and norepinephrine.*	inhibidor de monoaminooxidasa
monoclonal *Asexual formation of a clone from a single cell.*	monoclonal
monocyte *A leukocyte with an oval nucleus and grey cytoplasm.*	monocito
monocytosis *An abnormal increase in the number of monocytes in the blood.*	monocitosis
monodiplopia *Double vision in only one eye.*	monodiplopía
monomania *A psychotic obsession about a single subject.*	monomanía
mononeuritis *Inflammation of a single nerve.*	mononeuritis
mononuclear *A cell having only one nucleus.*	mononuclear
mononucleosis *An infectious disease exhibited by malaise and lymphadenopathy.*	mononucleosis
monoplegia *Paralysis of a single limb.*	monoplejía
mons pubis *The fleshy protuberance over the symphysis pubis.*	mons pubis
mood	humor
morbid	mórbido
morgue	morgue
moribund *Near death.*	moribundo
morning sickness *Nausea associated with pregnancy.*	enfermedad matinal Náuseas del embarazo.
morphea *A condition exhibited by an elevated or depressed patch of pink skin with a purple border.*	morfea
morphine *An opioid analgesic.*	morfina
morphology *The study of living organisms and the correlation between their structure.*	morfología
morula *A solid mass created by the splitting of an ovum.*	mórula
mosquito net	mosquitero
mossy fiber *Nerve fibers that surround the nerve cells of the cerebellar cortex.*	fibra musgosas
motion sickness *Nausea associated with travel.*	enfermedad del movimiento
motor	motor, motora
motor end plate *The expansions on a motor nerve where the branches terminate on muscle fiber.*	placa terminal motora
motor unit *The complex of one motor cell and its attached muscle fibers.*	unidad motor
mottling *An irregular arrangement of patches of color.*	moteado
mourning *A period of grieving.*	luto
mouth	boca
mouth to mouth *A manner of artificial respiration.*	resucitación boca a boca

English	Spanish
mouth to mouth resuscitation *A form of emergency management of respiratory failure.*	respiración boca a boca
mouthful	bocado
mucilage *1. A viscous bodily fluid. 2. A polysaccharide used in medicines and glue.*	mucílago
mucin *A glycoprotein that is the primary constituent in mucous.*	mucina
mucocele *An accumulation of mucous in a dilated cavity.*	mucocele
mucoid *Referring to mucous.*	mucoide
mucolytic *A substance that breaks down mucous.*	mucolítico
mucopolysaccharidosis type I *Also referred to as Hurler syndrome, persons cannot make lysosomal alpha-L-iduronidase which breaks down glycosaminoglycans.*	síndrome de Hurler
mucopolysaccharidosis type II *Also referred to as Hunter syndrome, persons with this inherited condition cannot produce iduronate sulfatase. There are mild to severe forms but all forms have deafness, coarse facial features, hypertrichosis and macrocephaly.*	síndrome de Hunter
mucopolysaccharidosis type III *Also referred to as Sanfilippo syndrome, persons cannot catabolize the heparan sulfate sugar chain. Symptoms include stiff joints, thick eyebrows, coarse facial features and developmental delays.*	síndrome de Sanfilippo
mucopolysaccharidosis type Is *Also referred to as Scheie syndrome, persons cannot produce lysosomal alpha-L-iduronidase. Symptoms include cloudy cornea, hirsutism, prognathism and stiff joints.*	síndrome de Scheie
mucopolysaccharidosis type IV *Also referred to as Morquio syndrome, persons do not produce galactosamine-6-sulfatase or in some cases beta-galactosidase. Symptoms include hypermobile joints, macrocephaly, short stature and wide spaced teeth.*	síndrome de Morquio
mucopolysaccharidosis type VI *Also referred to as Maroteaux-Lamy syndrome. It is characterized by hydrocephalus, macroglossia and coarse facial features but normal intelligence.*	síndrome de Maroteaux-Lamy
mucopurulent *That which contains both mucous and pus.*	mucopurulento
mucosa *A mucous membrane like the buccal mucosa.*	mucosa
Mucune-Albright syndrome *Polyostotic fibrous dysplasia with cutaneous brown patches, endocrine dysfunction that exhibits in females as precocious puberty.*	enfermedad de Albright
mucus *A substance secreted by mucous membranes.*	moco
multigravida *A woman who has been pregnant more than once.*	multigrávida
multilocular *The presence of more than one cell within a cavity.*	multilocular
multipara *A woman with more than one live births.*	multípara
multiple sclerosis *A chronic neurologic disease exhibited by numbness, vision and speech problems, and motor incoordination.*	esclerosis múltiple
mumble, to	mascullar
mumps *A contagious viral disease that is exhibited by parotid swelling and puts males at risk for sterility.*	paperas
murmur *An abnormal heart sound heard with a stethoscope.*	solpo
muscle	músculo
muscle weakness	debilidad
muscular	muscular
muscular dystrophy *A hereditary condition exhibited by progressive muscular weakness and muscle atrophy.*	distrofia muscular
mutation *A gene alteration that can be passed to the next generation.*	mutación

English	Spanish
mute	mudo
mutism *Inability to speak.*	mutismo
myalgia *Muscle pain.*	mialgia
myasthenia gravis *An autoimmune disease characterized by fluctuating weakness of the ocular, limb and respiratory muscles.*	miastenia grave
mycetoma *Persistent inflammation of the tissues caused by an infection.*	micetoma
mycosis *A disease caused by a fungal infection.*	micosis
mycotoxin *A substance toxic to fungus.*	micotoxinas
mydriasis *Pupillary dilation.*	midriasis
myelin *The substance that forms a sheath around some nerve fibers.*	mielina
myelitis *Inflammation of the spinal cord.*	mielitis
myelocele *Protrusion of the spinal cord through a defect in the bony structure.*	mielocele
myelogram *CT scan or roentgenography of the spinal canal after injection of contrast media.*	myelograma
myeloid *Referring to the bone marrow or spinal cord.*	mieloide
myeloma *Malignant tumor of the bone marrow.*	mieloma
myelomatosis *A leukemic disease in which there is an abnormally high amount of myeloblasts in the blood.*	mielomatosis
myelomeningocele *A protrusion of the spinal cord and its meninges through a defect in the vertebral canal.*	mielomeningocele
myelopathy *A condition of the spinal cord.*	mielopatía
myocardial *Referring to the muscular tissue of the heart.*	miocárdico
myocardial infarction *The death of myocardial tissue as a result of an interruption in flow to the region supplied by a coronary vessel.*	infarto miocardio
myocarditis *An inflammation of the heart.*	miocarditis
myocardium *The middle layer of the heart wall.*	miocardio
myoclonus *Contraction or spasm of a group of muscles.*	mioclono
myoglobin *A protein within muscle that carries and stores oxygen.*	mioglobina
myoma *A benign neoplasm of muscular tissue.*	mioma
myomectomy *Surgical resection of a myoma.*	miomectomía
myometrium *The smooth muscle layer of the uterus.*	miometrio
myopathy *Muscle disease.*	miopatía
myope *A person who is nearsighted.*	miope
myopia *Nearsightedness.*	miopía
myosarcoma *A mass with myoma and sarcoma characteristics.*	miosarcoma
myosin *A protein that when coupled with actin form the contractile complex of a muscle cells.*	miosina
myosis *Profound pupillary constriction.*	miosis
myositis *Inflammation of muscle tissue.*	miositis
myositis ossificans *Inflammation of muscle tissue with presence of bony deposits.*	miositis osificante
myotic *Referring to miosis.*	miotásico
myotomy *The surgical removal of muscle tissue.*	miotonía
myotonia dystrophica; Steinert's disease *A condition exhibited initially by hypertonic muscles followed by atrophy of the facial and neck muscles.*	miotonía distrófica
myringitis *Inflammation of the tympanic membrane.*	miringitis
myringoplasty *Surgical repair of tympanic membrane defects.*	miringoplastia

104

English	Spanish
myringotomy *Surgical opening of the tympanic membrane.*	miringotomíe
mysophobia *Severe fear of dirt or contamination from common objects.*	misofobia
myxedema *Diffuse edema with a wax-like appearance of the skin; this condition is associated with hypothyroidism.*	mixedema
myxoma *A tumor composed of mucous tissue.*	mixoma
myxosarcoma *A sarcoma that also has mucous tissue.*	mixosaroma
nail	uña
nailing *Referring to placement of an intramedullary rod in a long bone in order to treat a fracture.*	clavar
name	nombre
nap	siesta
narcissism *Abnormally excessive self-interest.*	narcisismo
narcolepsy *A condition exhibited by a strong desire to sleep and by sudden onset of sleep at increased intervals.*	narcolepsia
narcosis *A reversible medication-induced condition of excessive drowsiness or unconsciousness.*	narcosis
narcotic *A medication that produces narcosis.*	narcótico
nasal *Referring to the nose.*	nasal
nasogastric tube *A tube that is inserted into the nose with the distal tip in the stomach; it is used for irrigation or drainage of gastric contents.*	tubo nasogástrico
nasogastric tube placement *Insertion of a tube that is placed in the stomach via the nostril; it is used for administration of fluid or to suction gastric contents.*	inserción tubo nasogástrico
nasolacrimal *Referring to the nose and tear apparatus.*	nasolagrimal
nasopharyngeal *Referring to the nose and pharynx.*	nasofaríngeo
nasopharynx *The part of the pharynx which lies superior to the soft palate.*	nasofaringe
nausea	náusea
navicular *1. boat shaped 2. Referring to the navicular bone of the hand or foot.*	navicular
navicular bone *The most lateral bone in the proximal row of carpal bones.*	hueso navicular de la mano
near	cercano
nebula *An opaque spot on the cornea causing impaired vision.*	nébula
nebulizer *A device used for transforming a liquid into a fine mist for inhalation as in nebulized albuterol for an acute exacerbation of asthma.*	nebulizador
nebulizer treatment *Administration of medication such as albuterol via a fine mist using a nebulizer.*	tratamiento nebulizador
neck	cuello
necropsy *Synonym of autopsy.*	necroscopia
necrosis *The death of most of the cells of the affected part.*	necrosis
necrotic *Referring to necrosis.*	necrótico
need	necesitar
needle	aguja
needle biopsy *Use of a needle to aspirate body contents for microscopic or pathologic examination.*	aguja para biopsia
needle for lumbar puncture	aguja para punción lumbar
needle holder *A surgical instrument used to grasp a needle during suturing.*	portaagujas
negation	negación

English	Spanish
nematode *An endoparasite belonging to the class of the Nemathelminthes including roundworms and threadworms.*	nematodo
neonatal *Referring to the first four weeks after birth.*	neonatal
neonate *The term for a newborn infant for the first four weeks.*	neonato
neoplasm *A new and abnormal growth.*	neoplasma
nephrectomy *Surgical removal of a kidney.*	nefrectomía
nephritis *A general term meaning inflammation of a kidney that is further categorized depending on the associated pathology.*	nefritis
nephroblastoma *Congenital tumor of the kidney, also called Wilms' tumor.*	nefroblastoma
nephrocalcinosis *A condition exhibited by calcium phosphate deposition in the renal tubules; a cause of renal insufficiency.*	nefrocalcinosis
nephrolithiasis *A calculus in the kidney.*	nefrolitiasis
nephrolithotomy *Surgical removal of a renal calculus.*	nefrolitotomía
nephroma *A renal tumor.*	nefroma
nephron *A functional unit of the kidney that consists of the glomerulus, the proximal and distal convoluted tubules, the loop of Henle and the collecting tubule.*	nefrona
nephropathy *Renal disease.*	nefropatía
nephropexy *The surgical fixation of a kidney that was previously floating.*	nefropexia
nephroptosis *Inferior displacement of the kidney.*	nefroptosis
nephrosclerosis *Hardening of the kidney.*	nefrosclerosis
nephrosis *A kidney disease exhibited by edema and proteinuria; also called nephrotic syndrome.*	nefrosis
nephrostomy *Surgical creation of an opening between the renal pelvis and an opening in the skin.*	nefrostomía
nephrotic *Referring to nephrosis.*	nefrótico
nephrotomy *Surgical incision of the kidney.*	nefrotomía
nerve	nervio
nerve impulse *A signal transmitted along a nerve fiber.*	impulso nervio
nerve-block anesthesia *Injection of an anesthetic agent near a nerve, thus blocking the sensation distal to the injection.*	anestesia troncular
neural *Referring to a nerve or nerve impulse.*	neural
neuralgia *Severe pain along the course of a nerve.*	neuralgia
neurapraxia *Paralysis from nerve injury but no degeneration of the nerve.*	neurapraxia
neurasthenia *A psychoneurosis exhibited by severe fatigue.*	neuroastenia
neurectomy *Excision of a section of a nerve.*	neurectomía
neurilemma *The membrane covering a myelinated nerve fiber or the axon of an unmyelinated nerve fiber.*	neurilema
neuritis *Inflammation of a nerve.*	neuritis
neuroblastoma *A nervous system malignant tumor composed of neuroblasts.*	neuroblastoma
neurodermatitis *A pruritic, thickened eruption in the axillary and inguinal thought to be exacerbated by emotions.*	neurodermatitis
neuroepithelium *Cells specialized to serve as sensory cells such as cells of the cochlea and tongue.*	neuroepitelio
neurofibroma *A tumor formed by excessive growth of perineurium and endoneurium.*	neurofibroma
neurofibromatosis *A hereditary condition exhibited by formation of multiple soft tumors scattered throughout the skin surface. Also known as von Recklinghausen disease.*	neurofibromatosis; Enfermedad de von Recklinghausen.

English	Spanish
neuroglia *A type of connective tissue of the nervous system.*	neuroglia
neuroleptic *A drug that causes neurologic symptoms.*	neuroléptico
neurologist *A physician who specializes in the study of the nervous system.*	neurólgo
neurology *The study of the nervous system.*	neurología
neuroma *A mass composed of nerve cells and fibers.*	neuroma
neuron *A nerve cell.*	neurona
neuropathic *Referring to neuropathy.*	neuropático
neuropathy *Structural of pathologic changes of the peripheral nervous system.*	neuropatía
neurosis *A mental disorder.*	neurosis
neurosurgery *Surgery of the brain or spinal cord.*	neurocirugía
neurosyphilis *Infection of the central nervous system with Treponema pallidum.*	neurosífilis
neurotmesis *The severing of a nerve.*	neurotmesis
neurotomy *Surgical incision into a nerve.*	neurotomía
neurotransmitter *A substance released at the end of a nerve fiber that facilitates transmission of an impulse.*	neurotransmisor
neutropenia *Diminished number of neutrophils in the blood.*	neutropenia
neutrophil *A polymorphonuclear leukocyte.*	neutrófilo
nevus *A benign, well-circumscribed growth of tissue of congenital origin.*	nevo
next	próximo
nick	cortadura
nicotinic acid *A deficiency of this substance results in pellagra.*	ácido nicotínico
night blindness	ceguera nocturna
night shift	turno nocturno
night sweats	sudor excesivo durante el sueño
night terror *Sensation of profound fear upon wakening.*	pavor nocturno
nightmare	pesadilla
nipple	pezón
nitrogen *A colorless, odorless gas used as a coolant in the liquid form.*	nitrógeno
nitrous oxide *An inhalant gas used as an anesthetic agent.*	óxido nitroso
nocturia *Urination at night.*	nocturia
nocturnal emission *Involuntary emission of semen at night.*	micciones nocturnas
nocturnal *Referring to events that happen at night.*	nocturno
node *A swelling or prominence.*	nudo
nodule	nódulo
non-rebreather mask *A type of oxygen mask used to deliver a higher oxygen concentration.*	máscara respiratoria única o de sentido único
non-resorbable suture (nylon) *Suture used to be permanent as it is not removed by normal body processes.*	sutura quirúrgica no absorbible
noon	mediodía
norepinephrine *A hormone secreted by the adrenal medulla and a synthetic drug used as a pressor agent.*	norepinefrina
normoblast *A precursor cell for erythrocytes.*	normoblasto
normocyte *A normal erythrocyte.*	normocito
Norway itch *A severe pruritis caused by scabies and is associated with immune disorders such as AIDS.*	prurito de Noruega
nose	nariz

107

English	Spanish
nosebleed *Common term for epistaxis.*	epistaxis
nosocomial infection *An infection occurring after admission to a hospital.*	nosocomial
nosology *The medical science of disease classification.*	nosología
nosophobia *Unwarranted, excessive fear of any disease.*	nosofobia
nostril	naris
noxious *Harmful or poisonous.*	nocivo
nuclear magnetic resonance (NMR) *A type a diagnostic body imaging utilizing electromagnetic radiation in a magnetic field.*	resonancia magnética nuclear
nuclear medicine *The branch of medicine associated with the use of radioactive material in the evaluation and treatment of disease.*	medicina nuclear
nuclear *Referring to a nucleus.*	nuclear
nucleic acid *An organic compound found in living cells; its molecules contain nucleotides linked in long chains.*	ácido nucleico
nucleoprotein *A substance composed of a nucleic acid and a protein.*	nucleoproteína
nulligravida *A woman who has never been pregnant.*	nuligrávida
nullipara *A woman who has never given birth.*	nulípara
numb chin syndrome. *Generally associated with metastatic breast or prostate cancer, it is characterized by unilateral sensory loss of the chin and lower lip.*	síndrome del mentón entumecido
numbness	entumecimiento
nummulated *Formed as round, flat discs.*	mummular
nurse	enfermera
nurse practitioner	practicante de enfermera
nursing care	enfermería
nutation *Referring to nodding of the head.*	nutación
nutrient	nutriente
nutrient foramen *A conduit for passage of nutrient vessels in the marrow of bone.*	agujero nutricio
nutrition	nutrición
nutritional status	estado nutrición
nystagmus *Rapid involuntary movement of the eyes; it can be horizontal, vertical or rotary.*	nistagmo
nyxis *Paracentesis or a puncture.*	nixis
obesity	obesidad
obsession *A pathologic preoccupation.*	obsesión
obsolete	obsoleto
obstetric *Referring to The management of pregnancy, labor and the peuperium.*	obstétrico
obstetrician *A physician who specializes in the management of pregnancy, labor and the peuperium.*	obstetra
obstructed *To be blocked or halted.*	obstrucción
obturator *A device used to close an artificial or natural opening.*	obturador
obtuse *Rather insensitive or hard to understand.*	obtuso
occipital *Referring to the back part of the head.*	occipital
occipitofrontal muscle *Raises the eyebrows.*	músculo occipitofrontal
occlusion	oclusión
occlusive dressing *A synthetic covering for a wound that has a semipermeable membrane.*	vendaje oclusivo
occult blood *Presence of blood from an unknown source.*	sangre oculta

English	Spanish
occupational therapy *Rehabilitation focusing on activities of daily living.*	terapia ocupación
ocular melanoma. *An aggressive cancer that, when involving the eye, is located in the choroid layer.*	melanoma de ojo
ocular *Referring to the eye.*	ocular
oculogyric *Referring to movement of the eye around the anteroposterior axis.*	oculógiro
oculomotor nerve *Referring to cranial nerve III which is one of the nerves responsible for extraocular movements.*	nervi motot ocular común
odiferous	odorífero
odontalgia *Tooth pain.*	odontalgia
odontoid *A prominence on the second cervical vertebra on which the first cervical vertebra pivots.*	odontoide
odontology *Synonym of dentistry.*	odontología
odor	odor
odynophagia *Pain associated with swallowing.*	odinofagia
odynophonia *Pain associated with speaking.*	odinofonía
offspring	descendencia
ointment	ungüento
old age	anciano
older	más viejo
olecranon *The bony protrusion at the proximal ulna at the elbow.*	olécranon
olfactory *Referring to the sense of smell.*	olfatología
oligodactyly *Presence of fewer than 5 digits on a hand or foot.*	oligodactilia
oligodendroglia *The ectodermal cells forming part of the central nervous system.*	oligodendroglia
oligohydramnios *Inadequate amount of amniotic fluid.*	oligohidramnios
oligomenorrhea *Infrequent menstruation or low volume menstrual flow.*	oligomenorrea
oligoptyalism *Insufficient secretion of saliva.*	oligoptialismo
oligospermia *Abnormally low sperm count.*	oligospermia
oligotrophia *Inadequate nutritional state.*	oligotrofia
oliguria *Abnormally low urine output.*	oliguria
ombrophobia *An abnormal fear of rain.*	ombrofobia
omentocele *A herniated protrusion of omentum.*	omentocele
omentopexy *Surgically fastening the omentum to an adjacent tissue it was not previously attached to.*	omentopexia
omentum *A fold of peritoneum fastening the stomach to other organs in the viscera.*	epiplón
omphalitis *Inflammation of the umbilicus.*	onfalitis
omphalocele *A large congenital, umbilical hernia with only a thin membranous covering.*	onfalocele
on going	continuo
oncologist *A phyisician specializing in the treatment of cancer.*	oncólogo
oncology *The study of cancer.*	oncología
onion bulb neuropathy *Also known as hypertrophic interstitial neuropathy which is a sensorimotor polyneuropathy.*	neuropatía en bulbo de cebolla
onset	inicio
onychia *Inflammation of the toenail or fingernail matrix.*	oniquia
onychia sicca *Brittle fingernails or toenails.*	oniquia seca

English	Spanish
onychocryptosis *Ingrown toenail.*	onicocriptosis
onychogryphosis *A deformed nail that is incurved or hooked.*	onicogrifosis
onychomycosis *Fungal disease of the toenails or fingernails.*	noicomicosis
onychomycosis *Fungal disease of the toenails or fingernails.*	tiña de las uñas
onychophagia *Habitually chewing on one's fingernails.*	onicofagia
oocyte *An ovarian cell that needs to undergo meiotic division to become an ovum.*	oocito
oogenesis *The initiation and development of an ovum.*	oogénesis
oophorectomy *Surgical removal of an ovary.*	ooforectomía
oophoritis *Inflammation of an ovary.*	ooforitis
oophoron *Synonym for ovary.*	oóforo
oophorosalpingectomy *Surgical removal of an ovary and fallopian tube.*	ooforosalpingectomía
ooze, to *To slowly leak.*	exudar
open reduction of fractures *The realignment of a fractured bone using a surgical approach.*	reducción abierta de fracturas
operative note *A detailed description of a surgical procedure performed on a specific patient.*	registro operación
ophthalmia *Profound inflammation of the eye or its structures.*	oftalmía
ophthalmic *Referring to the eye.*	oftálmico
ophthalmologist *A physician specializing in diseases of the eye.*	oftalmólogo
ophthalmology *The study of diseases of the eye.*	oftalmolgía
ophthalmoplegia *Paralysis of the eye muscles.*	oftalmoplejía
ophthalmoscope *A device used to visually inspect the interior eye.*	oftalmoscopio
opiate *Referring to opium.*	opiáceo
opioid *A substance similar to opium that binds to at least one of the opium receptors in the body.*	opioide
opisthotonos *A profound spasm in which the head/neck is hyperextended, the feet are touching the bed and with the patient supine the body arched upward.*	opistótonos
opium *An addictive drug derived from opium poppy; synthetic versions are used as analgesics.*	opio
opponens *Synonym for opponent muscle.*	oponente
opsonin *An antibody used to facilitate phagocytosis of a bacterium.*	oposonina
optic *Referring to the eye.*	óptico
optic disk *The area of the retina where the optic nerve enters.*	disco óptico
optician *A person who makes eyeglasses.*	el óptico
optometrist	opometrista
optometry *The profession of examination of the eyes for disease (not a medical doctor).*	optometría
oral	oral
oral contraceptive *Tablet taken by mouth to prevent pregnancy.*	pildora anticonceptiva
oral hygiene	higiene bucal
orally	oralmente
orbicular *Rounded or circular.*	orbicular
orbit *The bony structure enclosing the eyeball.*	órbita
orbital *Referring to the orbit.*	orbitario
orchialgia *Testicular pain.*	orquialgia
orchidectomy *Synonym of orchiectomy; removal of one or both testes.*	orquidectomía

English	Spanish
orchidopexy *Surgical repair of an undescended testis.*	orquiopexia
orchiepididymitis *Inflammation of the testis and epididymis.*	orquiepididimitis
orchitis *Inflammation of one or both testes.*	orquitis
organ	órgano
organomegaly	organomegalia
oriental sore *A stigmata of cutaneous leishmaniasis caused by a bite from a sand fly.*	leishmaniasis cutánea
orifice *Synonym of foramen.*	orificio
ornithosis *A viral infection transmitted by birds that is manifested by chills, headache, photophobia, fever, nausea and vomiting.*	ornitosis
oropharynx *The portion of the pharynx between the soft palate and the superior aspect of the epiglottis.*	orofaringe
orthodontics *A subspecialty of dentistry concerned with treatment of dental irregularities and malocclusion, including the use of braces.*	ortodoncia
orthopedics *A surgical specialty concerned with treatment of skeletal problems.*	ortopédico
orthopnea *The inability to breath comfortably except in the upright position.*	ortopnea
orthosis *Straightening of a malaligned part with the use of braces and other supportive devices.*	ortosis
orthostatic *Referring to the standing position. Orthostatic hypotension is low blood pressure in the standing position.*	ortostático
oscillating nystagmus *Abnormal movement of the eyes in a wave-like pattern.*	oscilliopsia
osmolality *The concentration expressed in total number of solute particles per kilogram.*	osmolaidad
osmole *The recognized unit of osmotic pressure.*	osmol
osmosis *The movement of a solvent from a solution of greater concentration to one of lower concentration through a semi-permeable membrane until the two solutions have equal concentration.*	ósmosis
osmotic *Referring to osmosis.*	osmótico
osseous *Possessing the quality of bone.*	óseo
ossicle *A small bone. The stapes is an auditory ossicle.*	huesecillo
ossification *The formation of bone.*	osificación
osteitis *Inflammation of the bone.*	osteítis
ostensibly *Synonym of apparently and seemingly.*	ostensiblemente
osteoarthritis *A long term, progressive degenerative joint disease.*	osteoartritis
osteoarthrosis *Arthritis without inflammation.*	osteoartrosis
osteoblast *A cell that matures from a fibroblast and produces bone.*	osteoblasto
osteochondral *Referring to bone and cartilage.*	osteocondral
osteochondritis *Inflammation of bone and cartilage.*	osteocondritis
osteochondroma *A tumor with bony and cartilaginous characteristics.*	osteocondroma
osteoclasis *The surgical fracture of a bone usually in order to restore proper alignment.*	osteoclasia
osteoclast *A large bone cell that is associated with bone reabsorption and removal.*	osteoclasto
osteoclastoma *A tumor composed of giant cells or osteoclasts.*	osteoclastoma
osteocyte *An osteoblast within the bone matrix.*	osteocito
osteodystrophy *Abnormal bone formation.*	osteodistrofia
osteogenesis *Development of new bones.*	osteogénesis
osteolytic *Referring to the removal or loss of calcium from the bone.*	osteolítico

English	Spanish
osteomalacia *Softening of the bones because of a deficiency of vitamin D, calcium or phosphorus.*	osteomalacia
osteomyelitis *Inflammation of the bone or bone marrow because of a microorganism.*	osteomielitis
osteopathy *1. Any disease of the bone. 2. Medical practice concerning treatment of disease by manipulation and massage of bones, joints, and muscles.*	osteopatía
osteopetrosis *Increased bone density with no change in modeling.*	osteopetrosis
osteophony *The sound conduction of bone.*	osteofonía
osteophyte *Abnormal growth of a bone protuberance.*	osteófito
osteoporosis *Loss of bone substance because the osteoblasts fail to produce bone matrix.*	osteoporosis
osteosarcoma *A tumor composed of a sarcoma and osseous material.*	osteosarcoma
osteosclerosis *Abnormal hardening of bone.*	osteosclerosis
osteotomy *Creation of a surgical opening in bone.*	osteotomía
ostium *A vessel or body cavity opening.*	ostium
ostogenesis imperfecta *A connective tissue disorder characterized by bone fragility, skeletal deformity, blue sclerae, ligament laxity, and hearing loss.*	osteogénesis imperfecta
otalgia *Ear pain.*	otalgia
otitis *Inflammation of the ear. (otitis media or otitis externa)*	otitis
otolaryngologist *Surgical specialist concerned with organs of the ears, nose and throat.*	otolaringólogo
otolith *A calcium based calculus in the inner ear.*	otolito
otology *Study of conditions and anatomy of the ear.*	otología
otomycosis *Fungal infection of the ear.*	otomicosis
otosclerosis *A hereditary condition exhibited by progressive hearing loss because of bone overgrowth in the inner ear.*	otosclerosis
otoscope *A device used for inspection of the tympanic membrane.*	otoscopio
ototoxic *A substance harmful to the ear or its nerve supply.*	ototóxico
outbreak	brote
outdated	anticuado
ovarian cysts *Generally used to describe benign tumors.*	quistes ováricos
ovaritis *Synonym for oophoritis.*	ovaritis
overdose *An above normal dose of a medication.*	dosis excesiva
overriding suture *The overlapping of cranial sutures noted on vaginal exam when the head is descended.*	cabalgamiento
overt *Not hidden.*	abierto
overweight	excesivamente pesado
oviduct *The channel which an ovum passes from the ovary.*	oviducto
ovulation *The release of an ova from the ovary.*	ovulación
ovule *An immature ovum.*	óvulo
owing to	debido a
oxaluria *Existence of oxalates in the urine.*	oxaluria
oxidation *The process of a chemical combining with oxygen.*	oxidación
oximeter *A medical device used to measure the percent of oxygen that is saturated in the blood (oxygen saturation).*	oxímetro
oxycephaly *The deformation of the skull so that it appears pointed.*	oxicefalia
oxygen	oxígeno
oxygen consumption *The body's utilization of oxygen per unit of time.*	consumo de oxígeno

English	Spanish
oxygen tent *A manner of giving supplement oxygen to a neonate.*	tienda de oxígeno
oxygen therapy *Utilization of supplemental oxygen.*	terapia con oxígeno
oxygenation *Saturated with oxygen.*	oxigenación
oxyhemoglobin *The combination of oxygen and hemoglobin using a covalent bond.*	oxihemoglobina
oxytocic *Referring to rapid parturition.*	oxitócico
oxytocin *A natural hormone released by the pituitary or a synthetic hormone that facilitates uterine contraction.*	oxitocina
ozena *Various nasal conditions, all of which include fetid discharge.*	ocena
ozone *A toxic chemical that has profound oxidizing properties. It has three atoms in its molecule compared with oxygen which has two.*	ozono
pace	paso
pacemaker *An electrical device used to stimulate the heart used for bradyarrhythmias.*	marcapaso
pachydermia *An abnormally thick skin.*	paquidermia
pachymeningitis *Inflammation of the dura mater.*	paquimeningitis
pad	almohadilla
pagophagia *Compulsive need to eat ice which is usually associated with iron deficiency anemia.*	pagofagia
pain	dolor
painful	doloroso
palatal myoclonus *An involuntary, persistent, rapid regular tremor of the soft palate and face.*	mioclono palatino
palate *The roof of the mouth.*	paladar
palatoplegia *Paralysis of the palate.*	palatoplejía
palliative *A treatment used to reduce pain when cure is not possible.*	paliativo
pallidectomy *Surgical resection of all or part of the palate.*	palidectomía
pallor *Unusually pale appearance.*	palidez
palm *The anterior aspect of the hand.*	palma
palmar *Referring to the palm.*	palmar
palpation *The assessment of the body with the use of one's hands.*	palpación
palpebra, palpebrae *Eyelid, eyelids.*	palpebra, palpebrae
palpitation *Sensation of a forceful, rapid, irregular heartbeat present after exercise or with anxiety.*	palpitación
palsy	parálisis
paludism *Synonym of malaria.*	paludismo
pamper, to	mimar
panarthritis *Inflammation of the joints.*	panartritis
pancarditis *Inflammation of pericardium, myocardium and endocardium.*	pancarditis
pancreas *A gland that secretes digestive enzymes into the duodenum and insulin and glucagon into the blood.*	páncreas
pancreatectomy *Surgical excision of part or all of the pancreas.*	pancreatectomía
pancreatitis *Inflammation of the pancreas.*	pancreatitis
pancreozymin *A duodenal mucosal enzyme that facilitates the secretion of amylase and other enzymes from the pancreas.*	pancreocimina
pandemic *When a disease is present over an entire region.*	pandémico
panhypopituitarism *Insufficiency of the anterior pituitary.*	panhipopituitarismo
panic attack *Sudden, profound anxiety.*	ataque de pánico

English	Spanish
panniculitis *Inflammation of a section of subcutaneous tissue containing large amounts of fat.*	paniculitis
panophthalmia *Inflammation of the eye and all its structures.*	panoftalmía
panotitis *Inflammation of each part of a bone.*	panotitis
papilledema *Swelling of the optic disc.*	papiledema
papillitis *Swelling of a papilla.*	papilitis
papilloma *A benign, lobulated tumor coming from epithelium.*	papiloma
papule *A small, well-circumscribed elevation of the skin.*	pápula
para-aminobenzoic acid *A natural product (not FDA approved) reportedly beneficial for Peyronie's disease and scleroderma. It is a component of folic acid.*	ácido p-aminobenzoico
para-aminohippuric acid (PAH) *A chemical used for calculation of renal plasma flow.*	ácido p-aminohipúrico
paracentesis *A procedure involving aspiration of fluid from the abdominal cavity.*	paracentesis
paracusia *Any abnormality in the sense of hearing.*	paracusia
paradoxical pupil *Constriction of the pupil when exposed to darkness.*	pupilo paradójica
paralysis agitans *Synonym of Parkinson's disease.*	parálisis agitante
paralytic *1. Referring to paralysis. 2. A person who is paralyzed.*	paralítico
paramedian *Situated toward the middle of the body.*	paramediano
paramedical *Hospital support staff excluding physicians.*	paramédico
parametritis *Inflammation of the parametrium.*	parametritis
parametrium *The connective tissue and smooth muscle between the broad ligament serous layers.*	parametrio
paramnesia *A condition exhibited by a person's belief they have memory for an event that never happened.*	paramnesia
paranasal sinuses *Any of the sinuses (ethmoidal, frontal, maxillary or sphenoidal) that communicate with the nasal cavity.*	seno paranasales
paranasal *Situated adjacent to the nose.*	paranasal
paranoia *A mental condition exhibited by delusions of persecution.*	paranoia
paranoid *A person who has paranoia.*	paranoide
paraphimosis *A condition in which the foreskin is retracted but cannot be replace because of a restricted foreskin.*	parafimosis
paraplegia *Paralysis of the lower extremities.*	paraplejía
parapraxis *1. Unable to perform purposeful movements. 1. Irrational behavior.*	parapraxia
pararectal *Adjacent to the rectum.*	pararectal
parasite *An organism that lives on or within another organism without benefit to the latter.*	parásito
parasympathetic *Part of the autonomic nervous system that opposes sympathetic stimulation.*	parasimpático
parathormone *Synonym for parathyroid hormone.*	parathormona
parathyroid *Positioned adjacent to the thyroid.*	paratiroides
paravertebral *Positioned adjacent to the vertebra.*	paravertebral
parenchyma *The functional elements of an organ.*	parenquimal
parenteral *Other than the alimentary canal.*	parenteral
paresis *Incomplete paralysis.*	paresia
paresthesia *An abnormal sensation usually described as pins and needles.*	parestesia
parietal *Referring to the wall of a part or cavity.*	parietal

English	Spanish
parietal cell *Acid secreting cells of the stomach.*	célula parietal
Parkinson's disease *A progressive neuromuscular disease exhibited by masklike facial expression, resting tremor, cogwheel rigidity and abnormal gait.*	parkinsonismo Enfermedad de Parkinson.
paronychia *Inflammation of the tissue bordering a fingernail*	paroniquia
parosmia *An alteration in the sense of smell.*	parosmia
parotid *A gland near the ear.*	parótida
parotiditis *Inflammation of the parotid gland.*	parotiditis
paroxysmal *Occurring in sudden attacks.*	paroxístico
parrot-beak nail *A curved fingernail.*	uña en pico de loro
parthenogenesis *Reproduction that occurs without an egg being fertilized by sperm.*	partenogénesis
parting	despedida
parturition *The process of giving birth.*	parturición
passive *Not achieved through active effort.*	pasivo
past history *Prior medical problems experienced by a patient.*	historia clínica previa
paste	pasta
patch test *A test used to determine which substances provoke an allergic response in a patient.*	prueba alérgica
patella *The bone situated in the anterior portion of the knee.*	rótula
patellectomy *Surgical excision of the patella.*	rotulectomía
patellofemoral stress syndrome *Overuse syndrome causing anterior knee pain from excessive lateral motion.*	rodilla de atleta
patent ductus arteriosus *A condition exhibited by failure of the ductus arteriosus (communication between the aorta the the pulmonary artery normally noted in a fetus) to close.*	conducto arterioso permeable
patent foramen ovale *A congenital anomaly in which there is a defect in the wall between the right and left atria; this can be a benign condition or result in cryptogenic strokes.*	agujero oval permeable
pathogenesis *The course of a disease.*	patogénesis
pathogenic *Referring to an organism that can cause disease.*	patogénico
pathognomonic *Characteristic of something.*	patognomónico
pathological *Referring to pathology.*	patológico
pathology *1. The branch of medicine dealing with the study of tissues and the forensic application. 2. Referring to a condition that is abnormal.*	patología
patient	paciente
patient chart	registro médico
peak flow *A measurement of lung function used in asthma.*	flujo espiratorio máximo
pectineal ligament *A continuation of the lacunar ligament along the pectineal line in the pubis.*	ligamento pectíneo
pectoral *Referring to the pectoral muscle.*	pectoral
pectoriloquy *The examiner's voice is clearly audible when the patient speaks as when the examiner listens to an area of consolidation in the lungs of the speaker.*	pectoriloquia
pediatrician *Physician who is a specialist in pediatrics.*	pediatra
pediatrics *Medical specialty concerned with the treatment and prevention of childhood disease.*	pediatría
pedicle *Part of a skin/tissue graft temporarily left connected to the original site.*	pedícle

English	Spanish
pediculate *Referring to pedicle.*	pediculado
pediculosis *Lice infestation.*	pediculosis
peduncle *1. A stalk-like protrusion. 2. A bundle of nerve fibers connecting two parts of the brain.*	pedúnculo
peenash *Clear rhinitis induced by larvae presence in the nasal passages.*	peenash
pellagra *A deficiency in nicotinic acid exhibited by diarrhea and dermatitis.*	pelagra
pelvic inflammatory disease *Generally a bacterial infection affecting a woman with potential invovlement of the uterus, fallopian tubes, ovaries and cervix.*	enfermedad pélvica inflamatoria
pelvic *Referring to the pelvis.*	pélvico
pelvimetry *Measurement of the dimensions of the pelvis to determine whether a patient is capable of natural childbirth.*	pelvimetría
pelvis *The bony structure at the base of the spine.*	pelvis
pemphigus *A skin disorder with large bullous lesions.*	pénfigo
penetration	penetración
penicillin *A synthetic antibiotic originally produced from blue mold.*	penicilina
penis *Male genital organ used for the transfer of sperm and elimination of urine.*	pene
pentosuria *The presence of pentose in the urine (a monosaccharide with five carbon atoms in the molecule).*	pentosuria
pepsin *A proteolytic gastric enzyme.*	pepsina
peptic *Referring to pepsin or concerning digestion.*	péptico
peptide *A compound with low molecular weight and containing two or more amino acids.*	péptido
percussion *A manual procedure involving tapping a body part to determine the size or density (liquid or air) of a part.*	percusión
perforation *Presence of a hole.*	perforación
periaqueductal gray matter *Refers to the brain gray matter adjacent to the periaqueductal.*	materia gris periacueducto
periarthritis *Inflammation of the tissues around a joint.*	periartritis
pericardial *Referring to around the heart.*	pericardíco
pericarditis *Inflammation of the pericardium.*	pericarditis
pericardium *The structure enclosing the heart which contains a fibrous outer layer and serous inner layer.*	pericardio
perichondritis *Inflammation of the perichondrium.*	pericondritis
perichondrium *The membrane that encloses a cartilage.*	pericondrio
pericolitis *Inflammation of the membrane covering the colon.*	pericolitis
pericorneal ring *Also known as Kayser-Fleischer rings exhibited by presence of brown or grey-green rings on the cornea. This is from the deposition of copper and seen in Wilson's disease.*	anillo de Kayser-Fleischer
perilymph *The fluid separating the membranous and osseous labyrinth.*	perilinfa
perinatology *The study of disease in the period just before and right after birth.*	perinatología
perineal *Referring to the perineum.*	perineal
perineorrhaphy *Surgical repair of the perineum.*	perineorrafia
perinephric *Around the kidney.*	perinéfrico
perineum *The area between the anus and scrotum or anus and vulva.*	perineo
periodontal disease *Present around to a tooth.*	enfermedad peridontal
periosteal *Referring to the periosteum.*	perióstico
periosteum *A layer of connective tissue covering the bones.*	periostio

English	Spanish
periostitis *Inflammation of the periosteum.*	periostitis
peripheral *Referring to an outward part or surface.*	periférico
periproctitis *Inflammation of the tissue encircling the anus and rectum.*	periproctitis
peristalsis *The contraction of the longitudinal and circular muscle fibers of the alimentary canal so food is propelled.*	peristalsimo
peritomy *Surgically creating an opening of the periosteum.*	peritomía
peritoneal *Referring to the peritoneum.*	peritoneal
peritoneum *The serous membrane covering the abdominal organs and lining the abdominal walls.*	peritoneo
peritonitis *Inflammation of the peritoneum.*	peritonitis
peritonsillar abscess	absceso periamigdalino
peritonsillar *Surrounding the tonsils.*	perotonsilitis
periurethral *Surrounding the urethra.*	periuretral
permanent teeth	dentición secundaria
pernicious *1. Having a detrimental effect. 2. Pernicious anemia is a reduced red blood cell count due to Vitamin B12 deficiency.*	pernicioso
peroneal *Referring to the fibula or the outer part of the leg.*	peroneo
peroneal atrophy *Progressive muscle atrophy in the peroneal region.*	atrofia peroneo
personality	personalidad
perspiration	perspiración
pertussis *Synonym for whooping cough.*	pertussis
pes cavus *Excessive height of the longitudinal arch of the foot.*	pes cavus
pes valgus *Abnormal longitudinal arch- it is flat.*	pes valgus
pessary *A supportive device placed in the rectum or vagina.*	pesario
pet	animal doméstico
PET scan Positron emission tomography.	tomografía por emisión de positrones
petechia *A small red or purple macule on the skin caused by bleeding.*	petequia
petrissage *Massage using a kneading action.*	pétrissage
petrous *Possessing a density of a stone.*	pétreo
Peyronie's disease *Curvature of the penis during an erection to to plaque.*	enfermedad de Peyronie
phagocyte *A cell capable of surrounding and digesting microorganisms.*	fagocito
phagocytosis *The action of a phagocyte.*	fagocitosis
phalanx	falange
phantom limb pain *Pain sensed in an area where one has had an amputation as though the limb is still present.*	dolor de extremidad fantasma
pharmacist *A professional who prepares and sells medicine through various systems, including governmental organizations like the Veterans Administration.*	farmacéutico
pharmacokinetics *The study of the distribution, absorption and excretion of drugs within the body.*	famrmacocinética
pharmacology *The study of all aspects of medicines.*	farmacología
pharmacy	farmacia
pharyngeal pouch *A lateral diverticulum of the pharynx.*	bolsa faríngea
pharyngeal *Referring to the pharynx.*	faríngeo
pharyngectomy *Surgical excision of part of the pharynx.*	faringectomía
pharyngitis *Inflammation of the pharynx.*	faringitis
pharyngolaryngectomy *Surgical removal of part of the pharynx and larynx.*	faringolaringectomía

117

English	Spanish
pharyngotympanic tube *Synonym for eustachian tube.*	trompa de Eustaquio
pharynx *The membranous cavity from the mouth to esophagus.*	faringe
phenotype *The visual expression exhibited by a person from the association of the genotype with the environment.*	fenotipo
phenylketonuria *A hereditary condition in which a person cannot excrete phenylalanine; untreated it causes brain and spinal cord dysfunction.*	fenilcetonuria
phimosis *Stricture of the prepuce preventing it from being pulled back over the glans penis.*	fimosis
phlebectomy *Surgical excision of a vein.*	flebectomía
phlebitis *Inflammation of a vein.*	flebitis
phlebothrombosis *Presence of a clot in a vein, without associated inflammation.*	flebotrombosis
phlegmasia alba dolens *Phlebitis of the femoral vein that can occur after pregnancy or typhoid fever.*	flemasia alba dolens
phlegmasia *Inflammation or fever.*	flegmasia
phlyctenular *Related to the formation of small vesicles on the cornea or conjunctiva.*	flicentular
phobia *An profound fear of something.*	fobia
phonation *The vocalization of sounds.*	fonación
phoniatrics *The treatment of speech abnormalities.*	foniatría
phosphaturia *Presence of phosphates in the urine.*	fosfaturia
phospholipid *A substance, such as lecithin, that when hydrolyzed produces fatty acids, glycerin, and a nitrogen compound.*	fosfolípido
phosphonecrosis *The breakdown of the mandible caused by excessive exposure to phosphorus.*	fosfonecrosis
photophobia *Abnormal sensitivity to light.*	fotofobia
photosensitization *The process of reacting to sunlight by developing edema and dermatitis.*	fotosensibilización
phrenic *Referring to the diaphragm.*	frénico
phrenicectomy *Surgical excision of the phrenic nerve.*	freniconeurectomía
phrenoplegia *Paralysis of the diaphragm.*	frenoplejía
physical exam	examen físico
physical therapy *Treatment of disease by heat, massage and exercise as opposed to medications.*	terapia físico
physician	médico
physiologic dead space *The combination of anatomic and alveolar dead space.*	espacio muerto fisiológico
physiological saline *0.9% normal saline.*	solución fisiológica
physiology *A subspecialty of biology that studies the normal functioning of the body.*	fisiología
physiotherapy *Physical therapy.*	terapia física
pia mater *The first layer of three covering the brain and spinal cord.*	piamadre
pica *A desire for unusual substances as occurs in pregnancy and some psychological conditions.*	pica
pill	píldora
pillow	almohada
pilonidal cyst *A small cone-shaped cluster of tissue situated posterior to the third ventricle of the brain.*	quiste pilonidal
pin; wire	perno

English	Spanish
pineal gland *A small body posterior to the third ventricle of the brain.*	glándula pineal
pinguecula *The yellow tissue on the bulbar conjunctiva adjacent to the sclerocorneal junction.*	pinguécula
pinocytosis *The absorption of fluid into a cell by the formation of vesicles on the cell membrane.*	pinocitosis
pinworm *Common term for Enterobius vermincularis; a nematode worm that is a parasite.*	oxiuro
pipet *A slender tube with a bulb used for transferring liquids.*	pipeta
pitting edema *Edema of the lower extremities characterized by an indentation being left when the examiner applies pressure with their thumb.*	edema de fóveo
pituitary gland *A gland at the base of the hypothalamus.*	glándula pituitaria
pityriasis rosea *A skin disease characterized by dry pink oval papulosquamous eruptions.*	pitiriasis rosea
placebo controlled *When a study is placebo controlled it means part of the group received an inactive treatment while the other group received active therapy.*	prueba controlada por placebo
placenta *The vascular tissue that nourishes a fetus through an umbilical cord.*	placenta
placenta praevia *A condition in which the placenta covers the cervical os.*	placenta previa
placental *Referring to the placenta.*	placentario
plagiocephaly *A condition characterized by an asymmetric skull because the cranial sutures do not close normally.*	plagiocefalia
plantar *Referring to the bottom of the foot.*	plantar
plantar fibromatosis *Deep fascia nodules on the plantar aspect of the feet.*	fibromatosis plantar
plantar wart *A viral epidermal growth on the bottom of the foot.*	verruga plantar
plasma cell *A cell that produces only one type of antibody.*	célula plasma
plasmacytosis *The existence of plasma cells in the blood.*	plasmacitosis
plasmapheresis *A method of removing blood and reinfusing it after the elimination of antibodies.*	plasmaféresis
plaster cast *Use of gypsum impregnated gauze to immobilize fractured extremities.*	tablilla de yeso
plaster *Dehydrated gypsum that has water added to it in order to immobilize fractured extremities.*	yeso de París
platelet *An oval cell without a nucleus used in coagulation; also called a thrombocyte.*	plaqueta
pledget *A small plug of cotton or other synthetic material inserted into a wound.*	pledget
pleomorphism *The ability of an organism or substance to attain distinct forms.*	pleomorfismo
plethora *An excess of something.*	plétora
plethysmograph *A device used to measure the amount of blood flowing through a body part; impedance plethysmography is used to check for deep venous thrombosis.*	pletismógrafo
pleura *The serous membrane lining each lung.*	pleura
pleural effusion *An abnormal collection of fluid between the internal chest wall and the pleura.*	derrame pleural
pleurisy *Inflammation of the pleura.*	pleursía
plica *A fold, as in a fold in the peritoneum.*	plica
pneumatocele *1. A hernia-like protrusion of lung tissue. 2. A collection of gas in a sac such as the scrotum.*	neumatocele
pneumaturia *Presence of air or gas in the urine.*	neumaturia

English	Spanish
pneumococcus *A bacterium causing pneumonia and meningitis. A common type is Streptococcus pneumoniae.*	neumococo
pneumoconiosis *Fibrosis of the lung due to dust inhalation.*	neumoconiosis
pneumocystis jiroveci pneumonia. *A pulmonary infection associated with AIDS. Formerly called pneumocystis carinii pneumonia*	neumonía por pneumocystis jiroveci
pneumonectomy *Surgical excision of all or part of a lung.*	neumonectomía
pneumonia *Inflammation of the lung due to an infection caused by a virus or bacterium.*	neumonía
pneumoperitoneum *Abnormal or induced presence of air or gas in the peritoneum.*	neumoperitoneo
pneumothorax *Abnormal presence of air between the lung and chest wall.*	neumotórax
poikilocytosis *The presence of abnormally shaped erythrocytes.*	poiquilocitosis
poikilothermy *A condition of cold-blooded animals in which their temperature varies based on the ambient temperature.*	poiquilotermia
poison	veneno
polioencephalitis *Polio infection of the brain.*	polioencefalitis
poliomyelitis *An infectious viral disease exhibited by constitutional symptoms that can lead to quadriplegia.*	poliomielitis
polyarteritis nodosa *A systemic necrotizing vasculitis that effects medium sized arteries.*	poliarteritis nodusa
polychondritis *Inflammation of the cartilage at more than one site.*	policondritis
polycystic *Possessing more than one cyst.*	poliquístico
polycythemia *Excess in the number of erythrocytes in the blood.*	policitemia
polycythemia vera *Condition characterized by increase in erythrocytes, thrombocytes and leukocytes, as well as, splenomegaly.*	policitemia vera (o rubra)
polydactyly *Congenital anomaly exhibited by more than 5 digits on the hands and/or feet.*	polidactilia
polydipsia *Profound thirst.*	polidipsia
polymenorrhea *Increase in the frequency of menstruation.*	polimenorrea
polymyositis *Inflammation of several muscle groups at once.*	polimiositis
polyneuritis *Inflammation of more than one nerve.*	polineuritis
polyneuropathy *A condition involving more than one nerve.*	polineuropatía
polyopia *A condition in which one object is seen abnormally as two or more.*	poliopía
polyposis *The formation of multiple polyps.*	poliposis
polypus *Synonym of polyp (a prominent growth from a mucous membrane).*	polypus
polysaccharide *A carbohydrate that upon hydrolysis forms more than ten monosaccharides.*	polisacárido
polysialia *Abnormal increase in saliva.*	poliscelia
polytrauma *A condition exhibited by multiple injuries from blunt or penetrating trauma.*	traumatismo múltiple
polyuria *Abnormal increase in volume of urine excreted.*	poliuria
pompholyx *A condition exhibited by interdigital vesicles of the hands and feet.*	ponfólix Dishidrosis.
pons *The part of the brainstem that connects the medulla oblongata with the thalamus.*	pons
pontine *Referring to the pons.*	pontino
popliteal *Referring to the posterior aspect of the knee.*	poplíteo
porphyria *A hereditary condition currently classified based on the specific enzyme deficiency. The most common form is porphyria cutanea tarda that causes blistering lesions.*	porfiria

English	Spanish
porphyrin *A class of pigments that contain a flat ring of four heterocyclic groups.*	porfirina
port-wine mark *Also called nevus flammeus, it is a vascular anomaly characterized by purplish skin discoloration.*	marca en vino de Oporto. Nevus flammeus
portal *Referring to an entrance such as porta hepatis.*	portal
positive	positivo
post-mortem changes	alteración post mortem
post-nasal drip *The descent of sinus drainage.*	goteo postnasal
post-term pregnancy *A pregnancy that has gone beyond the expected length of time.*	embarazo prolongado
posterior	posterior
posterior chamber of the eye *An aqueous filled space between the cornea and the lens.*	cámara posterior
posterior columns *The dorsal portion of the gray matter of the spinal cord.*	columna posterior
postictal *The period of time after a seizure.*	posictal
postmaturity *Generally referring to a pregnancy that goes beyond the due date.*	postmadurado
postpartum psychosis *A episode of abnormal thought or hallucinations following delivery.*	psicosis del postpartum
postpone	posponer
postural hypotension *A significant drop in blood pressure when going from the supine or sitting position to standing.*	hipotensión postural
postural *Referring to position or posture.*	postural
potassium *A chemical of the alkali metal group.*	potasio
potency *Strength or power.*	fuerza
Pott's disease *Also referred to as tuberculous spnodylitis it is caused by a spinal deformity caused by a tuberculosis infection of the spine.*	enfermedad de Pott
poultryman's itch *Pruritis associated with the mite Dermanyssus gallinae.*	prurito de avicultor
powder	polvo
pox *A general term for fluid filled papules that upon rupturing leave pockmarks.*	pox
preauricular *Anterior to the ear.*	preauricular
precancerous *Referring to an early stage in cancer development.*	precanceroso
precipitin *An antibody-antigen reaction producing a precipitate.*	precipitina
precordialgia *Pain in the precordium.*	precordialgia
precordium *The area occupying the epigastrum and lower sternum.*	precordio
preeclampsia *Hypertension with proteinuria and/or edema in the setting of pregnancy.*	preeclampsia
pregnancy	embarazo
premature *Occurring earlier than expected.*	prematuro
premenstrual *Occurring prior to the onset of menstruation.*	premenstrual
premenstrual syndrome *A cluster of emotional, behavioral, and physical symptoms that occur in the premenstrual phase of the menstrual cycle and resolve with the onset of menstruation.*	síndrome premenstrual
premolar *The teeth anterior to the molars.*	premolar
prenatal care *Medical care received while one is pregnant.*	cuidado prenatal
prenatal *Referring to the time prior to birth.*	prenatal
presbyacusia *An age related, progressive hearing loss.*	presbiacusia
presbyopia *Farsightedness associated with aging.*	presbiopía

121

English	Spanish
prescription	receta
presenting symptom *The initial subjective complaint that initiated a visit.*	síntoma presente
pressure reducer *Anti-hypertensive agent.*	antihipertensivo
pressure ulcer *Loss in skin integrity due to a portion of the body being in the same position for too long and possibly other factors.*	úlcera de decúbito
presystole *The time just before systole.*	presístole
prevent, to	prevenir
priapism *A painful and abnormally prolonged erection.*	priapismo
prickly heat *A rash with small vesicles that is pruritic and associated with a warm moist environment.*	salpullido
primipara *A woman giving birth for the first time.*	primípara
prior status *Referring to a person's previous state of health.*	estado antecesor
probe *A device used for exploration.*	sonda
problem	problema
proctalgia *A chronic high, dull rectal pain worse with sitting position.*	proctalgia
proctectomy *Surgical excision of the rectum.*	protectomía
proctitis *Inflammation of the rectum.*	proctitis
proctocele *A hernia-type protrusion of the rectum into the vagina.*	proctocele
proctoscopy *Inspection of the rectum with a scope.*	proctoscopia
progeria *A childhood disorder exhibited by signs of aging including gray hair, wrinkled skin and short height.*	progeria
progesterone *A steroid hormone that prepares the uterus for pregnancy.*	progesterona
proglottis *Any segment of a tapeworm.*	proglotis
prognathism *Protrusion of the mandible which can cause malocclusion.*	prognatismo
prognosis	pronóstico
progressive	progresivo
prolactin *A pituitary hormone that facilitates milk production.*	prolactina
prolapse of the umbilical cord *Refers to the umbilical cord protruding from the cervix during active labor.*	prolapso del cordón umbilical
prolapse *The slipping downward of a body part, such as rectal prolapse.*	prolapso
promonocyte *An intermediate cell stage between monocyte and monoblast.*	promonocito
promontory *A protruding eminence.*	promontorio
pronation *Turning posteriorly. When the hand is pronated, it is turned medially until the palm is facing posteriorly (when the body was initially in the anatomic position).*	pronación
prone *Lying with the abdomen and face downward.*	prono
prophylaxis *That which is done to prevent disease.*	profiláctico
proprioceptor *A receptor that responds to sensory input including position sense.*	propioceptor
proptosis oculi *Synonym of exophthalmos; bulging of the eye.*	proptosis
prostacyclin *A prostaglandin that functions as an anticoagulant and vasodilator.*	prostaciclina
prostaglandin *A compound first found in semen (thus "prosta" in the name from prostate) with many effects including uterine contraction.*	prostaglandina
prostate *A gland found in men that surrounds the neck of the urethra and bladder.*	próstata
prostatectomy *Surgical excision of the prostate.*	prostatectomía
prosthesis *An artificial body part.*	prótesis

English	Spanish
prostration *Profound exhaustion.*	prostración
protein *A class of nitrogenous organic compound.*	proteína
proteinuria *The presence of protein in the urine.*	proteinuria
proteolysis *Enzyme action on proteins to form amino acids.*	proteólisis
prothrombin *A compound converted to thrombin during coagulation of blood.*	protrombina
protoplasm *The cytoplasm, organelles and nucleus of a living cell.*	protoplasma
protozoa *A single celled microscopic organism including amoebas among others.*	protozoario
provoke, to	provocar
proximal *Situated closer to the center of the body (opposed to that which is farther away, as in distal).*	proximal
prurigo *A chronic, pruritic papular skin eruption.*	prurigo
pruritis *A general term for conditions exhibited by itching.*	prurito
pseudarthrosis *Deossification of weight bearing long bones.*	seudoartrosis
pseudobulbar palsy *Sudden outbursts of laughter or tearfulness sometimes seen in amyotrophic lateral sclerosis.*	parálisis seudobulbar
pseudomnesia *Sensing the memory of an event that has never happened.*	seudomnesia
psittacosis *A chlamydial pneumonia that is transmitted by birds.*	psitacosis
psoriasis *A chronic papulosquamous dermatosis characterized by silver plaques.*	psoriasis
psychasthenia *Essentially any non-hysterical neuroses.*	psicastenia
psychiatry *A branch of medicine specializing in the treatment of mental disorders.*	psiquiatría
psychologist *A professional specializing in psychology.*	psicólogo
psychology *The study of the human mind and emotions.*	psicología
psychoneurosis *A mental disorder that could include depression or anxiety but does not include hallucinations.*	psiconeurosis
psychopathology *Scientific examination of mental disease.*	psicopatología
psychosis *A profound mental disorder that can include delusions and hallucinations.*	psicosis
psychosomatic *Physical ailments arising from mental disease.*	psicosomático
psychotherapy *Treatment of mental disease with cognitive-behavioral approaches.*	psicoterapia
pterygium *A membrane in the interpalpebral fissure present from the conjunctiva to the cornea.*	pterigión
ptosis *Drooping of the upper eyelid usually due to paralysis of the third cranial nerve.*	ptosis
ptyalin *An enzyme found in saliva.*	ptialina
puberty *The time when adolescents become capable of sexual reproduction.*	pubertad
pubic hair *Hair present in the perineal area.*	vello púbico
pubis *The anterior inferior part of the hip bone on each side that articulates at the pubic symphysis.*	pubis
pudendal *Referring to the female genitalia*	pudendo
pudendum *The mons, pubis, labia majora, labia minora and the vagina.*	vulva
puerpera *A woman who just gave birth.*	puérpera
puerperium *The six week period after childbirth.*	pueperio
puffiness	hinchazón
pull, to	tirón de la ingle

English	Spanish
pulmonary edema *Characterized by abnormal fluid buildup in the lungs.*	edema pulmonar
pulmonary embolism *A sudden blockage of a lung artery frequently eminating from a blood clot in one's leg.*	embolismo pulmonar
pulmonary *Referring to the lungs.*	pulmonar
pulmonary stenosis *A stricture between the pulmonary artery and the right ventricle.*	estenosis pulmonar
pulp *The tissue filling the root canals of a tooth.*	pulpa
pulpitis *Dental pulp inflammation.*	pulpitis
pulsatile	pulsátil
pulsation	pulsación
pulse *The rhythmic throbbing of arteries felt at major vessels.*	pulso
pulsus alternans *A regular alternation of weak and strong beats of the pulse.*	pulso alternante
pupil *The opening at the center of the iris.*	pupila
purpura *The presence of patches of ecchymosis or petechiae.*	púrpura
purulent *Referring to pus.*	purulento
pus	pus
putrefaction *The rotting or decaying of organic matter.*	putrefacción
pyelitis *Renal pelvis inflammation.*	pielitis
pyelography *Roentgenography of the renal pelvis and ureters after administration of contrast media.*	pielografía
pyelolithotomy *Surgical excision of a calculus from the renal pelvis.*	pielolitotomía
pyelonephritis *Inflammation of the renal parenchyma usually due to bacterial infection.*	pielonefritis
pyelonephrosis *Term, rarely used anymore,used to describe disease of the renal pelvis.*	pielonefrosis
pyemia *Sepsis characterized by the presence of secondary abscesses.*	piemia
pyknic *Possessing a short, stocky physique.*	pícnico
pyknosis *The degeneration of a cell with the nucleus shrinking.*	picnosis
pyloric *Referring to the pylorus.*	pilórico
pyloroplasty *Surgical enlargement of a pylorus that previously was stenotic.*	pilorplastia
pylorus *The opening at the distal stomach that opens into the duodenum.*	píloro
pyoderma *A purulent skin infection.*	pioderma
pyogenic liver abscess *A pus filled fluid collection in the liver.*	absceso hepático piógeno
pyogenic *Referring to the formation of pus.*	piogénico
pyonephrosis *Injury to the renal parenchyma due to pus.*	pionefrosis
pyorrhea *Emission of pus.*	piorrea
pyosalpinx *Purulent material in the oviduct.*	piosálpinx
pyramidal *A term that is used to describe various spinal tracts that originate in the cerebral cortex.*	piramidal
pyrexia *Fever.*	pirexia
pyridoxine *Synonym for vitamin B6.*	pirodoxina
pyrogen *A fever producing substance released by bacteria.*	pirógen
pyrosis *Synonym for heartburn.*	pirosis
pyuria *Presence of purulent material in the urine.*	piuria
Q fever *A disease caused by rickettsiae from the ingestion of unpasteurized milk.*	fiebre Q

English	Spanish
quadriceps jerk (reflex) *Also referred to as th patellar reflex.*	reflejo del cuádriceps
quadriceps *The anterior thigh muscle composed of four muscles.*	cuádriceps
quadrigeminal bodies *The cranial and caudal colliculi.*	cuerpos cuadrigéminos
quadriplegia *Paralysis of all four extremities.*	cuadriplejía
qualify	calificar
quarantine *A place of isolation for infectious persons until it can be certain it is safe to let them mingle.*	cuarentena
querulousness *Whining or complaining.*	quejarse continuamente
quiescent *A time of inactivity.*	quiescente
quiet	tranquilo
quinsy *Peritonsillar inflammation or abscess.*	quinsy
rabbeting *The interlocking of two sections of a fractured bone.*	enclavamiento
rabies *An infectious viral disease transmitted through the bite of a mammal. Symptoms include hydrophobia, pharyngeal spasms and hyperactivity.*	rabia
racemose *A gland having the form of a cluster.*	racemoso
radial *Referring to the radius.*	radial
radiation *1. The emission of energy in the form of electromagnetic waves. 2. Divergence from a common point.*	radiación
radiculitis *Inflammation of a spinal nerve root.*	radiculitis
radioactive *Referring to the emission of ionizing particles or radiation.*	radiactivo
radioactive isotope *An isotope with an unstable nucleus that is used in diagnostic imaging.*	radioisótopo
radiobiology *The study of the effects of radiation on organisms.*	radiobiología
radioepithelitis *The injury to epithelial cells due to effects of radiation.*	radioepitelitis
radiography *The department where images are produced on sensitive film by x-rays.*	radiografía
radiologist *A physician specializing in radiology.*	radiólogo
radiology *The branch of medicine concerned with roentgenography and other high-energy radiation.*	radiología
radionuclide *A radioactive nuclide.*	radionúclido
radiosensitivity *The susceptibility of the skin to radiation.*	radiosensibilidad
radiotherapy *Treatment of cancer with radiation.*	radioterapia
rage	ira
raise, to	levantar
rale *An abnormal lung sound noted during auscultation.*	rales
ramus *A branch; a term used to describe a smaller vessel branching off from a larger one.*	ramus
ranula *A retention cyst formed because of obstruction of a salivary gland in the floor of the mouth.*	ránula
rape *Forced sexual relations.*	violar
Rapid Eye Movement *The movement of a person's eyes during this period of sleep.*	movimiento ocular rápido
rash	erupción
rat bite fever *As the name implies, it is a condition exhibited by fever, nausea and skin erythema after one is bitten by a rat.*	fiebre por mordedura de rata
reaction	reacción
reactive	reactivo
rebound *A term used to describe a type of tenderness found with peritonitis.*	rebote

125

English	Spanish
receptor *A cell or organ that accepts stimuli and transmits data to a sensory nerve.*	receptor
recessive *This refers to genetic controlled traits that are only inherited when code from both parents is the same.*	recesivo
recollection *Memory.*	recuerdo
recovery room	sala de recuperación
rectal digital examination *Use of a gloved finger to assess the rectal vault.*	examen rectal digital
rectal *Referring to the rectum.*	rectal
rectocele *A herniation of the wall between the rectum and vagina.*	rectocele
rectoscopy *Visualization of the rectum with a scope.*	rectoscopia
rectosigmoidectomy *Surgical resection of the rectum and sigmoid colon.*	rectosigmoidectomíe
rectovesical septum *The wall between the rectum and the urinary bladder.*	tabique rectovesical
rectus abdominis muscle *The pair of long, flat muscles that connect the sternum with the pubis.*	músculo recto del abdomen
recumbent *Lying down.*	recumbente
red nucleus *A collection of gray matter near the subthalamus that receives data from the superior cerebellar peduncle.*	núcleo rojo
reduction *Return of a dislocated joint or fractured bone to its proper position.*	reducción
referred pain *Pain felt in an area distinct from the original source.*	dolor referido
regardless of	sin tener en cuenta
regurgitation *1. Backflow of blood in the heart. 2. Movement of gastric contents into the mouth.*	regurgitación
relapse *The return to a prior state of ill health.*	recidiva
relapsing fever *A recurrent bacterial infection, with fever, caused by Spirochetes.*	fiebre recurrente
related to	relacionado
relation *1. A person who has a blood or marriage connection.*	pariente
relaxant *Term generally used to refer to a muscle relaxant.*	relajante
relaxin *A hormone secreted by the placenta which dilates the cervix.*	relaxina
releasing hormone *Hormones that come from one gland such as the thalamus that cause release of hormones from another gland such as the pituitary.*	hormona estimulante
reliable	confiable
relief	alivio
relieve, to (pain)	aliviar (dolor)
REM (rapid eye movement) sleep *This period of sleep is associated with irregular respirations and heart rate, involuntary movements and dreaming.*	movimiento ocular rápido (MOR)
remission *A decrease in severity or a temporary resolution.*	remisión
removal	eliminación
renal *Referring to the kidney.*	renal
renal colic *Pain caused by passage of a calculus through the ureter.*	cólico nefrítico
renal failure *Diminution of kidney function.*	insuficiencia renal
renal pelvis *The kidney collecting system.*	pelvis renal
renin *A renal enzyme that facilitates the production of angiotensin.*	renina
resection *The removal of tissue.*	resección
residual urine *The amount of urine remaining in the bladder after a person voids.*	orina residual
residual volume (RV) *The amount of air left in the lung after a maximal exhalation.*	volumen residual

126

English	Spanish
resin *An organic substance that is insoluble in water. There are many types. Cholestyramine resin is used for hypercholesterolemia.*	resina
resorbable suture (chromic) *Suture that is not intended to be permanent as it is dissolved by normal body processes.*	sutura quirúrgica absorbible
respirator *A device used to artificially ventilate a patient.*	respirador
respiratory *Referring to respiration or the organs of respiration.*	respiratorio
respiratory distress syndrome *A disease in infants that is caused by a surfactant deficiency.*	síndrome de dificultad respiratoria
respiratory rate *The number of breaths per minute.*	tasa respiratoria
rest	descanso
restless legs *Associated with a syndrome exhibited by continuous movement of the legs from uncertain etiology.*	síndrome de las piernas inquietas
retching *Spasm of the stomach without presence of gastric material.*	arcadas
reticular *Referring to a matrix of membranous tubules inside the cytoplasm of a eukaryotic cells.*	reticular
reticulo-endothelial *Referring to the system of phagocytes involved in the immune system.*	reticuloendotelial
reticulocyte *A red blood cell without a nucleus.*	reticulocito
reticulocytosis *An abnormal increase in circulating reticulocytes.*	reticulocitosis
retina *The innermost of three layers of the eyeball; it surrounds the vitreous body and is continuous with the optic nerve.*	retina
retinal detachment *A tear or hole in the retina caused by vitreous traction.*	retina desprendida
retinitis *Inflammation of the retina.*	retinitis
retinoblastoma *A tumor consisting of retinal germ cells.*	retinoblastoma
retinopathy *Any one of a number of retinal inflammatory conditions.*	retinopatía
retraction *Being drawn back.*	retracción
retractor *A device for pulling back tissue during surgery.*	retractor
retrobulbar optic neuritis *An inflammatory, demyelinating condition in the retrobulbar region.*	neuritis retrobulbar
retroflexed uterus *Bending back of the uterus so that the top portion pushes against the rectum.*	útero retroflexionado
retrograde *Referring to backward movement.*	retrógrado
retroperitoneal *Situated or referring to the area posterior to the peritoneum.*	retroperitoneo
retropharyngeal abscess *A collection of purulent material posterior to the pharynx.*	absceso retrofaríngeo
retropharyngeal *Referring to the area posterior to the pharynx.*	retrofaríngo
Rett syndrome. *A rare inherited disorder causing developmental delays and is seen mostly in girls.*	síndrome de Rett
rhabdomyolysis *A acute destruction of muscle documented by myoglobinemia and myoglobinuria.*	rabdomiólisis
rhagade *Fissures in the skin, particularly adjacent to body orifices.*	rágade
rheumatic *Referring to rheumatism.*	reumático
rheumatic fever *A febrile streptococcal disease causing pain and joint swelling.*	fiebre reumática
rheumatic heart disease *A manifestation of rheumatic fever, frequently causing valvular dysfunction.*	enfermedad cardíaca reumática
rheumatism *Any condition exhibited by inflammation and pain in the joints and muscles.*	reumatismo
rheumatoid arthritis *A symmetric peripheral polyarthritis.*	artritis reumatoide

English	Spanish
rhinitis *A viral infection or allergic reaction exhibited by nasal mucosal inflammation.*	rinitis
rhinoplasty *Plastic surgery performed on the nose.*	rinoplastia
rhinorrhea *Abundant nasal mucosal drainage.*	rinorrea
rhinoscopy *Examination of the nasal passages.*	rinoscopia
rhizotomy *Interruption of the spinal nerve roots within the spinal canal.*	rizotomía
rhodopsin *A reddish purple light sensitive pigment in the human retina.*	rodopsina
rhomboid *A back muscle that elevates, retracts and adducts the scapula.*	romboide
rhonchus *A coarse, dry sound heard on auscultation of the lungs.*	ronquido
rhythm	ritmo
rib	costilla
riboflavin *Also called vitamin B2, this essential vitamin is present in food such as eggs and is synthesized in the small bowel.*	riboflavina
ribonucleic acid *An acid present in all living cells, it is a messenger for DNA.*	ácido ribonucleico (RNA)
ribosomal RNA *Four chains designated by their appropriate coefficients.*	RNA robosómico
rickets *A condition exhibited by softening and bowing of the long bones; caused by Vitamin D deficiency.*	raquitismo
rickettsia *A disease transmitted by ticks or fleas, caused by a bacterium from the genus Rickettsieae. Rocky Mountain Spotted fever is one of many diseases caused by this bacterium.*	rickettsias
right	derecho
rigor mortis *The normal stiffening of the muscles and joints that occurs a few hours after death.*	rigor mortis
ring	anillo
ringing in the ears *Common term for tinnitus.*	sonido en oídos
ringworm *A fungal skin infection exhibited by pruritic well circumscribed patches on the scalp or feet.*	tiña
risus sardonicus *A spasm of the facial muscles causing what appears to be a smile on one's face.*	risa canina
Ritgen's maneuver *A procedure that controls the rate of delivery of the infant's head during childbirth.*	maniobra de Ritgen
rodent	roedor
Roentgen *One unit of ionizing radiation named after the German physicist Wilhelm Conrad Röntgen.*	roentgen
room; chamber	cuarto
root	raíz
rosacea *Erythema of the cheeks and nose caused by chronic vascular and follicular dilation.*	rosácea
rotation	rotación
rotator cuff *The structure around the capsule of the shoulder joint formed by the infraspinatus, supraspinatus, teres minor and subscapularis muscles.*	manguito rotatotio del hombro
round ligament *The supporting structure of the uterus.*	ligamento redondo del útero
rub	roce
rubefacient *A substance that reddens the skin.*	rubefaciente
rubella *Also called German measles, it is characterized by a rash, fever, headache.*	rubéola
rude	grosero

English	Spanish
rugine *A surgical instrument that resembles a rasp.*	raspadera
ruling out	desechar
running suture *A method of sewing a wound in which there is a knot at each end and continuous otherwise.*	sutura continua
rupia *A sign of tertiary syphilis in which there are bullae or vesicles formed on the skin that erupt and form crusts.*	rupia
rupture	ruptura
sacral *Referring to the sacrum.*	sacral
sacral canal *The portion of the vertebral canal that progresses into the sacrum.*	conducto sacro
sacralization *The fusion of the fifth lumbar vertebra to the sacrum.*	sacralización
sacrum *The bone formed by five fused vertebrae that is situated between the two hip bones.*	sacro
saddle joint *A joint that exhibits two saddle type surfaces at a 90 degree angle to each other, such as the carpometacarpal joint.*	articulación en silla de montar
sadness	tristeza
sagittal suture *The line where the two parietal bones meet.*	sutura sagital
Saint Ignatius' itch *Pruritis noted with a cluster of symptoms related to niacin deficiency. Generally referred to as pellagra.*	prurito de San Ignacio. Pelagra.
saline *A solution of sodium chloride.*	salino
saliva	saliva
salivary gland *The parotid, submandibular and sublingual glands that secrete saliva.*	glándulas salivales
salivation *The process of secreting saliva.*	salivación
salpingectomy *Surgical resection of the fallopian tubes.*	salpingectomía
salpingitis *Inflammation of the fallopian tubes.*	salpingitis
salpingography *Roentgenography of the fallopian tubes after administration of contrast media.*	salpingografía
salpingostomy *A surgical procedure involving cutting the fallopian tube.*	salpingostomía
salt	sal
saluretic *An agent that promotes excretion of sodium and chloride in the urine.*	salurético
sampling	muestreo
sandfly fever *A febrile illness transmitted by a sandfly, from the genus Phlebotomus, and found in the Mediterranean.*	fiebre por flebótomos
sanitary napkin	paño higiénico
saphena *Referring to either of the two superficial saphenous veins.*	safena
saponify *The creation of soap from oil using an alkali.*	saponificar
saprophyte *Any organism living on dead organic material.*	saprofito
sarcoid *Referring to sarcoidosis.*	sarcoide
sarcoidosis *A chronic disease characterized by lymphadenopathy and widespread granulomas.*	sarcoidosis
sarcolemme *The sheath that covers skeletal muscle fibers.*	sarcolema
sarcoma *A non-epithelial malignant tumor.*	sarcoma
sartorius muscle *The thigh muscle that runs from the pelvis to the proximal, medial aspect of the tibia.*	sartorio
saturation *An amount, expressed in a percentage, that expresses the degree something is absorbed versus the maximal absorption possible.*	saturación
saw	sierra

English	Spanish
scabies *A skin condition exhibited by intense pruritis and a macular rash commonly in the perineal and interdigital spaces.*	sarna
scalding *A burn injury from extremely hot water.*	escaldaura
scale *A device to check a person's weight.*	balanza
scalp	cuero cabelludo
scalp laceration *A linear opening of the dermis on the cranium.*	laceración de cuero cabelludo
scalpel *A knife used during surgery for incision of skin and tissue.*	escalpelo
scaphocephaly *A condition exhibited by a long narrow skull because of early closure of the sagittal sutures.*	escafocefalia
scaphoid bone *The most lateral of the carpal bones; it articulates with the radius.*	escafoide
scapula *Medical term for the shoulder blade.*	escápula
scapulalgia *Scapular pain.*	escapulagia
scarification *Multiple small scratches of the skin, as is sometimes used for vaccine administration.*	escarificación
scarlet fever *A condition caused by streptococci that is exhibited by fever and a bright red (scarlet) rash.*	fiebre escarlatina
scatter	dispersión
scheme	esquema
schistocyte *Part of a red blood cell seen in hemolytic anemia.*	esquistocito
schistosomiasis *A condition, sometimes known as bilharzia, which involves infestation with flukes of the genus Schistosoma.*	esquistosomiasis
schizophrenia *A chronic mental condition exhibited by delusions, hallucinations, and faulty perception.*	esquizofrenia
schmorl's nodule *Protrusion of the nucleus pulposus through the vertebral body endplast into the adjacent vertebra.*	nódulo de Schmorl
sciatica *Pain radiating from the buttock down the back of the leg; it is caused by a compressed spinal nerve root.*	ciática
scimitar sign *An abnormal radiologic finding associated with anomalous pulmonary venous drainage.*	signo de la cimitarra
scirrhus *A cancer that is hard to palpation.*	escirro
scissors	tijeras
sclera *The white outer covering of the eyeball.*	sclera
scleritis *Inflammation of the eyeball.*	escleritis
sclerodactylia *Scleroderma of the digits.*	esclerodactilia
scleroderma *A systemic disease of the connective tissues.*	esclerodermia
sclerotomy *Surgical incision of the sclera.*	esclerotomía
scolex *The front end of a tapeworm.*	escólex
scoliosis *A lateral curvature of the spine.*	escoliosis
scopophilia *Sexual please attained by viewing sexual organs.*	escopofilia
scotoma *A blind spot within an otherwise normal visual field.*	escotoma
scrape	raspadura
scratch	rasguño
screening	escrutinio
scrofula *Cervical tuberculous lymphadenitis.*	escrófula
scrotal *Referring to the scrotum.*	escrotal
scrotal hydrocele *A benign collection of fluid in the scrotum.*	hidrocele escrotal

English	Spanish
scrotum *The sac which contains the testes.*	escroto
scurvy *A disease of vitamin C deficiency exhibited by bleeding gums.*	escorbuto
scutulum *A crust of tinea capitis.*	escútulo
scybalum *A hard, dry formation of stool in the bowel.*	escíbalo
seal	sellado
sebaceous *Referring to a sebaceous gland or what it secretes.*	sebáceo
sebaceous gland *A gland in the skin that secretes sebum.*	glándula sebácea
seborrhea *Abnormal amount of sebum production.*	seborrea
secretin *A hormone that increases secretion from the pancreas and liver.*	secretina
secretion *The discharge of substances from cells or glands.*	secreción
sedative *A medication used to facilitate sleep or calm a person.*	sedante
seizure *An episode of tonic/clonic movement noted in epilepsy.*	convulsión
semen analysis *Evaluation of semen used as part of a fertility workup.*	análisis semen
semicircular canal *The anterior, posterior and lateral canals in the inner ear that assist in balance control.*	conducto semicircular
seminiferous tubules *Used for transport of semen.*	túbulos seminíferos
seminoma *A malignant tumor of the testis.*	seminoma
senescence *The normal process of deterioration with age.*	senescencia
senile *Generally referring to mental deterioration associated with aging.*	senil
senility *The process of being senile.*	senilidad
sensation *A perception when one is touched.*	sensación
sensation of warmth or heaviness	sensación de calor o pesadez
sensibility *Ability to feel or perceive.*	sensibilidad
sensible	sensible
sensitization *The change in an organ by a hormone so it will respond to another stimulus.*	sensibilización
sensitized *Being abnormally sensitive to a substance.*	sensibilizar
sensory nerve *A nerve that receives input from various receptors.*	nervio sensitivo
sepsis *A condition exhibited by overwhelming inflammation due to infection.*	sepsis
septic *Referring to a state of sepsis.*	séptico
septicemia *A systemic disease in which microorganisms or their toxins are in the blood stream.*	septicemia
septum *A wall separating two chambers, the nasal septum for example.*	tabique
sequela *A medical problem related to an initial injury or disease.*	secuela
sequestrum *Necrotic bone present in an injured or diseased bone.*	secuestro
serial	serie
serotonin *A neurotransmitter that constricts blood vessels.*	serotonina
serous *Referring to serum or similar to serum.*	seroso
serpiginous *A skin lesion having wavy margin.*	serpiginoso
serum *The fluid that isolates out when blood coagulates.*	suero
sessile *Having a broad base with no stalk.*	sésil
severe	serio
sex	sexo
sexual intercourse *The act of copulation.*	relaciones sexuales
sexually transmitted disease (STD) *A condition one obtains from another during sexual relations.*	enfermedad transmitida sexual

English	Spanish
shake, to	temblar
sharp (pain)	agudo
sheath *A covering.*	vaina
sheet (bed)	sábana
shellfish	mariscos
shield	escudo
shin *Refers to the anterior tibial region.*	espinilla
shingles *A reactivation of herpes zoster.*	culebrilla
shiver	estremecimiento
shock *A condition characterized by systemic hypoperfusion.*	shock
shoe	zapato
shortening	acortamiento
shoulder	hombro
shunt *An alternate path for blood or fluid.*	shunt
sialadenitis *Inflammation of a salivary gland.*	sialadenitis
sialogogue *A substance that increase salivary flow.*	sialogogo
sialolith *A calculus in a salivary duct.*	sialolito
sibling	hermano
sickle-cell anemia *A hereditary type of anemia characterized by crescent shaped red blood cells.*	anemia drepanocítica
sickness	enfermedad
side	costado
side effect	efecto secundario
siderosis *Excess iron in the blood or a pulmonary disease from iron inhalation called Pneumoconiosis.*	siderosis
sigh, to	suspirar
sigmoid flexure *The S shaped curve located between the descending colon and rectum.*	flexura sigmoidea
sigmoid *Referring to the portion of the colon that leads into the rectum.*	sigmoide
sigmoidoscopy *Visualization of the sigmoid colon with a scope.*	sigmoidoscopia
sigmoidostomy *Formation of an opening in the sigmoid colon that communicates with the outside of the body.*	sigmoidostomía
silent	callado
silicosis *Grinders's disease; fibrotic lung disease caused by inhalation of silica.*	silicosis
silly	tonto
silver	plata
silver nitrate stick *A medical device used to treat hypergranulation tissue.*	nitrato de plata
simultaneous	simultáneo
single	individual
single (not married)	soltero
sinistrocardia *Location of the heart toward the left (more than normally seen).*	sinistrocardia
sinistrotorsion *Distorsion toward the left; in reference to the eye generally.*	sinistrotorsión
sinoatrial *Referring to the cardiac node of the same name.*	sinoauricular
sinoatrial node *A mass of cardiac tissue that acts as the pacemaker.*	nudo sinoauricular
sinus arrhythmia *Cardiac dysrhythmias related to sinoatrial nodal dysfunction.*	arritmia sinusal
sinusitis *Inflammation of the sinuses.*	sinusitis

132

English	Spanish
sinusoid *An irregular vessel having almost no adventitia that is found in the liver, heart, parathyroid, spleen and pancreas.*	sinusoide
sip, to	sorber
Sister Mary Joseph nodule *A nodule at the umbilicus associated with metastatic abdominal cancer.*	nódulo de la hermana Joseph
site	sitio
size	tamaño
Sjogren's syndrome. *Characterized by dryness of the mouth and eyes, it is sometimes linked to rheumatoid arthritis.*	síndrome de Sjogren
skeletal traction	tracción esquelética
skeleton	esqueleto
skin	piel
skin fold	pliegue piel
skin lesion	lesión piel
skin rash	erupción
sleep	sueño
sleep apnea *Episodic apnea during sleep that is exhibited by daytime symptoms of fatigue, difficulty concentrating and sleepiness.*	apnea del sueño
sleeping sickness *Also called Trypanosomiasis, this disease is caused by a parasitic protozoa and transmitted by the tsetse fly.*	enfermedad del sueño
slice	rebanada
slide *A thin, rectangular piece of glass used for viewing specimen under a microscope.*	portaobjeto
slight	pequeño
sling *A device used to give support to an injured extremity.*	cabestrillo
slow	lento
sludge *A viscous fluid.*	sedimento
slurring *Indistinct yet comprehensible speech.*	tragarse
smallpox *Variola.*	viruela
smear *Used to refer to a specimen smeared on a slide.*	frotis
smegma *A thick curdled secretion found around the clitoris and the prepuce.*	esmegma
smoke, to	fumar
sneeze, to	estornudar
sniffing	aspiración por la nariz
snore, to	ronquido
soap	jabón
sob, to	sollozar
socket *An anatomical hollow that is part of an articulation or where the eyeball rests.*	alvéolo
socks (as in footwear)	calcetín
sodium chloride	cloruro de sodio
soft	blando
solar plexus *A cluster of ganglia and nerves, located at the base of the sternum, that surround the celiac trunk.*	plexo solar
sole of foot *Common term for plantar aspect of the foot.*	planta de pie
soleus muscle *Assists with ankle plantar flexion.*	sóleo
solvent *Able to dissolve with other chemicals.*	solvente

133

English	Spanish
somatic *Referring to the body.*	somático
somnambulism *Sleepwalking.*	sonambulismo
somnolence *Drowsiness.*	somnolencia
soporific *Promoting drowsiness or sleep.*	soporífico
sore throat *Common term for pharyngitis.*	faringitis
sorrow	pesar
soul	alma
sound	sano
sour	agrio
span	alcance
sparing	parco
spasm *An involuntary contraction of muscles.*	espasmo
spasmolytic *A substance that diminishes spasms.*	espasmolítico
spastic *Stiff, awkward movement of the muscles.*	espástico
spasticity *Refers to continuous spastic movement.*	espasticidad
specific	específico
specimen	muestra
spectrometry *The use of a device to measure spectra.*	espectrometría
spectroscope *A device for producing and recording spectra.*	espectroscopio
speculum *A device used to open a canal, like the vagina, for inspection.*	espéculo
speech	habla
speech therapist	terapeuta habla
sperm	esperma
spermatic cord *The structure containing the ductus deferens, testicular artery, and nerves that goes from the inguinal ring to the testis.*	cordón espermático
spermatocele *A cyst in the epididymis containing spermatozoa.*	espermatocele
spermatogenesis *The production of spermatozoa.*	esperatogénesis
spermatozoon *A mature male germ cell that is capable of fertilizing an ovum.*	espermatozoide
spermicide *A substance capable of killing sperm.*	espermicida
sphenoidal sinus *Part of the sphenoid bone; it communicates with the most superior aspect of the nasal meatus.*	seno esfenoidal
spherocyte *An erythrocyte without the usual central pallor; it is noted in spherocytosis and some hemolytic anemias.*	esferocito
spherocytosis *The presence of spherocytes in the blood.*	esferocitosis
sphincter *A muscle the surrounds an orifice or duct so it closes when the muscle contracts.*	esfínter
sphincterotomy *Surgical incision of the anal sphincter.*	esfinterotomía
sphygmomanometer *Device for measuring blood pressure.*	esfigmomanometría
spica *A figure of eight bandage.*	spica
spicule *A sharp, slender part.*	espícula
spider nevus *A papule with telangiectases radiating from the center.*	nevo araña
spinal *Referring to the spine.*	espinal
spinal cord abscess *A localized collection of purulent material in or adjacent to the spinal cord.*	absceso de la médula espinal
spinal cord *The bundle of nerves that with the brain comprise the central nervous system.*	médula espinal
spinal ganglion *The ganglion located on the dorsal root of each spinal nerve.*	ganglio espinal

English	Spanish
spinal nerve *The term for each of the thirty pairs of nerves that originate in the spine and traverse between the vertebrae. There are eight cervical, twelve thoracic, five lumbar, five sacral and one coccygeal nerve pairs.*	nervios espinales
spinal reflex *A reflex that has an arc passing through the spine.*	reflejo espinal
spinal shock *Hypotension related to injury or intervention of the spine.*	shock espinal
spine *The spinal column or a thorny protrusion.*	espina
spirograph *A device used to record respiratory movements.*	espirógrafo
spirometer *A device used to measure pulmonary capacity.*	espirómetro
spitting	expectoración
splanchnic nerves *The nerves supplying the abdominal viscera and blood vessels.*	nervio esplánico
spleen *The visceral organ that is involved with production and removal of blood cells.*	bazo
splenectomy *Surgical excision of the spleen.*	esplenectomía
splenic flexure of the colon *The portion of the colon that turns from the transverse to the descending colon.*	flexura esplénica
splenic *Referring to the spleen.*	esplénico
splenomegaly *An abnormally enlarged spleen.*	esplenomegalia
splint *A rigid support used to immobilize and extremity.*	férula
splinter *A small, thin object; usually refers to the object being imbedded in the body.*	astilla
spoiled (for food to go bad)	echarse a perder
spondylitis *Inflammation of the vertebrae.*	espondilitis
spondylolisthesis *The overlapping of one vertebra over another.*	espondilolistesis
spondylolysis *Dissolution of the vertebra.*	espondilólisis
sponge	esponja
spongiosis *Edema of the spongy layer of the skin.*	espongiosis
spontaneous *Occurring without provocation.*	espontáneo
spoon nail *Also referred to as koilonychia, the nail is concave and is generally associated with anemia.*	uña en cuchara
spoonful	cucharada
sporotrichosis *A Sporotrichum schenckii infection manifested by formation of lymphatic and subcutaneous nodules.*	esporotricosis
sprain	torcedura (los ligamentos)
spray	aerosol
sputum *A mixture of respiratory tract secretions and saliva.*	esputo
squama *A scale or platelike body.*	escama
squamous *Scaly.*	escamoso
square root	raíz cuadrada
squeeze, pressure (hand shake)	apretón (apretón de manos)
squint	bizquera
squirt, to	lanzar un chorro
stab wound *An injury occurring with a sharp object.*	herida de arma blanca
stabbing pain	dolor penetrante
staggering	asombroso
staging *Refers to a stratification of cancer for example.*	estadificación

135

English	Spanish
stamina *Ability to maintain physical or mental exertion for a long period.*	resistencia
stammering *The impulse to repeat the first letter of words and involuntary pauses while speaking.*	tartamudeo
standing	de pie
stapedectomy *Surgical excision of the stapes.*	estapedectomía
stapedius muscle *Located in the tympanic interior, it reduces stapedial movement.*	estapedio
stapes *This auditory ossicle is the innermost of three ossicles and is shaped like a stirrup.*	estribo
staphyloma *Protrusion of the cornea due to inflammation.*	estafiloma
staphylorrhaphy *Surgical repair of a defect between the soft palate and uvula.*	estafilorrafia
starvation	inanición
stasis *Lack of movement.*	estasis
state	estado
statement	declaración
static *Not changing.*	estático
status	estado
status of illness	estado de condición
steady state *In equilibrium.*	equilibrio
steatoma *A sebaceous cyst or lipoma.*	quiste sebáceo
steatorrhea *Excrement with an abnormally high fat content.*	esteatorrea
steatosis *Fatty degeneration; when referring to the liver it involves invasion of fat into hepatocytes.*	esteatosis
stellate ganglion *Formed by the seventh cervical, eighth cervical and first thoracic ganglia.*	estrellado
stenosis *Narrowing of an orifice.*	estenosis
stercobilin *A substance created by the reduction of bilirubin and gives excrement the brown hue.*	estercobilina
stereognosis *The ability to identify an object by touch.*	estereognosis
sterile *1. Infertile 2. Refers to equipment that is free of contamination.*	estéril
sterilization *A procedure done to prevent production of offspring.*	esterilización
sternal *Referring to the sternum.*	esternal
sternocleidomastoid *The pair of muscles that connect the sternum, clavicle and mastoid process.*	esternocleidomastoideo
sternum	esternón
sterol *Unsaturated steroid alcohols such as cholesterol.*	esterol
stethoscope *Device used to auscultate the heart, lungs and over arteries to assess for abnormalities.*	estetoscopia
stiff	rígido
stiff-neck	cuello rígido
stillborn *Refers to a newborn that died in utero.*	nacido muerto
sting	picadura
stippling	punteado
stirrup *An attachment to an exam table where a woman puts her legs to assist examination of the genitalia.*	estribo
stomach	estómago
stomach cramps	retorcijones de estómago

English	Spanish
stomach pain	estomacalgia
story	historia
strabismus *An anomaly of ocular movement.*	estrabismo
strain *As in a muscle strain.*	estirón (los músculos y los tendones)
strait-jacket *A device used to temporarily restrain the arms of patients who are psychotic and violent.*	camisa de fuerza
strange	extraño
straw itch *Pruritis associated with exposure to straw that is infested with the mite Pyemotes ventricosus. Also referred to as dermatitis pediculoides ventricosus.*	prurito de paja
stream	corriente
strength	fuerza
stress	tensión
stress fracture *A long bone fracture caused by repetitive mechanical stress.*	fracción por tensión
stretcher *A device used to carry a patient in the supine position.*	parihuela
stria *A narrow bandlike body.*	estría
stricture	estrechez
stride	zancada
stridor *An abnormal, high-pitched, musical sound caused by an obstruction in the largynx or stenosis of the vocal cords.*	estridor
string	cordel
stroke *Common term for cerebrovascular accident.*	accidente cerebrovascular
stroke volume *The amount of blood ejected from the ventricle with each contraction.*	volumen sistólico
stroma *A term used to describe the framework of an organ.*	estroma
strong	fuerte
stump *Term used to designate what remains of an amputated extremity.*	muñón
stupor *A reduced level of consciousness.*	estupor
stuttering *Involuntary repetition of the first consonant.*	tartamudez
stylet *A thin wire within a catheter that is removed after the catheter is in place.*	estilete
subacute *A stage between acute and chronic.*	subagudo
subarachnoid *The layer of the brain covering between the arachnoid and pia mater.*	subaracnoideo
subareolar abscess *A purulent fluid collection in the areolar gland.*	absceso subareolar
subclavian *Refers to the area under the clavicle; the subclavian vein runs below the clavicle.*	subclavio
subclavian steal syndrome *Retrograde vertebral artery flow due to ipsilateral subclavian artery stenosis.*	síndrome del robo de la subclavia
subdural *The area between the dura mater and the arachnoid membrane.*	subdural
subdural hematoma *Formation of a blood clot between the dura mater and the arachnoid membrane.*	hematoma subdural
suberosis *A type of hypersensitivity pneumonitis related to inhalation of moldy cork dust.*	suberosis
sublingual *Situated under the tongue.*	sublingual
submaxillary *Situated below the maxilla.*	submaxilar
subphrenic *Referring to below the diaphragm.*	subfrénico

English	Spanish
success	éxito
succussion *The presence of a splashing sound when a body cavity is moved indicating presence of both air and fluid.*	sucusión
suck, to *As in, to suction fluid.*	succionar
suckle, to	amamantar
sudamina *White vesicles noted because of retained sweat in the layers of the epidermis.*	sudamina
sudden infant death syndrome *A leading cause of death of infants from one month to one year; the etiology is unknown.*	síndrome de la muerte súbita del lactante
suffer, to	sufrir
suffocation	sofocación
sugar	azúcar
suicide	suicida
sulcus *A groove, like in the brain.*	surco
sulfonamide *A class of drugs derived from sulfanilamide that are antibacterial.*	sulfonamidas
sulfur	azufre
summer itch *Pruritis noted upon exposure to hot weather, also known as pruritis aestivalis.*	prurito de verano o prurito estival.
superciliary arch *The area superior to the upper border of each orbit.*	arco superciliar
superfecundation *The fertilization of two different ova by spermatozoa of two different males.*	superfetación
superficial inguinal ring *The opening of the aponeurosis of the external oblique muscle for the round ligament or spermatic cord.*	anillo subcutáneo
superior	superior
supination *Turning the sole of the foot or the palm of the hand upward..*	supinación
supine	supino
supplies	provisiones
suppository *A delivery system for medication placed in an orifice.*	supositorio
suppuration *Formation of purulent material.*	supuración
supranuclear ophthalmoplegia *A disorder that effects the extraocular movements especially limiting the upward movement of the eyes.*	oftalmoplejía supranuclear
supraorbital *Situated above the orbit.*	supraorbitario
suprapubic *Situated above the pubis.*	suprapúbico
sural *Referring to the calf of the leg.*	sural
surfactant *A substance that reduces surface tension in the lungs.*	surfactante
surgeon	cirujano
surgery	cirugía
surgical *Referring to surgery.*	quirúrgico
surname	apellido
sustain, to	sostener
sustained release tablet *Describes a medicine that is slowly dispersed so it has a lasting effect.*	tableta de acción sostenida
suture	sutura
swab	hisopo
swallow, to	deglutir
sweat	sudor
sweat, to	sudar

English	Spanish
swelling	tumefacción
swimmer's itch *Pruritis caused by exposure to schistosomes.*	prurito del nadador
swollen (distended) abdomen	abdomen inflamado
sycosis *A bacterial infection affecting the hair follicles on a person's face.*	sicosis
Sydenham chorea *Historically known as Saint Vitus' dance, it is a childhood chorea associated with rheumatic fever.*	corea de Sydenham
symbiosis *The living together of two organisms.*	simbiosis
symmetry *Being equally bilaterally.*	simetría
sympathectomy *The surgical resection of a sympathetic nerve to reduce undesired effects.*	simpatectomía
sympathetic nervous system *The nerves responsible for the flight or fight response.*	sistema nerviso simpático
symptom	síntoma
synapse *The intersection of two nerve cells.*	sinapsis
synarthrosis *Adjacent bones connected by a joint but the joint is fixed.*	sinartrosis
synchondrosis *A joint with little motion that uses cartilage such as the vertebral bodies.*	sincondrosis
syncope *Sudden loss of consciousness.*	síncope
syncytial knot *Aggregation of syncytiotrophoblastic nuclei in the villi of the placenta during early pregnancy.*	nudo sinctitial
synechia *The adhesion of two body parts, such as synechia vulvae in which the labia minora are congenitally adherent.*	sinequia
synovectomy *Surgical resection of a synovial membrane.*	sinovectomía
synovial fluid *The fluid that surrounds, for example, the knee within a capsule.*	fluido sinovial
synovitis *Inflammation of the synovium.*	sinovitis
syphilis *A infectious disease caused by Treponema pallidum that causes a painless penile ulcer in the primary stage but can lead to irreversible brain damage in the untreated tertiary stage.*	sífilis
syringe	jeringa
syringomelia *A condition exhibited by fluid-filled cavities in the spinal cord.*	siringomielia
syrup	jarabe
systole *The phase of the cardiac cycle in which the ventricles contract.*	sístole
systolic *Referring to systole or that which occurs during systole.*	sistólico
tablespoon	cucharada
tablet	tableta
tachycardia *Heart rate higher than physiologic normal.*	taquicardia
tachypnea *Breathing faster than normal.*	taquipnea
tactile *Able to be felt.*	táctil
talipes calcaneus *A foot deformity exhibited by abnormal dorsiflexion.*	talipes calcáneo
talipes equinovaro *Medical term for what is commonly known as club foot.*	talipes equinovaro
talipes equinus *A foot deformity exhibited by abnormal plantar flexion.*	talipes equino
talon *The ball of the ankle joint.*	garra
talus *The most superior tarsal bone that articulates with the tibia.*	astrágalo
tampon *Disposible intravaginal product used to collect blood from menstruation.*	tampón
tamponade *1. Stopping bleeding during surgery with a cotton pledget. 2. When referring to cardiac tamponade, it is the limitation of cardiac contraction because of blood or fluid accumulation in the pericardial sac.*	taponamiento

English	Spanish
tap	punción
tape measure	cinta métrica
tapeworm *A parasitic, intestinal flatworm.*	tenia
tarantula	tarántula
target	blanco
target cell *An abnormal cell that is present in liver disease and certain hemoglobinopathies.*	célula blanco
tarsal *Referring to any bone in the tarsus.*	tarsal
tarsal tunnel syndrome *Characterized by impingement of various nerves of the ankle.*	túnel tarsiano
tarsalgia *Pain in any of the tarsal bones.*	tarsalgia
tarsectomy *Surgical excision of all or part of the tarsus.*	tarsectomía
tarsorrhaphy *Suturing the eyelids in order to tighten the palpebral fissure.*	tarsorrafia
tarsus *The group of seven bones of the ankle or foot (three cuneiform bones, talus, calcaneus, navicular, cuboid bones).*	tarso
task	tarea
taste	gusto
tattoo	tatuaje
taurocholic acid *A bile acid composed of cholic acid and taurine.*	ácido taurocólico
tear *As in, to shed a tear.*	lágrima
tear *Referring to a vaginal tear after childbirth.*	desgarramiento
teaspoon	cucharadita
tectum *A roof-like body.*	tectum
tectum mesencephali *The posterior portion of the mesencephalon including the sup. and inf. colliculi and tectal lamina.*	lámina del techo del mesencéfalo
telangiectasis *A condition exhibited by red, dilated capillaries on the skin.*	telangiectasia
telemetry *Use of radio signals to transmit patient data. The most common form is for electrocardiography in a patient who is ambulatory.*	telemetría
temperature	temperatura
temporomandibular joint *The hinged joint of the temporal bone and mandible.*	articulación temporomandibular
tendinitis *Inflammation of a tendon.*	tendinitis
tendon *Fibrous tissue that connects muscle to bone.*	tendón
tendon reflex *A deep reflex elicited by gently tapping the tendon.*	reflejo tendón
tenesmus *The attempt to defecate but attempts elicit pain and are ineffective.*	tenesmo
tennis elbow *Inflammation at the lateral aspect of the epicondyle where the muscle and tendon join; lateral epicondylitis.*	codo de tenista Epicondilalgia externa.
tenoplasty *Surgical repair of a tendon.*	tenoplastia
tenorrhaphy *The surgical repair with suture of a separated tendon.*	tenorrafia
tenosynovitis *Inflammation and swelling of an articulation.*	tenosinovitis
tenotomy *Incision of a tendon as is done for strabismus.*	tenotomía
tepid *Lukewarm.*	tibio
teratogen *A substance that induces fetal anomalies.*	teratógeno
teratoma *A tumor made up of tissue not usually at the location (a mass of hair, teeth and gingival tissue in a leg tumor for instance).*	teratoma
terebrant *Having a piercing quality.*	terebrante
terminal illness	enfermedad maligna

English	Spanish
tertian fever *A febrile syndrome caused by Plasmodium vivax which produces a fever spike every 48 hours.*	fiebre terciana Fiebre de Paludismo vivax.
tertiary	terciario
test tube	tubo de ensayo
testicle *One of a pair of organs in the male scrotum that produces sperm.*	testículo
testicular torsion	torsión de los testículos
testosterone *This steroid hormone produces secondary male sexual characteristics.*	testosterona
tetanus *A condition caused by Clostridium tetani which produces spasm and rigidity of voluntary muscles.*	tétanos
tetany *A condition caused by the hypocalcemic effect of hypoparathyroidism, exhibited by periodic muscle spasms, convulsions, and peri-oral numbness.*	tetania
tetracycline *An antibiotic used for gram positive and gram negative infections.*	tetraciclina
tetradactylous *Referring to a condition of having only four digits on a hand or foot.*	tetradáctilo
thalamus *A paired structure located adjacent to the third ventricle.*	tálamo
thalassemia *A hereditary hemolytic anemia first observed in people from the Mediterranean area.*	talasemia
thalidomide *A drug used originally as a sedative, after it was found to cause congenital anomalies, its use was restricted. Now it is used for a few conditions such as multiple myeloma.*	talidomida
theca *A tendon or ovarian follicle sheath.*	teca
thecoma *A tumor composed of theca cells.*	tecoma
thenar eminence *Formed by the bellies of the abductor pollicis brevis, flexor pollicis brevis and opponens pollicis.*	eminencia tenar
therapeutic range	límite terapéutico
thermometer	termómetro
thiamine *Also called vitamin B1; a deficiency causes beriberi.*	tiamina
thigh	muslo
thin	delgado
thirst	sed
thoracentesis *Insertion of a needle into the pleural space to drain and or obtain a specimen for analysis.*	toracentesis
thoracic *Referring to the thorax.*	torácico
thoracoplasty *Surgical removal of ribs.*	toracoplastia
thoracoscopy *Visualization of the thoracic cavity with a scope.*	toracoscopia
thoracotomy *Surgical incision of the thorax.*	toracotomía
thorax *The part of the body between the neck and abdomen.*	tórax
three way foley *A urinary tube used for irrigation of the bladder.*	catéter de triple canal
threonine *An amino acid needed for the growth in infants.*	treonina
throat	garganta
throb, to	latir
thrombectomy *Excision of a thrombus from a vein or artery.*	trombectomía
thrombin *An enzyme that is a catalyst for the conversion of fibrinogen to fibrin in the formation of a clot.*	trombina
thromboangiitis *Inflammation and thrombosis in a blood vessel.*	tromboangitis
thromboarteritis *Thrombosis of an inflamed artery.*	tromboarteritis
thrombocytopenia *Abnormal decrease in the number of blood platelets.*	trombocitopenia

English	Spanish
thrombophlebitis *Inflammation of a venous wall associated with a thrombus.*	tromboflebitis
thrombosis *Formation of a clot in a vein or artery.*	trombosis
throughout	lo largo de
thrush *Candida albicans*	muguet
thumb	pulgar
thymectomy *Surgical excision of the thymus.*	timectomía
thymine *A chemical with a pyrimidine base found in DNA.*	timina
thymocyte *A lymphocyte located in the thymus.*	timocito
thymoma *A tumor composed of thymic tissue and is sometimes associated with myasthenia gravis.*	timoma
thymus *A body organ located in the neck and it produces T cells to improve immune function.*	timo
thyroglossal cyst *A common congenital growth in the thyroglossal duct.*	quiste tirogloso
thyroid *A gland in the neck that secretes hormones regulating metabolism.*	tiroides
thyroid stimulating hormone (TSH) *A thyroid secreted by the pituitary that regulates the thyroid.*	hormona tiroideoestimulante
thyroidectomy *Surgical resection of all or part of the thyroid.*	tiroidectomía
thyrotoxic periodic paralysis *Weakness associated with an elevated TSH.*	parálisis periódica tirotóxica
thyrotoxicosis *Abnormal increase in thyroid activity exhibited by thinning hair, hypertension, tachycardia and at times atrial fibrillation.*	tirotoxicosis
thyroxine *An iodine containing hormone, referred to T4.*	tirotoxina
tibia *The larger of two long bones in the lower leg.*	tibia
tic	tic
tic douloureux *Also referred to as trigeminal neuralgia.*	tic doloroso Neuralgia del trigémino
tick bite	picadura de garrapata
tick-borne fever *A relapsing fever caused by a spirochete of the genus Borrelia.*	fiebre por garrapata
tickle	cosquilleo
tidal volume *The amount of air inspired with each breath. One can set a ventilator to deliver a preset number of milliliters of oxygenated air with each breath.*	volumen corriente pulmonar
tight junction *An intercellular junction with an impermeable membrane.*	unión estrecha
tincture *1. A very small amount of something. 2. A medicine dissolved in alcohol.*	tintura
tinea barbae *Ringworm on the face in the region a man shaves.*	tiña de la barba
tinea capitis *Ringworm of the scalp, a fungal infection.*	tiña del cuero cabelludo
tinea corporis *Ringworm of the body, a fungal infection.*	tiña del cuerpo
tinea cruris *Ringworm in the inguinal region, a fungal infection.*	tiña de la región genitocrural
tinea *Medical term for ringworm.*	tiña
tinea pedis *Ringworm of the feet, a fungal infection.*	tiña de los pies
tingling	hormigueo; el zumbar
tinnitus *Medical term for ringing in the ears. It is associated with Meniere's syndrome among other conditions.*	tinnitus
tired	consado
tissue	tejido
tocopherol *Vitamin E.*	alpha-tocoferol

English	Spanish
toe	dedo del pie
toenail	uña del pie
tongs *A medical device used for holding or grasping.*	tenazas
tongue	lengua
tongue depressor; tongue blade *As the name implies, the stick pushes the tongue down so the posterior aspect of the mouth can be viewed more readily.*	depresor de lengua
tonometer *A device used to measure ocular pressure in glaucoma.*	tonómetro
tonsil *A rounded mass of lymphoid tissue, most commonly referring to the pharyngeal tonsil.*	amígdala
tonsillectomy *Excision of the tonsils.*	tonsilectomía
tonsillitis *Inflammation of the tonsils.*	tonsilitis
tooth	diente
toothache	dolor de dientes
toothless *Edentulous.*	edentado
torn	roto
torpor *Unresponsiveness to normal stimuli.*	torpor Embotamiento.
torsade de pointe *Ventricular cardiac rhythm disturbance.*	taquicardia ventricular polimorfo
torsion *Refers to twisting. Testicular torsion is the twisting of the spermatic cord that can lead to ischemia and gangrene of the testicle.*	torsión
torsion spasm *Also called dystonia musculorum deformans, a genetic condition exhibited by twisting contortions sideways and forward while walking.*	espasmo de torsión
torso *The trunk of the body.*	torso
torticollis *A condition exhibited by the head being turned to one side continuously.*	tortícolis
touch	tacto
tourniquet *A device tied tightly around an extremity to diminish blood flow or blood loss.*	torniquete
toxemia *The release of toxic substances into the blood stream from a local infection. Toxemia of pregnancy is a synonym for preeclampsia.*	toxemia
toxic	tóxico
toxicology *The study of the nature, effects and detection of poisons.*	toxicología
toxin *A poison of plant or animal origin.*	toxina
toxoid *A chemically modified toxin that can be used as a vaccine.*	toxoide
toxoplasmosis *A disease caused by an organism from the genus Toxoplasma. One can have simple malaise to central nervous system involvement.*	toxoplasmosis
trabecule *A connective tissue strand that goes from a capsule to the enclosed organ.*	trabécula
trabeculotomy *A surgery for open angle glaucoma.*	trabeculectomía
trachea *The ringed canal between the pharynx and bronchi.*	tráquea
tracheitis *Inflammation of the trachea.*	traqueítis
trachelorrhaphy *Surgical repair of a lacerated cervix.*	traquelorrafia
tracheobronchitis *Inflammation of the trachea and bronchi.*	traqueobronquitis
tracheostomy *Creation of a surgical opening in the trachea so a tube could be placed in the trachea.*	traqueostomía
tracheotomy *Surgical incision of the trachea.*	traqueotomía
trachoma *An infection of the cornea and conjunctiva caused by Chlamydia.*	tracoma
tract	tracto

English	Spanish
traction	tracción
tragus *The fleshy prominence anterior to the opening of the ear.*	trago
tranquilizer *A medication used to diminish anxiety.*	tranquilizante
transabdominal *Through the abdominal wall.*	transabdomino
transaminase *An enzyme that facilitates the transfer of an amino group to an amino acid.*	transaminasas
transdermal *Through the skin.*	transdérmico
transfusion *Administration of blood products intravenously.*	transfusión
transient ischemic attack *Cerebral ischemic changes resulting from transitory hypoperfusion.*	accidente isquémico transitorio
transpire, to *To release vapor from the skin or respiratory mucosa.*	transpirar
transplant *To move a body part from one location to another.*	trasplantar
transplantation *The grafting of tissues.*	trasplante
transrectal ultrasound	ultrasonido transrectal
transudation *The movement of body tissue through a membrane that is usually the result of inflammation.*	trasudación
transvaginal ultrasound	ultrasonido transvaginal
trapezium *The lateral bone in the distal row of carpal bones.*	trapecio
trapezius muscle *The muscle with an origin of occipital bone and seventh cervical vertebra, insertion of clavicle and scapula, and it draws the scapula backward.*	trapezius
trapezoid *The bone between the trapezium and capitate bones.*	trapezoide
trauma	trauma
treadmill	rueda de andar
treatment	tratamiento
treatment regimen	método de tratament
trematoda *A parasitic fluke such as Schistosoma.*	trematodo
tremor *Involuntary contraction and relaxation of small muscle groups.*	temblor
trench mouth *Inflammation and ulceration of the gingivae.*	boca de trinchera Gingivitis ulcerosa necrosante.
trephining *Cutting away a circular disc of bone or the cornea.*	trefina
triceps *Referring to something having three heads like the triceps muscle.*	tríceps
triceps reflex *A tendon reflex causing extension of the arm when the triceps tendon is gently tapped.*	reflejo del tríceps
trichiasis *Inversion of the eyelashes.*	triquiasis
trichinosis *A disease caused by meat infected by Trichinella spiralis causing fever and gastrointestinal effects.*	triquinosis
trichomoniasis vaginitis	tricomoniasis vaginitis
trichophytosis *A skin or nail fungal infection caused by Trichophyton.*	tricofitosis
tricuspid valve *The cardiac valve located between the right atrium and right ventricle.*	válvula tricúspide
trigeminal *Generally refers to the fifth cranial nerve.*	trigeminal
trigeminal nerve *The fifth cranial nerve which supplies the motor function of mastication and has three sensory branches, the ophthalmic, maxillary and mandibular.*	nervio trigémino
trigeminal neuralgia *Pain in the region of one or more branches of the fifth cranial nerve sensory branches.*	neuralgia del trigémino

144

English	Spanish
trigger	gatillo
trigger finger *A condition in which one's finger gets stuck in the flexed position and when extended it snaps like a trigger. Also called stenosing tenosynovitis.*	dedo en gatillo
trigone of bladder *Refers to the area at the base of the bladder between the openings of the ureters and the urethra.*	trígono vesical
triplegia *Paralysis of three extremities.*	triplejía
triplets	trídimo
triploid *Referring to a cell with three homologous sets of chromosomes.*	triploide
trismus *Commonly called lockjaw, it is a spasm of the muscles supplied by the trigeminal nerve and is an early symptom of tetanus.*	trismo
trisomy 21 *A congenital anomaly in which chromosome 21 is effected and results in Down's syndrome.*	síndrome de trisomía 21
trisomy *A general category of congenital anomalies in which there is an extra set of chromosomes in the cell nucleus.*	trisomía
trivial	trivial
trocar *A device enclosed in a catheter that is used to withdraw fluid from a body cavity.*	trocar
trochanter *Refers to the greater or lesser trochanter; the prominences on the femoral neck.*	trocánter
trochlea *A pulley-shaped structure such as the groove at the distal humerus.*	tróclea
trochlear *Referring to a trochlea.*	troclear
trochlear nerve *The fourth cranial nerve that supplies the superior oblique muscle of the eyeball.*	nervio troclear
trophoblast *A layer of endodermal tissue that helps attach an ovum to the uterine wall.*	trofoblasto
truncal *Referring to the trunk of a body or a nerve.*	troncal
truss *A synthetic device for containing a hernia within the abdomen.*	braguero
truth	verdad
trypanosomiasis *A disease caused by a protozoa of the genus Trypanosoma that can cause sleeping sickness and Chagas' disease.*	tripanosomiasis
trypsin *An enzyme whose precursor is secreted by the pancreas that breaks down proteins in the intestine.*	tripsina
trypsinogen *The precursor to trypsin that is secreted by the pancreas.*	tripsinógeno
tryptophan *An amino acid that is a precursor of serotonin. If present in the body in appropriate levels it can prevent pellegra even if niacin levels are low.*	triptófano
tsetse fly *An insect that transmits the protozoa trypanosoma and can cause sleeping sickness.*	mosca tsetse
tubal *Referring to a tube, as in fallopian tube.*	tubario
tubercle *1. A granulomatous nodule produced by Mycobacterium tuberculosis. 2. A small prominence on a bone.*	tubérculo
tuberculin *A solution containing M. tuberculosis or M. bovis that is used to test for tuberculosis by injecting the solution intradermally and looking for a reaction.*	tuberculina
tuberculoma *1. A tuberculous growth in the brain. 2. A mass that is produced from enlargement of a caseous tubercle.*	tuberculoma
tuberculosis *Any infectious disease caused by Mycobacterium.*	tuberculosis
tuberculous *Referring to tuberculosis.*	tuberculoso
tuberosity *A protuberance. For instance the iliac tuberosity is a prominence on the surface of the ilium.*	tuberosidad

English	Spanish
tuberous sclerosis *An inherited neurocutaneous disorder exhibited by benign hamartomas of the brain, lung, kidney, skin and other organs.*	esclerosis tuberosa
tubo-ovarian *Referring to the fallopian tube or ovary.*	tuboovárico
tubular *Referring to a hollow, round-shaped organ.*	tubular
tularemia *An infectious disease caused by Francisella tularensis. The symptoms range from mild constitutional complaints to septic shock.*	tularemia
tumefaction *An area of swelling.*	tumefacción
tumor *A benign or malignant overgrowth of tissue.*	tumor
tunica *Generally a covering of a body part or organ. The tunica mucosa nasi is the mucous membrane lining the nasal cavity.*	túnica
tuning fork *A device used to distinguish between perceptive and conductive hearing loss.*	diapasón
tunnel vision	visión en túnel
turbinate bones *The three curved shelves in the nasal cavity.*	huesos cornete
turbinectomy *Surgical excision of a turbinate bone.*	turbinectomía
turgid *Congested and swollen.*	túrgido
turgor *Referring to the elasticity of skin. If one pinches skin and it remains in place the patient is dehydrated.*	turgor
twins	gemelos
twitch	espasmo muscular
two times	dos veces
tympanic *Referring to the tympanic membrane or having a resonant quality to percussion.*	timpánico
tympanic membrane *The membrane between the external and middle ear.*	membrana timpánica
tympanoplasty *Restoration of the tympanic membrane's continuity.*	timpanoplastia
typhoid fever *A condition caused by ingestion of food or water containing salmonella typhi that is exhibited by fever and abdominal signs and symptoms.*	fiebre tifoidea
typhus fever *A rickettsiae infection exhibited by rash, fever, headache and myalgia.*	fiebre tifus
tyrosine *An amino acid important in the synthesis of hormones.*	tirosina
ulcer *A concave wound caused by a break in the integrity of skin or mucous membrane.*	úlcera
ulcerative *Referring to ulceration.*	ulceroso
ulcerative colitis *Recurrent episode of inflammation of the membranous layer of the colon.*	colitis ulceroso
ultrasonography *Visualization of body structures with the echoes of ultrasound pulses.*	ultrasonografía
ultrasound *A sound or vibration of ultrasonic frequency.*	ultrasonido
ultraviolet rays *Electromagnetic radiation with wavelength longer than x rays.*	rayos ultravioletas
umbilicated *Referring to depressed areas that resemble the umbilicus.*	umbilicado
umbilicus *The scar that denotes the end of the umbilical cord.*	umbilicus
unciform *Another term for hamate bone in the wrist.*	unciforme
uncinariasis *Hookworm infestation of genus Uncinaria.*	uncinariasis
uncinate bone *Hamate bone.*	uncinado
unconsciousness *Unable to respond to sensory stimuli.*	inconsciencia
under; infra *Sometimes used when indicating a patient is "under treatment" for a condition (active treatment).*	debajo
underlying	subyacente

English	Spanish

undulant *Wave-like appearance.* — undulado

unexpected — inesperado

unicellular *A term describing organisms like protozoans that only have cell.* — unicelular

unigravida *Term used to describe a woman's first pregnacy.* — unigrávida

unilateral *One side only.* — unilateral

uniovolar *Referring to one fertilized ovum.* — uniovular

uniparous *Refers to a single birth.* — unípara

unknown — desconocido

unstable knee *A condition with giving way of the knee due to ligamentous or cartilaginous dysfunction.* — rodilla inestable

unsteady — variable

upper limb — extremidad superior

upper respiratory tract *Generally considered the part of the respiratory tract superior to the vocal cords.* — aparato respiratorio superior

upright — erguido

urachus *A connection between the bladder and the allantois in the fetus.* — uraco

urate *The salt of uric acid.* — urato

urea *A nitrogenous product of protein metabolism; excreted in urine.* — urea

uremia *An excess of urea and creatinine in the blood.* — uremia

ureter *The conduit between each kidney and the urinary bladder.* — uréter

ureteral *Referring to one of two tubes from the kidneys to the bladder that carry urine.* — ureteral

ureterectomy *Surgical resection of one or both ureters.* — ureterectomía

ureteritis *Inflammation of the ureter.* — ureteritis

ureterocele *Protrusion of the distal portion of the ureter into the bladder.* — ureterocele

ureterolith *Presence of a stone in the ureter.* — ureterolito

ureterolithotomy *Removal of a ureteral stone.* — ureterolithotomía

ureterovaginal *Referring to the ureter and vagina.* — ureterovaginal

ureterovesical *Referring to the ureter and urinary bladder.* — ureterovesical

urethra *The canal connecting the urinary bladder with the outside of the body.* — uretra

urethral *Referring to the urethra.* — uretral

urethritis *Inflammation of the urethra.* — uretritis

urethrocele *A prolapse of the urethra through the meatus.* — uretrocele

urethrography *Imaging of the urethra after instillation of contrast media.* — uretrorrafía

urethroplasty *Surgical repair of the urethra.* — uretroplastia

urethroscope *A scope used to visualize the inside of the urethra.* — uretroscopia

urethrotomy *A surgical opening of the urethra.* — uretrotomía

urgency — urgencia

uric *Uric acid is a purine-derived product of nitrogen metabolism that can increase the risk of gout and calculi.* — úrico

urinalysis *Chemical and microscopic examination of the urine.* — análisis de orina

urinary *Referring to the urine.* — urinario

urinary bladder *The organ collecting urine from the ureters prior to discharge via the urethra.* — vejiga urinaria

urinary casts *A protein precipitated from renal tubules and excreted in the urine.* — cilindros urinarios

English	Spanish
urinary sediments *The debris that settles in a urine sample when left undisturbed.*	sedimento urinario
urinary tract *The organs and canals associated with urine secretion including the kidneys, ureters, bladder and urethra.*	vías urinarias
urine	aguas menores; orina
urinometer *A device for measuring urine specific gravity.*	urinómetro
urobilin *A brownish pigment that is an oxidized form of urobilinogen.*	urobilina
urobilinogen *A colorless substance produced in the intestines when bilirubin is reduced.*	urobilinógeno
urochrome *A yellow pigment in the urine that gives urine its color.*	urocromo
urodynamics	urodinamia
urogenital *Referring to the urinary and genital systems.*	urogentital
urography *Roentgenography of the urinary tract after administration of contrast media.*	urografía
urolith *Urinary calculi.*	urolito
urology *Surgical specialty involving medical and surgical treatment of the urogenital system.*	urología
urticaria *A diffuse pruritic macular rash, caused by an allergy.*	urticaria
usual	usual,normal
uterine *Referring to the uterus.*	uterino
uterine bleeding	sangrado uterino
uterine fibroids *Benign tumors made up of muscular and fibrous tissue in the uterus.*	miomas uterinos Tumores no cancerosos que aparecen en el útero.
uterine prolapse *Protrusion of the uterus out the vagina.*	prolapso del útero
uterovesical *Referring to the uterus and urinary bladder.*	uterovesical
uterus *The hollow organ in the female pelvis where a fertilized ovum embeds and grows.*	útero
utricle *A small sac. It can refer to a division of the membranous labyrinth.*	utrículo
uveitis *Inflammation of the uvea.*	uveítis
uvula *A fleshy pendent at the back of the soft palate.*	úvula
uvulectomy *Excision of the uvula.*	uvulectomía
uvulitis *Inflammation of the uvula.*	uvulitis
vaccination *The act of receiving a vaccine.*	vacunación
vaccine *A solution of attenuated microorganisms given to prevent or treat a disease.*	vacuna
vaccine status	status vacuna
vacuole *A cavity that develops in a cell.*	vacuola
vagal *Referring to the vagus nerve.*	vagal
vagina *The canal in a female that extends from the vulva to the cervix.*	vagina
vaginal *Referring to the vagina.*	vaginal
vaginismus *Involuntary contraction of the vagina muscles that causes a painful spasm.*	vaginismo
vagitus *An infant cry that can be further defined as vagitus vaginalis in which the infant cries while its head is in the vaginal canal.*	vagido uterino
vagotomy *Incision of the vagus nerve.*	vagotomía

148

English	Spanish
vagus nerve *The tenth cranial nerve that supplies the heart, lungs visceral organs; its function is tested by assessment of elevation of the uvula.*	nervio neumogástrico
valgus *Refers to a joint being abnormally angulated away from the midline of the body.*	valgus
valine *An essential amino acid that assists with nitrogen equilibrium.*	valina
Valsalva's maneuver *A technique in which one attempts to exhale with the mouth and nose closed; this equalizes pressure in the ears.*	maniobra de Valsalva
valvulotomy *Surgical incision of a valve.*	valvultomía
varicella *A virus that causes chickenpox and shingles. Also called herpes zoster.*	varicela
varicocele *A cluster of varicose veins in the scrotum.*	varicocele
varicose *Referring to an abnormally distended, irregular vein.*	varicoso
varix *A twisted, distended vein, artery or lymph vessel.*	várice
varus *Refers to a joint being abnormally angulated toward the midline of the body.*	varus
vascular *Referring to a blood vessel.*	vascular
vasculitis *Inflammation of a blood vessel.*	vasculitis
vasectomy *The surgical separation of each vas deferens with the intent of producing a sterile person.*	vasectomía
vasoconstriction *The process of making the blood vessels smaller which increases blood pressure.*	vasoconstricción
vasodilatation *The process of making the blood vessels larger which decreases blood pressure.*	vasodilatación
vasomotor *Referring to the constriction or dilation of vessels.*	vasomotor
vasopressin *A hormone secreted by the pituitary that facilitates the retention of sodium and water and also increases blood pressure.*	vasopresina
vasospasm *The abrupt constriction of a blood vessel.*	vasoespasmo
vasovagal *Referring to overstimulation of the vagus nerve, exhibited by hypotension, pallor, nausea and diaphoresis.*	vasovagal
vector *An organism that transmits disease.*	vector
vegetation *Abnormal growth, such as cardiac valve vegetations as found in endocarditis.*	vegetación
vein	vena
velum *A veil-like part.*	velo
vena cava *The large vein that carries deoxygenated blood to the right atrium.*	vena cava
venereal disease *A condition transmitted via sexual intercourse.*	enfermedad venéreo
venereal wart	verruga venérea Condiloma acuminado.
venography *Roentgenography of a vein after administration of contrast media.*	venografía
venom *A term used to describe the toxin injected via a bite or sting.*	veneno
venous *Referring to the veins.*	venoso
ventilation *The movement of air into the lungs; generally meant to suggest by an artificial process.*	ventilación
ventral *Referring to the underside but in humans, a ventral hernia, for example, refers to an abdominal hernia.*	ventral
ventricle *1. One of two chambers of the heart. 2. The four inter-connected cavities in the center of the brain.*	ventrículo
ventricular septal defect *An abnormal communication between the right and left ventricles via a hole in the septum.*	defecto del tabique ventricular

English	Spanish
ventriculography *Roentgenography of the ventricles after administration of contrast media.*	ventriculografía
ventriculostomy *A tube placed into the third ventricle to relieve increased intracranial pressure.*	ventriculostomía
venula *The vessels that connect the capillary plexuses to veins.*	venula
verminous *Referring to presence of worms.*	verminoso
verruca *A hyperplastic epidermal lesion, sometimes referred to as plantar wart.*	verruga
vertebra *A term for each bone surrounding the spine.*	vértebra
vertebral column	columela vertebral
vertebrobasilar insufficiency *Diminished flow to the vertebral and basilar arteries causing posterior fossa symptoms.*	insuficiencia vertebrobasilar
vertex *The crown of the head.*	vértice
vertigo *A sensation of imbalance with many possible causes.*	vértigo
vesical *Referring to the urinary bladder.*	vesical
vesicovaginal *Referring to the urinary bladder and vagina.*	vesicovaginal
vesiculitis *Inflammation of the urinary bladder.*	vesiculitis
vestibular *Referring to a vestibule.*	vestibular
vestigial *Rudimentary.*	vestigial
viable *Referring to a fetus that can survive childbirth.*	viable
vial	vial
vibration	vibración
villous *Covered with many villi.*	velloso
villus *A small vascular prominence from a membrane surface.*	vellosidad
virilization *The result of androgen; a process of development of masculine characteristics.*	virilización
virology *The study of viruses.*	virología
virulence *The potential severity of a disease or poison.*	virulencia
viscera *Referring to the organs in the abdominal or thoracic cavity.*	vísceras
viscometer *A device used to measure viscosity.*	viscosímetro
viscous *Having a thick, sticky consistency.*	viscoso
vision	visión
vision, blurred	visión velada
visual field *The complete area a person can see with their eyes in a fixed position.*	campo visual
vital capacity (VC) *The maximal amount of air exhaled after a maximal inhalation.*	capacidad vital
vital signs *The designation for blood pressure, pulse, respirations and temperature.*	signos vitales
vitamin B12 neuropathy *Abnormal sensation related to a chronic deficiency of cyanocobalamin.*	neuropatía por vitamina B12
vitelline *Referring to the yolk of an egg or ovum.*	vitelino
vitreous *Glass appearance; used to describe the vitreous body of the eye.*	vítreo
vivisection *Animal surgery done for purposes of research.*	vivisección
vocal	vocal
vocal cords *Paired folds of mucous membranes stretched across the larynx.*	cuerdas vocales
voice	voz
void	evacuar

English	Spanish
voiding cystography *Roentgenography of the bladder and urethra after administration of contrast media.*	cistograma urinaria
volunteer	ofrecer
volvulus *Twisting of the bowel leading to obstruction and sometimes perforation.*	vólvulo
vomit, to	vómito
vulval cleft *The area between the labia majora where the vagina and urethra rest.*	hendidura vulvar
vulvectomy *Surgical resection of the vulva.*	vulvectomía
vulvitis *Inflammation of the vulva.*	vulvitis
vulvovaginitis *Inflammation of the vulva and vagina.*	vulvovaginitis
waddling gait *Walking in short steps in a swaying fashion.*	andar coma un pato
walker	andador
walking cast *A cast used for simple fractures of the lower leg.*	molde para andar
ward	sala de hospital
wart *A flesh colored growth that is also called verruca.*	verruga
wasp	avispa
water	agua
wax	cera, cerumen
weak	débil
weakness	debilidad
weekly	semanal
weep, to	supurar
wet	mojado
wheal *A circumscribed urticarial lesion.*	roncha
wheelchair	silla de ruedas
wheeze *A whistling or musical sound made by air passing through a narrowed airway.*	silbilancia
whiplash *Common term for cervical strain following a sudden deceleration.*	traumatismo cervical
whipworm *A parasitic, intestinal nematode worm of the genus Trichuris.*	gusano látigo Trichuris trichiura.
whisper	susurro
whisper, to	surrar
whistle, to	silbar
white	blanca
white matter *The brain tissue consisting of myelin sheaths and nerve fibers.*	sustancia blanca
whitlow *An abscess occurring on the palmar surface of the fingertips.*	panadizo
whooping cough *Pertussis*	tos ferina
wick; drain	mecha
widespread	extendido
width	anchura
wisdom tooth *Third molar.*	tercer molar
wise	sabio
withdrawal	supresión
withhold	retener
wooden belly *A rigid abdomen.*	rigidez abdominal

English	Spanish
World Health Organization (WHO)	Organizació Mundial de la Salud
worm	gusano
worry, to	inquietar
worsen, to	empeorar
wound	herida
wound care	cuidado de heridas
wrist	muñeca
wrist drop *The inability to hyperextend the wrist due to radial nerve injury.*	mano péndula
xanthine *A purine derivative that is found in the blood and urine after the metabolism of nucleic acids to uric acid.*	xantina
xanthochromia *A yellow tone to the skin or spinal fluid.*	xantocromía
xanthoma *A lipid deposition on the skin exhibited by an irregular yellow patch.*	xantoma
xerodermia *A mild form of ichthyosis.*	xeroderma
xerophthalmia *A manifestation of Vitamin A deficiency exhibited by dryness of the cornea and conjunctiva.*	xeroftalmía
xeroradiography *A form of radiography using photoelectric cells.*	xerradiografía
xerosis	xerosis
xerostomia *A dry mouth from salivary gland hypofunction.*	xerostomía
xiphoid process *The inferior segment of the sternum.*	apéndice xifoide
yawn	bostezo
yaws *A tropical disease characterized by ulcers on the extremities, caused by Treponema pertenue.*	frambesia
year	año
yearly	anualmente
yeast	levadura
yell, to	gritar
yellow	amarillo
yellow fever *A viral, hemorrhagic fever transmitted by mosquitos.*	fiebre amarilla
young	joven
youth	juventud
zeiosis *Resembling a bubbling activity.*	zeiosis
zero	cero
Ziehl-Neelsen carbolfuchsin stain *A stain used to detect acid-fast bacilli that appear red on the methylene blue background.*	coloración de Ziehl-Neelsen
zinc	cinc
zonula *A small zone or junction.*	zónula
zoology *The study of animals.*	zoología
zoonosis *An animal-born disease that can be transmitted to humans, such as rabies.*	zoonosis
zygomatic bone *The triangular cheek bone.*	cigomático
zygote *A fertilized ovum.*	cigoto
zymogen *An inactive compound that is metabolized to an active state.*	cimógeno

Spanish	English
abajo	down
abajo de	below
abasceo intraabdominal	intraabdominal abscess
abasia, movimiento incierto	abasia Inability to walk due to impaired coordination
abdomen inflamado	swollen (distended) abdomen
abdomen, vintre	abdomen The portion of the body bordered by the diaphragm and the pelvis.
abdominocentesis, punción abdominal	abdominocentesis Puncturing of the abdominal wall for drainage purposes.
abducente	abducent Abducting or to separate.
aberrante Desviado del curso normal.	aberrant Different than normal.
abierto	gaping Wide open.
abierto	overt Not hidden.
ablación	ablation Surgical removal or amputation.
ablatio placentae	ablatio placentae Abruption or detachment of the placentae.
aborto espontáneo	miscarriage Spontaneous abortion.
aborto Expulsión prematura.	abortion Premature expulsion of the fetus from the uterus.
aborto inducido	induced abortion Surgical or medical evacuation of the fetus.
abrazadera	bracing
abrojo	burr
abruptio placentae	abruptio placentae The premature detachment of a normally implanted placenta resulting in maternal decompensation.
abrupto, abrupta	abrupt
absceso	abscess A localized collection of pus.
absceso anorrectal	anorrectal abscess
absceso de la médula espinal	spinal cord abscess
absceso hepático amebiano	amebic liver abscess
absceso hepático piógeno	pyogenic liver abscess A pus filled fluid collection in the liver.
absceso hígado	liver abscess
absceso o quiste de Bartolino	Bartholin's cyst or abscess This is a purulent fluid collection in the Bartholin cysts which are located in the perivaginal area.
absceso periamigdalino	peritonsillar abscess
absceso retrofaríngeo	retropharyngeal abscess
absceso subareolar	subareolar abscess A purulent fluid collection in the areolar gland.
absoluto	absolute
absorción (absorción entérica)	absorption (intestinal absorption)
abuso	abuse
abuso de drogas	drug dependence Addiction to a substance.
acabar, realizar	accomplish

Spanish	English
acalasia	achalasia Inability to relax the smooth muscle fibers of the gastrointestinal tract. In the case of esophageal achalasia one has dilatation and hypertrophy of the esophagus.
acalculia	acalculia The inability to perform mathematical calculations.
acantoma	acanthoma An adult cornyfying squamous carcinoma.
acantosis	acanthosis Hypertrophy of the prickle cell layer of the skin.
acantosis pigmentaria	acanthosis nigricans A skin disorder characterized by dark, thick, velvety skin in the body folds and creases.
acapnia	acapnia A condition of lower than normal carbon dioxide level in the blood.
acariasis	acariasis Mite infestation.
acaricida	acaricide A treatment for mite infestation.
acarus	acarus A mite.
acatalasia	acatalasia A condition characterized by the congenital absence of the enzyme catalase.
acatisia	acathisia The inability to sit quietly or to have motor restlessness.
acatisia	akathisia A condition exhibited by motor restlessness and inability to sit quietly.
accesorio, accesoria	accessory Complimentary or concomitant.
accidente	accident
accidente cerebrovascular	stroke Common term for cerebrovascular accident.
accidente cerebrovascular con amnesia	amnesiac stroke Cerebral infarct exhibited by loss of memory.
accidente isquémico transitorio	transient ischemic attack Cerebral ischemic changes resulting from transitory hypoperfusion.
acedía	heart burn Synonym of pyrosis.
acelerar (Acelerar la cura.)	accelerate (To accelerate the healing process).
acetabular	acetabular Referring to the acetabulum.
acetabulo	acetabulum The cup-shaped cavity with which the head of the femur articulates.
acetaminofeno	acetaminophen Mild analgesic drug used for pain relief.
acetilcolina	acetylcholine A reversible acetic acid ester of choline.
acetonemia	acetonemia The presence of acetone in the blood.
acetonuria	acetonuria The presence of acetone in the urine.
acéfalo	acephalous A absence of a head.
acidemia	acidemia A lower than normal pH in the blood.
acidez	acidity Referring to an acid state.
acinitis	acinitis The inflammation of the acini.
aclaramiento	clearance
aclimatación	acclimatization The process of becoming adapted to a new environment.
acné	acne Inflamed or infected sebaceous glands.
acné rosácea	acne rosacea A chronic disease characterized by the presence of flushing of the skin of the nose, forehead and cheeks.
acné vulgar o común	acne vulgaris Chronic acne occurring on the face, chest and back of youth.
acocear	kick, to
acolia	acholia The lack of bile.

Spanish	English
acomodación	accommodation A term used to describe the ability of the eye to adjust to various distances.
acondroplasia	achondroplasia A congenital inadequacy of enchondral bone formation resulting in a type of dwarfism.
acorea	acorea The absence of the pupil of the eye.
acortamiento	shortening
acrocefalia	acrocephaly A condition characterized by a pointed head.
acrocianosis, enfermedad de Raynaud	acrocyanosis, Raynaud's disease A benign condition in which the feet and hands are cyanotic, cold and sweating.
acrodermatitis Inflamación de los pies y las manos.	acrodermatitis Inflammation of the skin of the hands and/or feet.
acrodinia	acrodynia An infantile condition exhibited by swollen bluish-red extremities and later polyarthritis..
acrofobia	acrophobia The morbid fear of heights.
acromatopsia	achromatopsia Inability to differentiate yellow, blue, red or their intermediates.
acromegalia	acromegaly Hyperplasia of the nose, jaw, fingers and toes.
acromioclavicular	acromioclavicular Referring to the junction of the acromion and clavicle.
acromión	acromion The flattened process extending laterally from the spineof the scapula which forms the most prominent point of the shoulder.
acrótico	acrotic Referring to the surface.
actina	actin A protein in the muscle that, along with myosin, facilitates muscle contraction and relaxation.
actinomicosis	actinomycosis A chronic bacterial infection that effects the face and neck and is caused by Actinomyces israelii. In rare cases it can cause a pulmonary infection.
actividad	activity
actomiosina	actomyosin Myosin and actin complex present in muscles.
actualmente	currently
acuerdo, pacto	agreement
acuoso, acuosa	aqueous Use of water as a solvent or medium.
acupuntura	acupuncture Traditionally an aspect of Chinese medicine involving insertion of needles into the skin.
acústico, acústica	acoustic Referring to the auditory system.
adactilia	adactylia A congenital condition exhibited by the absence of toes and fingers.
adaptación a la luz	light adaptation The pupillary adjustment after going from a dark environment to one of bright light.
adaptacióna la oscuridad	dark adaptation Adjustment to low light by reflex dilation of the pupil.
adecuado,adecuada	adequate
adenectomía	adenectomy The removal of a gland.
adenitis	adenitis The inflammation of a gland.
adenoacantoma	adenocanthoma Malignant tumor comprised of glandular tissue.
adenocarcinoma	adenocarcinoma Cancer from glandular tissue.
adenofibroma	adenofibroma Connective tissue with glands that form a tumor.
adenohipófisis	adenohypophysis The anterior portion of the pituitary gland.
adenoidectomía	adenoidectomy Removal of the adenoids.

155

Spanish	English
adenoideo	adenoid Referring to a gland.
adenoides	adenoids Pharyngeal tonsils.
adenoiditis	adenoiditis Inflammation of the adenoids.
adenolinfoma	adenolymphoma A salivary gland tumor, also called Warthin's tumor.
adenomioma	adenomyoma A tumor characterized by the overgrowth of endometrial and uterine muscle tissue.
adenomiosis	adenomyosis A condition characterized by the overgrowth of endometrial and uterine muscle tissue.
adenopatía	adenopathy Generally referring to a condition of the lymphatic glands.
adenosina difosfato	adenosine diphosphate A product of hydrolysis of ATP.
adenosina trifosfato	adenosine triphosphate (ATP) A chemical that represents the energy reserve of the muscle.
adenosine monofosfato	adenosine monophosphate A nucleotide, it is produced when ATP is converted to ADP.
adenovirus	adenovirus A type of a virus that can cause upper respiratory tract infections.
adesión	adhesion The abnormal adherence of tissue exposed to inflammation or after surgery.
adherencia	adherence
adiadococinesia	adiadochokinesia The inability to perform rapid alternating movements.
adicción	addiction
adicción inhalación de cemento	glue sniffing addiction
adicción cocaína	cocaine addiction Physical habituation to cocaine.
adiposa	adipose Referring to fat.
adipsia	adipsia Absence of thirst which can be caused by SIADH, hydrocephalus or injury/tumor to/of the hypothalamus.
aditus	aditus The entrance to an organ or part.
adjutor	adjuvant Term used to describe the medical treatment after initial therapy, as in adjuvant radiation therapy after initial chemotherapy.
admisión	admission
adolescenia	adolescence
adrenalectomía	adrenalectomy Excision of the adrenal gland.
adrenalina	adrenaline (epinephrine) A hormone secreted by the adrenal glands and a synthetic medication used for treatment of allergic reactions and cardiac arrest.
adrenocorticotropina	adrenocorticotrophic hormone (ACTH) A hormone that influences the cortex of the adrenal glands.
adrenogénico	adrenergic That which is activated or transmitted by epinephrine.
aducción	adduction To bring toward the midline.
adventicia	adventitia Outermost.
advertir, recomendar	advise, to
aerobio	aerobe An organism that grows in the presence of oxygen.
aerodontalgia	aerodontalgia The dental pain that occurs with low atmospheric pressure, like during airflight.
aerofagia	aerophagy or aerophagia A condition associated with hysteria in which one swallow repeatedly swallows air and then belches.
aerosol	spray
afagia	aphagia The lack of eating.
afaquia	aphakia The congenital absence of the lens of the eye.

Spanish	English
afasia	aphasia Diminished ability to communicate via speech or writing.
afebril	afebrile Absence of fever.
afectado, afectada	affected
afectar	affect
aferente	afferent Moving toward the center.
afibrinogenemia	afibrinogenemia Marked deficiency of fibrinogen in the blood.
afido	aphid A minute insect that feeds on plants.
afinidad	affinity To have a natural liking for.
aflaxotin	aflatoxin A toxin produced by Aspergillus flavus.
afonía	aphonia The loss of voice.
afta	canker sore An ulceration, usually of the mouth or lips.
agar	agar Media used for bacterial cultures.
agenesia gonadal	anorchous The absence of testicles.
agente quelación	chelating agent A compound used to bind with metal typically used in the treatment of poisoning.
agentes antiinflamatorios	anti-inflammatory agents Medications used to reduce inflammation.
agénesis	agenesis The absence of an organ.
agitación	agitation
aglutición	aglutition The inability to swallow.
aglutinación	agglutination The process of adherence of a mass.
agnatia	agnathia Congenital abnormality characterized by the absence of the mandible.
agnosia	agnosia A condition exhibited by the loss of sensory stimuli.
agnosia del dedo	finger agnosia
agnosia gustativo	gustatory agnosia The loss of the sense of taste.
agonista	agonist A synthetic compound that activates cells normally activated by natural chemicals.
agonía	agony Anguish or torment.
agorafobia	agoraphobia The fear of being in a large open space.
agrafia	agraphia The inability to express one's thoughts in writing.
agranulocitosis	agranulocytosis A condition characterized by leukopenia and neutropenia.
agresión	aggression
agrio	sour
agua	water
agua potable	drinking water
aguas menores; orina	urine
agudeza, precisión	acuity 1. Relating to accuracy of hearing, as in hearing acuity. 2. Severity of illness as in, "What is the patient's acuity?"
agudo	sharp (pain)
agudo, aguda	acute Abrupt onset.
ague	ague A term used to describe recurrent fever typically associated with malaria.
aguja	needle
aguja para biopsia	needle biopsy Use of a needle to aspirate body contents for microscopic or pathologic examination.
aguja para punción lumbar	needle for lumbar puncture

157

Spanish	English
agujero de buril	burr hole A treatment of subdural hematoma that involves drilling a hole into the cranium to release the hematoma.
agujero nutricio	nutrient foramen A conduit for passage of nutrient vessels in the marrow of bone.
agujero oval permeable	patent foramen ovale A congenital anomaly in which there is a defect in the wall between the right and left atria; this can be a benign condition or result in cryptogenic strokes.
ahogamiento	drowning
aire	air
aislamiento	isolation A ward where patients with infectious disease are housed.
ajustar	adjust
ajuste	adjustment
al azar	at random
alantoides	allantois A posterior portion of the hind-gut of an embryo.
alargamiento	lengthening
albinismo	albinism Congenital absence of pigment in the eyes, skin and hair.
albino, albina	albino A person who lacks pigment in the eyes, skin and hair.
albuminuria	albuminuria The presence of albumin in the urine.
albúmina	albumin A protein that is soluble in water and coagulates if heated.
alcalino	alkaline Referring to something with properties of an alkali.
alcalinuria	alkalinuria The urine in an alkaline state.
alcaloide	alkaloid Plant derived nitrogenous organic compound.
alcalosis	alkalosis A condition in which the pH is increased.
alcance	span
alcaptonuria	alkaptonuria A condition exhibited by the urine turning dark upon standing because of the presence of alkapton bodies in it.
alcohol	alcohol
alcoholismo	alcoholism An addiction to alcohol.
alcohólico, alcohólica	alcoholic
alcohómetro	breath test (for alcohol)
aldehído	aldehyde A substance derived by oxidizing and containing a CHO group from alcohol.
aldosterona	aldosterone A steroid secreted by the adrenal cortex that regulates electrolytes.
aldosteronismo	aldosteronism A condition characterized by the excessive secretion of aldosterone.
alelo	allele A type of a gene; in humans there are two alleles per chromosome pair.
alergia	allergy An immune response by the body to a compound it is hypersensitive to.
alerta	alert
aleteo	flutter Used to describe a cardiac rhythm disturbance, as in atrial flutter.
aleteo auricular	atrial flutter
alexia	alexia Inability to read due to a central brain lesion.
alérgenos	allergens Compounds that cause an allergic reaction.
alfa-fetoproteína	alpha-fetoprotein A glycoprotein that has a high serum level in hepatocellular and nonseminomatous germ cell tumors.
algas	algae
algodón	cotton wool
algogénico	algogenic Pain causing.

158

Spanish	English
algoritmo	algorhithm Any procedure designed to solve a problem in a step-by-step or mechanical fashion.
alimenticio, alimenticia	alimentary
alimento	food
alimentos bajos en grasas	low-fat foods
aliviar	alleviate
aliviar (dolor)	relieve, to (pain)
alivio	relief
allanar	flatten, to
alma	soul
almohada	pillow
almohadilla	pad
aloinjerto	allograft A tissue transplant of from someone of the same species but different genotype.
alopatía	allopathy Treatment of disease with minute amounts of natural substances.
alopecia	alopecia The absence of hair in areas where it normally exists.
alorhidria	achlorhydria The absence of hydrochloric acid in gastric secretions.
alpha-tocoferol	tocopherol Vitamin E.
alteración	alteration
alteración post mortem	post-mortem changes
alto	high
alto nivel de colesterol	high cholesterol
altura	height
alucinógeno	hallucinogen A substance that elicits hallucinations.
aluncinación	hallucination A perception that is not based on reality.
alveolar	alveolar Referring to the alveolus.
alvéolo	alveolus A small sac like structure commonly used for the pulmonary alveolus.
alvéolo	socket An anatomical hollow that is part of an articulation or where the eyeball rests.
amalgama	amalgam An alloy that includes mercury as one ingredient.
amalgamar	amalgamate To make an amalgam by dissolving a metal in mercury.
amamantar	suckle
amargo	bitter
amarillo	yellow
amastia	amastia A development condition exhibited by the absence of breasts.
amaurosis	amaurosis Blindness that occurs without an ocular lesion but may include the optic nerve.
amaurosis fugax	amaurosis fugax This transient monocular blindness is considered a sign of an impending stroke.
ambidextro, ambidextra	ambidextrous Ability to use both hands equal ability.
ambigüedad genital	genital ambiguity
ambisexual	ambisexual Referring to both sexes.
ambliopía	amblyopia Decreased vision without an ocular lesion.
ambulatorio, ambulatoria	ambulatory Referring to one's ability to walk.

Spanish	English
ameba	ameba A one-celled protozoan.
amebiasis	amebiasis A condition in which one is infected with amebae, mostly commonly Entamoeba histolytica.
amebicida	amebicide A compound used to treat amebiasis.
ameboma	ameboma A mass caused by inflammation as seen in amebiasis.
amelia	amelia A congenital anomaly exhibited by the absence of limbs.
amencia	amentia The absence of mental ability.
amenorrea	amenorrhea The absence of menses.
ametria	ametria Congenital absence of the uterus.
ametropía	ametropia Abnormal refractive ability of the eyes resulting in hypermetropia, myopia or astigmatism.
amilasa	amylase An enzyme involved in the hydrolysis of starch.
amiloidosis	amyloidosis The accumulation of amyloid in body tissues.
aminoácido	amino acid A compound containing a carboxyl and an amino group.
aminos	amnion The membrane lining the placenta which produces the amniotic fluid.
amiotonía	amyotonia A condition associated with the lack of muscle tone.
amiotrofia	amyotrophy Atrophy of muscle tissue.
amígdala	amygdala Any almond shaped structure such as the tonsil
amígdala	tonsil A rounded mass of lymphoid tissue, most commonly referring to the pharyngeal tonsil.
amnesia	amnesia The inability to remember past events.
amnesia anterógrada	amnesia, antegrade The inability to remember events which occurred after the insult that caused the condition.
amniocentesis	amniocentesis Transabdominal aspiration of amniotic fluid.
amniografía	amniography X-ray of the gravid uterus after insertion of opaque dye.
amoníaco	ammonia A colorless alkaline gas.
amorfo, amorfa	amorphous A fetus with no heart and no definitive shape.
ampolla	ampulla The dilated end of a duct.
ampolla	blister Common term for bulla.
ampolla	bulla A large cutaneous serous filled vesicle.
ampolla del quilo	ampulla chyli Also called cisterna chyli; it is a dilated area of the thoracic duct that collects lymph from several areas.
anabolismo	anabolism The formation of molecules in organisms from simpler molecules.
anacrótico	anacrotic Referring to a prominent bulge on the ascending portion of a pulse recording.
anaeróbico	anaerobe An organism that lives in the absence of oxygen.
anafase	anaphase A stage in mitosis following metaphase.
anafilaxis	anaphylaxis An exaggerated response to a foreign substance.
anaforesis	anaphoresis Reduced activity of the sweat glands.
anal	anal
analéptico	analeptic A medication used as a stimulant to the central nervous system.
analfabeto, analfabeta	illiterate
analgesia	analgesia The absence of pain.
analgesia espinal	epidural analgesia Medication into this space produces analgesia for surgical procedures.
analgésico	analgesic A medication used to remove pain.
anaplasia	anaplasia The loss of normal differentiation of tumor cells.

160

Spanish	English
anastomosis	anastomosis Surgical formation of a connection between two previously separate parts.
anatomía	anatomy The study of body structure.
anatómico, anatómica	anatomical Referring to the anatomy.
análisis de orina	urinalysis Chemical and microscopic examination of the urine.
análisis semen	semen analysis Evaluation of semen used as part of a fertility workup.
análogo	analogous To resemble or be similar to.
anchura	width
anciano	old age
andador	walker
andar coma un pato	waddling gait Walking in short steps in a swaying fashion.
androginoide	androgynous Referring to a female pseudohermaphroditism (a genetic female with masculine characteristics).
androsterona	androsterone A hormone excreted in the urine of men and women.
andrógeno	androgen A compound that produces masculinizing characteristics.
anejos	adnexa The appendages, for example, of the uterus are the ovaries, fallopian tubes and the ligaments of the uterus.
anemia	anemia Lower than normal red blood cell count.
anemia aplásica	aplastic anemia Bone marrow failure causing a decrease in all types of blood cells.
anemia drepanocítica	sickle-cell anemia A hereditary type of anemia characterized by crescent shaped red blood cells.
anemia ferropénica	iron-deficiency anemia A microcytic anemia.
anemia hemolítica	hemolytic anemia Reduced number of erythrocytes due to shortened survival and inability of the bone marrow to compensate.
anencefalia	anencephaly The congenital absence of the cranial vault and cerebral hemispheres.
aneroide	aneroid The absence of liquid.
anestesia	anesthesia Loss of sensation.
anestesia en guante	glove anesthesia Absence of sensation of the hand and wrist.
anestesia troncular	nerve-block anesthesia Injection of an anesthetic agent near a nerve, thus blocking the sensation distal to the injection.
anestestista	anesthetist A person who administers anesthesia.
anestésico	anesthetic A chemical that produces anesthesia.
aneurisma	aneurysm A condition exhibited by the dilatation of the walls of an artery or vein to form a blood-filled sac.
aneurisma di-secante	dissecting aneurysm A condition in which blood is present between the layers of an artery.
angiectasia	angiectasia Dilation of a blood or lymph vessel.
angiitis	angitis or angiitis The inflammation of a lymph or blood vessel.
angina de esfuerzo	exercised induce angina
angina de pecho	angina pectoris Exercise induced myocardial ischemia.
angiocardiografía	angiography Roentgenographic imaging of blood vessels.
angioedema	angioedema Also called angioneurotic edema, it is caused by a histamine reaction. It can produce welts in mild cases but in severe cases can cause swelling of the lips and tongue.
angioespasmo	angiospasm A spasm of a blood vessel.

161

Spanish	English
angiofibroma juvenil	juvenile angiofibroma A noncancerous growth in the nose or pharyngeal region.
angiografía coronaria	coronary angiography Roentgenographic visualization of the coronary vessels after injection of dye.
angiograma	angiogram Radiologic imaging of blood vessels.
angioma	angioma A tumor comprised of blood or lymph vessels.
angioneurótico	angioneurotic Caused by a neurosis affecting the blood vessels, like vasospasm.
angioplastia	angioplasty Surgical alteration of blood vessels.
angiosarcoma	angiosarcoma A sarcoma comprised of blood vessels.
angiotensina	angiotensin A blood protein that increases aldosterone secretion.
angiotensina	angiotensin converting enzyme inhibitors (ACEI) A class of medicines that prevent conversion of angiotension I to angiotensin II, a potent vasoconstrictor.
angustia	anguish
anhidro	anhydrous Lacking water.
anhidrosis	anhidrosis A condition exhibited by reduced quantity of sweat.
anhidrótico	anhidrotic Something the reduces the quantity of sweat.
anieblado	hazy
anillo	ring
anillo de Kayser-Fleischer	pericorneal ring Also known as Kayser-Fleischer rings exhibited by presence of brown or grey-green rings on the cornea. This is from the deposition of copper and seen in Wilson's disease.
anillo subcutáneo	superficial inguinal ring The opening of the aponeurosis of the external oblique muscle for the round ligament or spermatic cord.
animal doméstico	pet
aniscoria	anisocoria Pupillary diameter inequality.
aniseiconía	aniseikonia A condition in which the ocular image of an object is viewed differently by each eye..
anisocitosis	anisocytosis Variation in size of erythrocytes.
anisomelia	anisomelia Unequal size of arms or legs.
anisometropía	anisometropia Refractive power inequality between the two eyes.
ano	anus The body opening distal to the rectum.
anomalía congénito	birth defect A congenital anomaly.
anomalía congénito cárdiaca	congenital heart disease A cardiac disorder present prior to birth.
anomia	anomia Inability to name or recognize familiar objects.
anoniquia	anonychia Congenital absence of fingernails or toenails.
anoperineal	anoperineal Referring to the anus and perineum.
anorexia	anorexia The loss of appetite.
anorexia nervosa	anorexia nervosa A mental disorder characterized by the desire to avoid eating and to lose weight.
anormal	abnormal
anorrectal	anorectal Referring to the anus and rectum.
anosmia	anosmia Lack of the sense of smell.
anovulación	anovulation Lack of ovulation.
anoxemia	anoxemia Reduction in blood oxygen concentration.
anoxia	anoxia Reduced oxygen levels in body tissues.

162

Spanish	English
anoxia por altitud	altitude sickness A general term used for an illness that occurs at high altitude.
anquiloglosia	ankyloglossia Limitation of tongue motion because of a short frenulum.
anquilosis	ankylosis Abnormal immobility of a joint.
anquilostomiasis	ancylostomiasis A type of nematode parasite, also called hookworm.
ansia	craving
ansiedad	anxiety Nervousness or unease.
ansioso, ansiosa	anxious Experiencing nervousness or unease.
antagonista	antagonist A muscle or agent that acts in counteract to effects of another muscle or agent.
antebrazo	forearm
antecedente	above
antecedente	former
antemortem	antemortem Refers to: before death.
antenatal	antenatal Refers to events before birth.
anterior	anterior Toward the front.
anteroinferior	anteroinferior Toward the front and lower part.
anterolateral	anterolateral Toward the front and away from the midline.
anteromediano	anteromedian Toward the front and toward the midline.
anteroposterior	anteroposterior From front to the back. (An AP x-ray has the beam directed from the front to the back.)
anterosuperior	anterosuperior Toward the front and the upper part.
anterógrado	anterograde Moving forward.
anterversión	anteversion The forward leaning of an organ.
antes	beforehand
antiácido	antacid A medication, usually with a calcium or magnesium base that binds with acid in the stomach.
antibióticos	antibiotic A medication that inhibits or kills microorganisms.
anticoagulante	anticoagulant Medication used to inhibit coagulation.
anticodón	anticodon A series of three nucleotides that form a unit of genetic code for transfer RNA.
anticolinesterasa	anticholinesterase Cholinesterase blocker.
anticolinérgico, anticolinérgica	anticholinergic Parasympathetic blocker.
anticonvulsivo	anticonvulsant Medication used to treat seizures.
anticuado	outdated
anticuerpo	antibody A protein that combines with and counteracts foreign substances.
antidepresivo	antidepressant Medication used to treat depression.
antidiurético	antidiuretic hormone Vasopressin.
antidoto	antidote A medication that neutralizes a toxin.
antiemético	antemetic A medication used to control nausea.
antiespasmódico	antispasmodic Medication used to treat muscle spasm.
antigeno	antigen A foreign substance, like bacteria, that induces an immune response.
antihelmíntico	anthelmintic An agent used to destroy worms.
antihipertensivo	pressure reducer Anti-hypertensive agent.
antihisamina	antihistamine Medication used to treat conditions exhibited by a histamine response
antilimfocite	antilymphocyte A serum globulin that has antibodies to lymphocytes.

Spanish	English
antimetabolito	antimetabolite A substance that impedes metabolism.
antimicótico	antimycotic Inhibition of fungal growth.
antimitótico	antimitotic Impeding mitosis.
antipalúdico	antimalarial Medication used to treat malaria.
antiperistáltico	antiperistaltic An agent that impedes normal peristalsis.
antipirético, antipirético	antipyretic Medication used to treat fever.
antipruriginoso, antipruriginosa	antipruritic Medication used to treat pruritus.
antiséptico	antiseptic A substance that inhibits microorganism growth.
antisuero	antiserum A substance that contains antibodies to specific antigens.
antitiroideo	antithyroid A substance inhibiting the effect of the thyroid.
antitoxina	antitoxin A substance that inhibits the effect of a toxin.
antitrombina	antithrombin A substance that inhibits thrombin, thus decreasing the body's ability to coagulate.
antiveneno	antivenin An antitoxin formulated for various types of snake bites.
antracosis	anthracosis Pneumoconiosis caused by coal dust.
antro	antrum Referring to a cavity or chamber.
antrotomía	antrotomy To cut open the antrum.
anualmente	yearly
anular	annular Referring to a ring.
anuria	anuria The lack of urine excretion.
añadir	add, to
año	year
aorta	aorta The large artery originating at the left ventricle and going to the pelvis where it bifurcates.
aórtico, aórtica	aortic Referring to the aorta.
aparato respiratorio superior	upper respiratory tract Generally considered the part of the respiratory tract superior to the vocal cords.
aparato yuxtaglomerular	juxtaglomerular apparatus Cells located in the tunica media of the afferent glomerular arterioles.
apariencia	appearance
aparte	apart
apatia	apathy
apellido	surname
apellido de soltera	maiden name
apendectomía	appendectomy Surgical excision of the appendix.
apendicitis	appendicitis Inflammation of the appendix.
apercepión	apperception The ability to interpret sensory impressions.
aperistalsis	aperistalsis Lack of intestinal peristalsis.
apertura	aperture An opening or hole, as in the hole the light passes through in a camera.
apex	apex The highest point of something.
apéndice	appendix An appendage of the cecum.
apéndice xifoide	xiphoid process The inferior segment of the sternum.
Apgar, test de	Apgar score A scoring system for newborns that utilizes heart rate, respiratory effort, muscle tone, responsiveness and skin color.

Spanish	English
apiceotomía	apicetomy Removal of the apex of the petrous portion of the temporal bone.
aplicación	application
aplicador	applicator
apnea	apnea Absence of respiration.
apnea del sueño	sleep apnea Episodic apnea during sleep that is exhibited by daytime symptoms of fatigue, difficulty concentrating and sleepiness.
aponeurosis	aponeurosis A tendinous expansion that connects with muscle to move a part.
apoplejía	apoplexy Extravasation of blood within an organ.
apófisis	apophysis Generally a bony outgrowth that forms a process or tubercle.
apófisis mastoides	mastoid process The posterior part of the temporal bone bordered by the parietal bone superiorly and the occipital bone posteriorly.
apraxia	apraxia The inability to carry out intentional movements when paralysis is not present.
aprehensión	apprehension A fear that something unpleasant will happen.
aprendizaje	learning
apretón	squeeze, to
aprieto, emergencia	emergency An urgent, life-threatening situation.
aprobasión	approval
aproximadamente	approximately
aproximado, aproximada	approximate
aptialismo	aptyalism Diminished or absence of saliva.
aptitud	aptitude A natural talent for something.
apto	apt Suitable in the circumstances.
aquilia	achylia The absence of chyle.
aquilobursitis	achillobursitis Inflammation around the calcaneal tendon.
aquilodinia	achilliodynia Pain arond the calcaneal tendon.
aquinesia	akinesia An absence of movement or sparsity of movement.
aquinestesia	akinesthesia Lack of perception of movement.
arachnoides	arachnoid Refers to that which resembles a spider web.
aracnodactilia	arachnodactyly A condition exhibited by abnormally long and slender fingers.
arbovirus	arbovirus Virus that is transmitted by arthropods; responsible for diseases such as Yellow fever and dengue fever.
arcadas	retching Spasm of the stomach without presence of gastric material.
arco superciliar	superciliary arch The area superior to the upper border of each orbit.
arcus	arcus Narrow opaque band.
areóla	areola The pigmented skin surrounding a nipple.
argininosuccinicoaciduria	argininosuccinicaciduria Presence of arginosuccinic acid in the urine; associated with mental retardation.
argiria	argyria The greyish discoloration of the skin and conjunctiva.
argumentar	argue, to
aritenoideo	arytenoid Referring to the cartilage in the posterior larynx.
arodillarse	kneeling
arrenoblastoma	arrhenoblastoma An ovarian tumor that results in masculine secondary sex characteristics.
arritmia	arrhythmia An abnormal heart rhythm.
arritmia sinusal	sinus arrhythmia Cardiac dysrhythmias related to sinoatrial nodal dysfunction.

Spanish	English
artefacto	artifact An aberration from the normal.
arteria	artery Vessel that carries oxygenated blood from the heart to the periphery.
arteria femoral	femoral artery
arteria braquial	brachial artery A continuation of the axillary artery and branches into the radial and ulnar among others.
arteria coronaria	coronary vessel Referring to a coronary artery.
arteria innominada	innominate artery The first branch off the aortic arch that branches into the right common carotid and right subclavian arteries.
arterial	arterial Referring to an artery.
arteriectomía	arteriectomy Surgical excision of an artery.
arterioesclerosis	arteriosclerosis Hardening and thickening of arterial walls.
arteriografía	arteriography Roentgenography of an artery after infusion of contrast media.
arterioplastia	arterioplasty Surgical repair of an artery.
arteriotomía	arteriotomy Creation of an opening in an artery.
arteriovenoso malformaciones	arteriovenous malformation A sac like structure created by the abnormal communication of an adjacent artery and vein.
arteritis	arteritis Inflammation of an artery.
arthrografía	arthrography Joint roentgenography.
articulación de la cadera	hip joint
articulación en silla de montar	saddle joint A joint that exhibits two saddle type surfaces at a 90 degree angle to each other, such as the carpometacarpal joint.
articulación temporomandibular	temporomandibular joint The hinged joint of the temporal bone and mandible.
articulación tobillo	ankle joint
articular	articular Referring to a joint.
artificial	artificial Not natural produced.
artralgia	arthralgia Joint pain.
artritis	arthritis Joint inflammation.
artritis gonorreico	gonorrheal arthritis
artritis reumatoide	rheumatoid arthritis A symmetric peripheral polyarthritis.
artrodesis	arthrodesis Surgical fusion of a joint.
artrodinia	arthrodynia Joint pain.
artropatía hemofílico	hemophilic arthropathy
artroplasia	arthroplasty Plastic surgery involving a joint.
artroscopia	arthroscopy Viewing of the inside of a joint with a specially designed scope.
artrotomía	arthrotomy Surgical opening of a joint.
asbesto	asbestos A heat resistant silicate material.
asbestosis	asbestosis Lung disease caused by the inhalation of asbestos.
ascaricida	ascaricide Agent that destroys ascaris.
Ascaris	ascaris A nematode from genus intestinal lumbricoid parasite, also called round worm.
ascitis	ascites Serous fluid in the abdominal cavity.
asegurer	ensure, to To make certain of.
asepsia	asepsis Lack of infection.
asesoramiento genético	genetic counseling

166

Spanish	English
asesoramiento matrimonial	marital counseling
asexual	asexual Without sex or sex organs.
aséptico, aséptica	aseptic Being free of septic matter.
asfixia	asphyxia A condition exhibited by a lack of oxygen and subsequent loss of consciousness or death.
asimetría	asymmetry Lack of symmetry.
asinclitismo	asynclitism Oblique presentation of the head during delivery.
asintomático, asintomática	asymptomatic
asistencia	assistance
asistente de salud	caregiver
asombroso	staggering
aspecto general	general appearance
Asperger, sindrome de	Asperger's syndrome A condition characterized by disturbed social interaction; if was named after the Austrian scientist who first described it.
aspermia	aspermia Absence of sperm.
aspiración	aspiration Taking air or matter into the lungs. Removal of fluid from a cavity.
aspiración médula ósea	bone marrow puncture The aspiration of marrow to look for pressure of disease.
aspiración por la nariz	sniffing
aspirador	aspirator A device used to remove fluid from a cavity.
aspirina	aspirin Common name for acetylsalicylic acid.
asta, cuerno	horn A keratinized outgrowth.
asteatosis	asteatosis A condition exhibited by diminished sebaceous secretion.
astenia	asthenia Diminished strength and energy.
astenopía	asthenopia Visual fatigue accompanied by ocular pain.
astereognosía	astereognosis Lack of ability to recognize objects by touching them.
astilla	splinter A small, thin object; usually refers to the object being imbedded in the body.
astrágalo	astragalus Synonym of talus.
astrágalo	talus The most superior tarsal bone that articulates with the tibia.
astringente	astringent An agent causing contraction of the skin.
astrocitoma	astrocytoma A tumor comprised of astrocytes.
astroglia	astroglia The neurologic tissue which is composed of astrocytes.
ataque	attack A fit or paroxysm.
ataque convulsivo	crisis Seizure.
ataque de pánico	panic attack Sudden, profound anxiety.
ataque epiléptico	epileptic seizure A convulsion related to abnormal brain activity (as opposed to being precipitated by hypoglycemia.)
ataque, acceso	access
atavismo	atavism The inheritance of characteristics from remote rather than immediate ancestors.
ataxia	ataxia Lack of muscular coordination.
atelectasis	atelectasis Incomplete expansion or collapse of a lung.
atentados con explosivos	blast injury Trauma from a wave of air pressure.
aterogénico	atherogenic Something that causes atheromatous lesions in arterial walls.

Spanish	English
ateroma	atheroma Degenerative arteriosclerosis.
atetosis	athetosis An involuntary symptom exhibited by continuous slow, writhing movements, mostly in the hands.
atipico, atipica	atypical Not usual.
atlas	atlas The first cervical vertebra.
atomizador	atomizer A device for propelling a fine mist.
atonía	atony Absence of normal muscle tone.
atontado	groggy
atragantarse	choke, to
atresia	atresia Closure of a body orifice as in atresia ani in which there is a congenital imperforate anus.
atresia coanal	choanal atresia A congenital condition characterized by blockage of the nasal passages by tissue.
atrio, atria	atrium Referring to a chamber used as an entrance, as in the entrance to the heart.
atrioventricular	atrioventricular Referring to the atrium and ventricle.
atrofia	atrophy A diminution in the size of a part.
atrofia muscular progresiva	amyotrophic lateral sclerosis A progressive neurodegenerative disorder.
atrofia peroneo	peroneal atrophy Progressive muscle atrophy in the peroneal region.
atropina	atropine A parasympathetic agent derived from Atropa belladonna.
atrófico	atrophic Referring to atrophy.
audición	hearing
audiograma	audiogram The recording of a one's hearing in decibels.
auditivo, auditiva	auditory Referring to hearing.
audífono	hearing aid
audiólogo, audióloga	audiologist A specialist in the field of hearing.
audiómetro	audiometer A device used to measure hearing.
aumento	enlargement Becoming bigger.
aumento, acrecentamiento	accretion The expected growth of tissue from the intake of nutrients.
aural, auricular	aural Referring to the ear.
aural, auricular	auricular Referring to the auricle.
auricula	auricle The external portion of the ear.
auricular	atrial Referring to the atrium.
auriculotemporal	auriculotemporal The area of the ear and temple.
auris externa	ear, external
auris interna	ear, inner
auris media	middle ear
auscultación	auscultation The act of listening to sounds emanating from the body.
ausencia	absence
ausente	away from
austistico, autistica	autistic Referring to autism.
autismo	autism A mental condition exhibited by difficulty in forming relationships, communicating and uses abstract thought.
autoanticuerpo	autoantibody An antibody that acts against the organism's own tissue.
autoantígeno	autoantigen A normal tissue constituent that prompts a cell-mediated response.

Spanish	English
autoclave	autoclave A device used for sterilization with the use of steam under pressure.
autogena	autogenous Self-generated.
autohipnosis	autohypnosis Self-hypnosis.
autoinjerto	autograft Grafting tissue from one part of person to another part of the same person.
autoinmunización	autoimmunization The body's ability to promote an immune response without external resources.
autopsia	autopsy Examination of a body post-mortem in an attempt to determine cause of death.
autosómico	autosomal Referring to an autosome.
autotranfusión	autotransfusion The reinfusion of one's own blood.
autólisis	autolysis A state of self destruction of cells within a body.
avanzado	advanced
avascular	avascular An area with no blood supply.
aventado, aventada	bloated Sensation of having an abnormally large amount of air in the viscera.
aviario	avian Referring to birds.
avispa	wasp
avitaminosis	avitaminosis A state of vitamin deficiency.
axila	axilla The hollow beneath the arm.
axilar	axillary Referring to the axilla.
axis	axis The second cervical vertebra.
axon	axon The structure along which nerve impulses are transmitted from the cell body to other cells.
ayuno	fasting Absence of caloric intake for a specified period.
azoospermia	azoospermia The absence of spermatozoa in the semen.
azotemia	azotemia Prerenal disease.
azoturia	azoturia An excess of urea in the urine.
azufre	sulfur
azul	blue
azúcar	sugar
àntrax	anthrax An infectious disease caused by Bacillus anthracis; there are cutaneous, inhalation and gastrointestinal syndromes.
ácido	acid Substance with a pH less than 7.
ácido desoxirribonucleico	deoxyribonucleic acid (DNA) The carrier of genetic information.
ácido desoxirribonucleico	DNA Deoxyribonucleic acid.
ácido fólico	folic acid Also called pteroylglutamic acid; a deficiency can cause megaloblastic anemia.
ácido nucleico	nucleic acid An organic compound found in living cells; its molecules contain nucleotides linked in long chains.
ácido acetilsalicílio	acetylsalicylic acid The chemical name for common aspirin.
ácido ascórbico	ascorbic acid Commonly known as vitamin C; a deficiency of this vitamin causes scurvy.
ácido clorhídrico	hydrochloric acid A solution with a low pH formed by dissolving hydrogen chloride in water.
ácido nicotínico	nicotinic acid A deficiency of this substance results in pellagra.

169

Spanish	English
ácido p-aminobenzoico	para-aminobenzoic acid A natural product (not FDA approved) reportedly beneficial for Peyronie's disease and scleroderma. It is a component of folic acid.
ácido p-aminohipúrico	para-aminohippuric acid (PAH) A chemical used for calculation of renal plasma flow.
ácido ribonucleico (RNA)	ribonucleic acid An acid present in all living cells, it is a messenger for DNA.
ácido taurocólico	taurocholic acid A bile acid composed of cholic acid and taurine.
ácidos biliares	bile salts Normally occurring salts of bile acids.
ácidos grasos	fatty acid A carboxylic acid occurring as a an ester in fats and oils.
álcali	alkali A class of compounds that form soluble carbonates.
álgido, álgida	algid cold
bacalao	cod
bacilar	bacillary Referring to bacilli.
bacilo	bacillus A rod-shaped bacterium.
bacin	bedpan
bacteriano, bacteriana	bacterial Referring to bacteria.
bactericida	bactericidal An agent that destroys bacteria.
bacteriemia	bacteremia The presence of bacteria in the blood.
bacteriostático	bacteriostatic An agent that impedes bacterial growth.
bacteriruia	bacteriuria The presence of bacteria in the urine.
bagazosis	bagassosis A pulmonary disorder contracted from inhalation of the waste of sugar cane (bagasse dust).
baipás	bypass
balanitis	balanitis Inflammation of the glans of the penis.
balanza	scale A device to check a person's weight.
balanza bebé	baby-scale
balón	flask
banco de sangre	blood bank
barrera hematoencefálica	blood brain barrier A matrix of capillaries that move blood between the blood and brain, as well as, limiting some substances from passing.
basal	basal Referring to the base.
basilar	basilar Referring to the base or lower segment.
basófilo	basophil A polymorphonuclear granulocyte.
bazo	spleen The visceral organ that is involved with production and removal of blood cells.
bálsamo	balm
beber	drink, to
bebé	baby
bemol	flat
berilosis	berylliosis A lung exhibited by granulomas and caused by inhalation of beryllium.
beta bloqueador	betablocker A substance that inhibits adrenergic stimulation. It is used to reduce pulse, blood pressure and to treat angina.
bezoar	bezoar A concretion composed of either hair, vegetable/fruit fibers or hair and vegetable/fruit fibers that is found in the stomach.
biauricular	binaural Referring to both ears.
biblioteca	library

170

Spanish	English
biceps	biceps A muscle with two heads usually referring to the biceps brachii which is used for forearm flexion.
bicho	bug
bicúspide	bicuspid Having two points as in bicuspid valve or a premolar tooth.
bifurcarse	bifurcate When one branch divides into two branches.
bilateral	bilateral
Bilharzia	Bilharzia Historical name of a genus of flukes or nematodes now known as Schistosoma.
biliar	biliary Referring to bile, bile ducts or gallbladder.
bilioso, biliosa	bilious Something that contains bile.
bilirrubina	bilirubin A pigment found in bile that is responsible for the yellow color seen in patients with elevated serum levels of bilirubin.
bilirubinuria	biliuria The presence of bile in the urine.
bilis	bile An alkaline fluid secreted by the liver to aid digestion.
biliverdina	biliverdin A green pigment formed by oxidation of bilirubin.
bimanual	bimanual Use of two hands, as in bimanual pelvic examination in which the right hand touches the cervix uteri and the left hand presses above the mons pubis.
binocular	binocular Referring to both eyes.
biodisponsibilidad	bioavailability The portion of a drug that is able to be utilized by the body after it is introduced to the body.
bioensayo	bioassay A laboratory test determination as compared to normal.
biologia	biology The study of living organisms.
biopsia	biopsy The removal and examination of bodily tissues or fluids.
biopsia por extracción	excisional biopsy Surgical removal of tissue for pathologic examination.
bioquímica	biochemistry The study of chemistry and physiochemical processes in living organisms.
biotina	biotin A vitamin involved in the synthesis of fatty acids and glucose.
biovular	binovular Derived from two different ova.
bisinosis	byssinosis A disease caused by inhalation of cotton dust; a type of pneumoconiosis.
bizquera	squint
bífido	bifid Presence of two branches.
blanca	white
blanco	target
blando	soft
blastomicosis	blastomycosis Infection caused by organisms of genus Blastomyces.
blefaritis	blepharitis Inflammation of the eyelids.
blefaroespasmo	blepharospasm A spasm of the orbicularis oculi muscle that causes closure of the eyelid.
blenorrea	blennorrhea Discharge from the mucous membranes, usually referring to gonorrhea.
bloque de rama	bundle branch block A cardiac dysrhythmia produced by a blockage of a branch of the bundle of His.
bloqueador de los canales de calcio	calcium channel blocker A medication used to treat angina, supraventricular arrhythmias and hypertension; it works by blocking calcium influx into myocytes and vascular smooth muscle cells.
bloqueo atrioventricular	atrio-ventricular block An interruption of the electrical conduction at the atrio-ventricular node.

Spanish	English
bloqueo del corazón	heart block An alteration in the cardiac electrical conduction system.
boca	mouth
boca de trinchera Gingivitis ulcerosa necrosante.	trench mouth
bocado	mouthful
bochornos o ruborización	flushing
bocio	goiter Swelling of the thyroid gland.
bolo	bolus A fluid bolus is a phrase used for rapid infusion of fluid.
bolsa de colostomía	colostomy bag A pouch attached to the skin with a mild adhesive that collects stool emitted from a colostomy.
bolsa faríngea	pharyngeal pouch A lateral diverticulum of the pharynx.
borde, margen	border; margin
borracho	drunk Inebriated.
bostezo	yawn
botella	bottle
bougienage	bougienage Passage of a bougie through a body orifice with the goal of increasing the diameter of the orifice.
bóveda craneal	calvaria The superior portions of the frontal, parietal and occipital bones.
brachium conjunctivum cerebelli	brachium cerebelli Synonym of pedunculus cerebellaris superior (upper portion the cerebellum).
bradicardia	bradycardia Lower than normal cardiac rate measured in beats per minute.
bradicinina	bradykinin A peptide that causes contraction of smooth muscle and dilation of blood vessels.
braguero	brace
braguero	truss A synthetic device for containing a hernia within the abdomen.
branquial	branchial Referring to or resembling the gills of a fish.
braquial	brachial Referring to the arm.
braquicefalia	brachycephaly The presence of a short broad skull.
brazo	arm
brazo fracturado	broken (arm)
bregma	bregma Located at the convergence of the coronal and sagittal sutures.
brillante	bright
bromhidrosis	bromidrosis Foul smelling perspiration.
bromismo	bromism Poisoning caused by excessive intake of bromine.
bronceospasmo	bronchospasm Bronchial smooth muscle spasm.
broncogénico (a)	bronchogenic Referring to the bronchi.
broncografía	bronchography Roentgenography of the bronchi after administration of contrast media.
bronconeumonía	bronchopneumonia Pneumonia that starts in the distal bronchioles.
broncoscopía	bronchoscopy Use of a scope to visualize the bronchi.
bronquial	bronchial Referring to the bronchus.
bronquiectasia	bronchiectasis The presence of abnormally wide bronchi or branches.
bronquio	bronchus The major air channels that bifurcate from the distal trachea.
bronquiolitis	bronchiolitis Inflammation of the pulmonary bronchioles.
bronquiolo	bronchiole A small branch that a bronchus divides into.

172

Spanish	English
bronquitis	bronchitis Inflammation of the mucous membranes of the bronchioles that causes bronchospasm and cough.
brote	flare A sudden intensity or dilatation.
brote	outbreak
brucelosis	brucellosis A gram-negative bacteria in cattle that causes persistent fever in humans.
bubón	bubo An inflamed, swollen lymph node in the axilla or inguinal region.
bucal	buccal Referring to the cheek.
buccinador	buccinator A thin, flat muscle in the cheek wall.
buceo	diving
bulimia	adephagia Insatiable hunger.
bulimia	bulimia Pathologic increase in hunger.
bunio	bunion Swelling of the bursa of the metatarsal head of the first metatarsal.
bursitis	bursitis Inflammation of the bursa.
cabalgamiento	overriding suture The overlapping of cranial sutures noted on vaginal exam when the head is descended.
cabello	hair (of head)
cabestrillo	sling
cabeza	head
caboxihemoglobina	carboxyhemoglobin A compound formed from hemoglobin when it is exposed to carbon monoxide.
cada dos días	every other day
cadáver	cadaver A dead body.
cadera	hip
caduceo	caduceus An ancient herald's wand with two serpents twined around that is a symbol of the medical arts.
café	brown
calambre	cramp
calcáneo	calcaneus Commonly called the heel bone.
calcáreo	calcareous Referring to something containing lime or calcium.
calcemia	calcemia The presence of an abundance of calcium in the blood.
calcetín	socks (as in footwear)
calciferol	calciferol It is formed when egesterol is exposed to ultraviolet light; a D vitamin.
calcificación	calcification Deposition of calcium salts causing hardening of an organic tissue.
calcio	calcium A chemical element that is an essential component in teeth and bone.
calcitonina	calcitonin A thyroid hormone that lowers serum calcium levels.
calibrado	calibration The process of calibrating an instrument.
calibrar	calibrate, to To adjust an instrument using a standard.
calibre	gauge The size or thickness of something. An 18gauge needle.
caliente	hot
calificar	qualify
callado	silent
callo	callus Thickened hardened skin.
callosidad	callosity Callus; thickened hardened skin.
calmante para la tos	antitussive Medication used to diminish a cough.

Spanish	English
calor	heat
caloría	calorie A unit of heat.
calvaría	calvaria The portion of the skull that is composed of the superior aspects of the occipital, parietal and frontal bones.
calyx	calyx A cup shaped organ or cavity.
cama	bed
camisa de fuerza	strait-jacket A device used to temporarily restrain the arms of patients who are psychotic and violent.
campo	drape The fabric used as a sterile covering in the OR.
campo visual	visual field The complete area a person can see with their eyes in a fixed position.
canabis	cannabis A plant from the Cannibidaceae family that is known for its psychotropic effects.
canal iónico	ion channel A selectively permeable cell membrane to certain ions.
canalículo	canaliculus A term for various small channels.
cancelar	cancel, to
cancellus	cancellous A bony mesh-like structure with many pores.
cancroide	cancroid A tumor occurring in the stomach, small or large bowel.
cancrum oris	cancrum oris Gangrenous stomatitis.
candela	candle
canino dientes	canine teeth Located between the incisors and premolars.
cantidad	amount
capa	layer
capa granular	granular layer A deep layer of the cerebellum.
capacidad vital	lung capacity The amount of air in the lungs after a maximal inhalation.
capacidad vital	vital capacity (VC) The maximal amount of air exhaled after a maximal inhalation.
capilar	capillary A vessel that connects arterioles to venules.
capitado	capitate bone The bone at the base of the palm that articulates with the third metacarpal.
capo del cuello uterino	cervical pleura The dome-like cap of the pleura.
capsulitis	capsulitis Inflammation of a capsule.
capsulitis adhesiva	adhesive capsulitis Also known as frozen shoulder.
capsulotomía	capsulotomy Incision of a capsule as in with eye surgery.
caput	caput The head.
caput succedaneum	caput succedaneum Edema that occurs in the scalp of an infant during child-birth.
caquexia	cachexia Generalized weakness and severe wasting.
carbohidrato	carbohydrate A group of organic compounds including sugar and starch.
carcinogénico, carcinogénica	carcinogenic That which causes cancer.
carcinoide	carcinoid A tumor occurring in the stomach, intestine and colon.
carcinoma	carcinoma A malignant growth.
carcinoma broncogénico	bronchial carcinoma A general term for a malignancy of the bronchi.
carcinomatosis	carcinomatosis Dissemination of cancer throughout the body.
cardias	cardia The superior aspect of the stomach at the opening of the esophagus.

174

Spanish	English
cardiología	cardiology A specialty of medical practice involve treatment and prevention of heart disease.
cardiomiopatía	cardiomyopathy Chronic cardiac muscle disease.
cardiovascular	cardiovascular Referring to the heart or circulatory system.
carditis	carditis Inflammation of the heart.
cardíaco, cardíaca	cardiac Referring to the heart.
caries	caries Referring to decay or death of a tooth.
caries dentales	dental caries Decay of teeth.
carina	carina The protrusion of the lowest tracheal cartilage.
cariocinesis	karyokinesis A part of mitosis involving the cell nucleus division.
cariotipo	karyotype The arrangement of chromosomes in a single cell.
carne	flesh
carne de gallina	goose bumps
caroteno	carotene A hydrocarbon that can be converted to vitamin A.
carótida	carotid The large artery in the neck.
carpo	carpus The joint between the hand and wrist.
carpometacarpiano	carpometacarpal Referring to the carpus and metacarpus.
carraspear	clear one's throat, to
carúncula	caruncle A small fleshy protuberance.
caseína	casein The principal protein in milk, a phospholipid.
caspa	dandruff Dead skin found in the hair.
castriación	castration Excision of the gonads.
catabolismo	catabolism The reduction of complex molecules to more simple ones in living organisms.
cataforesis	cataphoresis The use of an electric field to move charged particles in fluid.
catalepesia	catalepsy A condition exhibited by rigidity and the person maintains the same position if he is moved by another.
cataplejía	cataplexy A condition exhibited by rigidity and immobility.
cataracta	cataract An opacity of an eye lens or the capsule.
catarro	catarrh Inflammation of a mucous membrane.
catarsis	catharsis The act of cleansing or purging, usually referring to thought.
catatonía	catatonia Seen in schizophrenia, it is a state of stupor or excitability and abnormal movements.
catártico	cathartic To be cleansed or evacuated, referring to thought or the cleansing of the bowels.
catéter de Foley	Foley catheter A drainage tube placed in the urinary bladder via the urethra.
catéter de Foley	indwelling foley A catheter inserted into the urinary bladder with an inflatable ballon on the tip.
catéter de triple canal	three way foley A urinary tube used for irrigation of the bladder.
catéter permanente	indwelling catheter Continuous use tube usually referring to a tube in the urinary bladder.
catéter, sonda	catheter A flexible tube inserted into the body.
caudado	caudate Referring to the caudate nucleus.
caudal	caudal Referring to a cauda.
causativo	causative
cauterio	cautery Application of an electric current to cut something.
cavidad	cavity Pouch or chamber.

175

Spanish	English
cálculo	calculus A stone of minerals that can lead to the blockage of the bile duct or ureters.
cálculo dentario	dental calculus Calcium phosphate and carbonate adhered to the teeth.
cálculos en la vesícula	gallstones Calculi produced in the bile duct or gallbladder.
cámara hiperbárica	hyperbaric chamber A device used to treat decompression illness.
cámara posterior	posterior chamber of the eye An aqueous filled space between the cornea and the lens.
cáncer	cancer; carcinoma A disease of uncontrolled abnormal cell growth.
cánula	cannula A tube inserted into the body.
cápsula	capsule
cárneo	carneous Synonym of fleshy.
cáustico, cáustica	caustic Abrasive or corrosive.
ceceo	lisping A speech problem in which "s" and "z" are pronounced "th".
cefalagia	headache
cefalagia de Horton	cluster headache A unilateral, severe, recurrent headache.
cefálico, cefálica	cephalic Towards the head.
ceguera	blindness
ceguera nocturna	night blindness
ceja	eyebrow Supercilium.
celíaco	celiac Referring to the abdominal cavity.
celulitis	cellulitis Infection characterized by diffuse, subcutaneous inflammation.
celulosa	cellulose A polysaccharide that occurs naturally in fibrous products.
centígrado	centigrade A scale with 100 gradations, usually referring to a temperature scale.
centímetro	centimeter One hundredth of a meter.
centrifugadora	centrifuge Machine used to separate substances of different weights.
centrípeto, centrípeta	centripetal The movement toward the center.
centro	center
centro	core
cepillo	brush
cera, cerumen	wax
cerca de	around
cercano	near
cercaria	cercaria Larval trematode worm that live in a molluscan.
cerebelo	cerebellum The part of the brain in the posterior portion of the skull that controls muscle coordination and movement.
cerebración	cerebration Operating activity of the cerebrum.
cerebral	cerebral Referring to the cerebrum.
cerebro	brain A common term for cerebrum.
cerebro medio Mesencéfalo.	midbrain
cerebro posterior	hindbrain The brainstem which includes the pons, medulla oblongata and cerebellum.
cerebrovascular accident El flujo de sangre a una parte del cerebro se detiene.	cerebrovascular accident (stroke) A decrease in level of consciousness and paralysis caused by a cerebrovascular thrombosis, hemorrhage or vasospasm.
cero	zero

Spanish	English
cerrado, cerrada	closed
cerumen	cerumen Waxy substance found normally in the external ear canals.
cervical	cervical Referring to the neck or the cervix.
cervicectomía	cervicectomy Excision of the cervix uteri.
cervicitis	cervicitis Inflammation of the cervix.
cestodo	cestode A class of parasitic flatworms.
cetoacidosis	ketoacidosis
cetone	ketone
cetonemia	ketonemia Presence of ketone in the blood.
cetonuria	ketonuria Presence of ketone in the urine.
cetosis	ketosis The presence of an abnormally high level of ketones in the blood and body tissues.
célula	cell The smallest functional unit of an organism.
célula blanco	target cell An abnormal cell that is present in liver disease and certain hemoglobinopathies.
célula parietal	parietal cell Acid secreting cells of the stomach.
célula plasma	plasma cell A cell that produces only one type of antibody.
célula calciforme	goblet cells They aid in the secretion of respiratory and intestinal mucous.
célula mastocito	mast cell A cell containing basophilic granules that releases histamine and other substances during allergic reactions.
célula pilosas	hair cell Epithelial cells with hairlike projections.
célula sangre	blood cell
chancro	chancre The initial ulcer that is the source of entry for a pathogen.
chancroide	chancroid A sexually transmitted disease caused by Haemophilus ducreyi that is exhibited by ulcers without indurated margins.
chasquido crujido	crepitus A noise heard when one auscultates the lungs that is similar to the sound of rubbing hair between one's fingers. It is also considered the sound of two broken bones rubbing together.
chicle	gum (chewing gum)
chinche	bedbug Cimex lectularius. A small insect that is parasitic and hides in clothing or bedding.
chloroformo	chloroform A colorless, sweet smelling liquid formerly used as a general anesthetic.
cianocobalamina	cyanocobalamin Also called B12; used to treat pernicious and other macrocytic anemias.
cianosis	cyanosis Bluish discoloration of the skin and mucous membranes.
ciática	sciatica Pain radiating from the buttock down the back of the leg; it is caused by a compressed spinal nerve root.
cicatriz	cicatrix (scar) New tissue in a healed wound.
cicatrizal	cicatricial Referring to cicatrix.
ciclica	cyclitis Inflammation of the ciliary body.
ciclo anovulatorio	anovulatory cycle A menstrual cycle in which no ovum is released.
ciclo del ácido tricarboxílico	Krebs cycle The process of aerobic respiration by which living cells generate energy.
ciclodiálisis	cyclodialysis The surgical creation of a communication between the anterior chamber of the eye and the suprachorodial space for the purpose of treating glaucoma.
cicloplejía	cycloplegia Paralysis of the ciliary muscle.

Spanish	English
ciclotimia	cyclothymia Manic-depressive tendencies.
ciclotomía	cyclotomy Surgically creating an opening in the ciliary body.
ciego	cecum The portion of the bowel between the ileum and and the ascending colon.
ciego, ciega	blind
cierre	clasp
ciertemente	indeed
cifoescoliosis	kyphoscoliosis An abnormal outward and lateral curvature of the spine.
cifosis	kyphosis Abnormal outward curvature of the spine.
cigomático	zygomatic bone The triangular cheek bone.
cigoto	zygote A fertilized ovum.
cilindro epitelial	epithelial cast Debris found in the urine composed of columnar renal epithelium.
cilindros urinarios	urinary casts A protein precipitated from renal tubules and excreted in the urine.
cilio	cilia The hairs growing on the eyelid or a motile extension of a cell surface.
cimógeno	zymogen An inactive compound that is metabolized to an active state.
cinasa	kinase An enzyme that facilitates movement of phosphate from ATP to another molecule.
cinc	zinc
cinconismo	cinchonism The toxic effects induced by ingestion of cinchona bark; it is exhibited by tinnitus, deafness and cognitive changes.
cineplastia	kineplasty An amputation done in a fashion to facilitate ambulation.
cinesia	kinesis Movement of a part in response to a stimulus.
cinta adhesiva	adhesive tape Tape used to secure dressings or intravenous lines to the body.
cinta métrica	tape measure
cintura pelviana Cíngulo de las extremidades inferiores	hip girdle The bony supporting structure for the legs.
cinturón	belt
circadiano	circadian Referring to a 24 hour period.
circonvolución	gyrus Convolutions of the brain where there is infolding.
circuncisión	circumcision Surgical excision of the foreskin.
circunferencia	circumference The distance around an object or part.
circunferencia abdominal	abdominal girth
circunscribir	circumscribe To have well defined borders.
cirrosis	cirrhosis A liver disease characterized by destruction of liver cells and increased connective tissue.
cirsoide	cirsoid Similar to a tortuous vein, artery or lymph vessel.
cirugía	surgery
cirugía de parto	cesarian section Incision of the abdominal and uterine walls in order to deliver a fetus when natural delivery is not possible.
cirujano	surgeon
cistadenoma	cystadenoma Adenoma associated with cysts of neoplastic origin.
cistectomía	cystectomy Surgical removal of a cyst or the bladder.
cisticercosis	cysticercosis The state of being infected with a type of tapeworm.
cistico, cistica	cystic Referring to a cyst.

178

Spanish	English
cistinosis	cystinosis A congenital disorder of increased cystine that leads to renal insufficiency, rickets and dwarfism.
cistinuria	cystinuria The presence of cystine in the urine.
cistitis	cystitis Inflammation of the urinary bladder.
cistocele	cystocele Protrusion of the urinary bladder through the vaginal wall.
cistografía	cystography Roentgenographic visualization of the urinary bladder after insertion of contrast media.
cistograma urinaria	voiding cystography Roentgenography of the bladder and urethra after administration of contrast media.
cistolitiasis	cystolithiasis Presence of a calculus in the urinary bladder.
cistoscopio	cystoscope A device used to visualized the urinary bladder.
cistoscopía	cystoscopy Direct visualization of the urinary bladder with a cystoscope.
cita	appointment
citología	cytology The study of cells, their function and structure.
citoplasma	cytoplasm The protoplasm of the cell except for the nucleus.
citotoxina	cytotoxin That which is harmful to cells.
citotóxica	cytotoxic Referring to being harmful to cells.
clamidiasis	chlamydiosis A disease caused by the species Chlamydia.
claro, clara	clear
claudicación	claudication; limp Intermittent claudication is a phrase used to describe pain experienced in the leg from arterial insufficiency.
claustrofobia	claustrophobia An unreasonable fear of being in an enclosed environment.
clavar	nailing Referring to placement of an intramedullary rod in a long bone in order to treat a fracture.
clavio	clavus A corn or horny protrusion.
clavícula	clavicle A bone that articulates with the sternum and scapula.
clavícula	collarbone
cleidotomía	cleidotomy A procedure used in difficult deliveries in which the clavicle is broken to facilitate childbirth.
clic	click A sound heard by the sudden closure of a heart valve.
clínica	clinic
clítoris	clitoris A small erectile body in the anterosuperior aspect of the vulva.
cloasma	chloasma Brown or black macula that occur on the face during pregnancy or when there is ovarian dysfunction.
clono tobillo	ankle clonus An abnormal response exhibited by alternating plantar- and dorsiflexion noted after the examiner rapidly dorsiflexes the foot.
clorhidrato	hydrochloride
cloroma	chloroma A malignant tumor associated with myelogenous leukemia.
cloruro de sodio	sodium chloride
clónico	clonic Referring to a spasm that alternates in rigidity and relaxation.
cnemial	cnemial Referring to the shin.
coagulación	coagulation The formation of a clot.
coana	choanae The two openings between the nasal cavity and the nasopharynx.
coartación	coarctation A stricture, as in narrowing of the aorta with coarctation of the aorta.
coágulo	clot A thrombus or embolus.
coágulo de sangre	blood clot
cobalto	cobalt A metal that with causes polycythemia with increased ingestion.

Spanish	English
cobre	copper
cocaína	cocaine A highly addictive opiate derivative.
coccidinia	coccydynia Coccygeal pain.
coche durante parto	coaching (during labor)
cociente de inteligencia (CI)	intelligence quotient (IQ) A number representing a person's ability to problem solve compared to a matched-control.
coco	coccus A spherical shaped bacterium.
codeína	codeine A morphine derived analgesic.
codo	elbow
codo de tenista Epicondilalgia externa.	tennis elbow Inflammation at the lateral aspect of the epicondyle where the muscle and tendon join; lateral epicondylitis.
codón	codon A series of three nucleotides that form a unit of genetic code.
cognición	cognition The process of acquiring thought or understanding.
coiloniquia	koilonychia Thin and concave fingernails.
coito	coitus Sexual intercourse between members of the opposite sex.
cojinete	cushion
cola equina	cauda equina The roots of the lower spinal nerves.
colagogo	cholagogue A compound used to stimulate flow of bile from the liver.
colangiografía	cholangiogram Radiologic imaging of the gallbladder and bile ducts.
colangitis	cholangitis Inflammation of the bile ducts.
colapso por calor	heat exhaustion A condition that occurs secondary to prolonged exposure to high ambient temperature; it is exhibited by subnormal temperature, dizziness and nausea.
colágeno	collagen The principal supportive protein bone, skin, tendon and cartilage.
colchón	mattress
colecistectomía	cholecystectomy Surgical excision of the gallbladder.
colecistenteronotomía	cholecystenterostomy Creation of a surgical anastomosis between the intestine and the gallbladder.
colecistitis	cholecystitis Inflammation of the gallbladder.
colecistolitiasis	cholecystolithiasis The presence of gallstones in the gallbladder.
colectomía	colectomy Surgical removal of part of the colon.
coledocolitomía	choledocholithotomy Creation of an incision in the bile duct for the purpose of removing a stone.
colelitiasis	cholelithiasis Presence or creation of gallstones.
colemia	cholemia Bile or bile products in the blood.
colesteatoma	cholesteatoma A cystic mass that has a lining made of keratinizing material and cholesterol.
colesterol	cholesterol A compound or its derivatives are found in cell membranes and precursors to hormones but high levels can cause atherosclerosis.
colesterol alto	hypercholesterolemia Higher than normal level of cholesterol in the blood.
colgado	flap A term used to describe a piece of tissue partially excised and placed over an adjacent surface.
colinesterasa	cholinesterase An esterase used to cleave acetylcholine into choline and acetic acid.
colinérgico	cholinergic Referring to the stimulation, activation or transmission of acetylcholine.
colitis	colitis Inflammation of the colon.

Spanish	English
colitis ulceroso	ulcerative colitis Recurrent episode of inflammation of the membranous layer of the colon.
coloboma	coloboma A congenital defect that involves a fissure of the eye.
coloboma	coloboma A congenital eye fissure.
colodión	collodion A product of the breakdown of colloid.
coloide	colloid A solution used for infusion, such as albumin or hetastarch, that are more likely to remain in the intravascular space than crystalloids.
colon	colon The portion of the large intestine that goes from the cecum to the rectum.
colon ascendente	ascending colon The portion of the colon between the cecum and the right colic flexure.
colonoscopía	colonoscopy Inspection the color, ideally to the cecum, with a lighted scope.
coloración de Ziehl-Neelsen	Ziehl-Neelsen carbolfuchsin stain A stain used to detect acid-fast bacilli that appear red on the methylene blue background.
colostomía	colostomy Surgically creating an opening in the colon that is extended to outside the abdominal wall.
colostro	colostrum The fluid secreted by the mammary glands a few days around parturition.
colpitis	colpitis; vaginitis Inflammation of the vagina.
colpocele	colpocele A hernia into the vagina.
colporrafia	colporrhaphy A surgical procedure that involves suturing the vagina.
colposcopio	colposcope A scope used to visualize the vagina.
colposcopía	colposcopy Use of a scope to visualize the vagina and cervix.
columela	modiolus A column located in the cochlea.
columela vertebral	vertebral column
columna posterior	posterior columns The dorsal portion of the gray matter of the spinal cord.
coluria	choluria Term indicating the presence of bile in the urine.
coma	coma A state of unconsciousness.
comatoso, comatosa	comatose Referring to a coma.
comedón	comedones The medical term for blackheads.
comensal	commensal Living in or on another organism without being a detriment.
comentario	comment
comer	eat, to
compatibilización	matching
compatible	compatible To coexist without problems.
compendio	compendium A concise summary about a subject.
comprensión	comprehension Understanding.
compresión	compression
compresión de la médula espinal	cord compression Pressure being applied to the spinal cord.
comprimido recubierto	coated tablet
compuesto	compound
común	common That which is usual.
concavidad	concavity The state of being concave.
concentración	concentration
concentración de alcohol en la sangre	blood alcohol level A quantitative measurement of the amount of alcohol in the blood.
concepción	conception The act of an egg being fertilized by sperm.

181

Spanish	English
concéntrico	concentric Referring to circles or arcs that share the same center.
concreción	concretion A hard solid mass.
concusión, conmoción cerebral	concussion Head trauma resulting in temporary loss of consciousness.
condiloma	condyloma A warty papule near the anus or vulva.
condón	condom A covering for the penis or the vagina (female condom) used during sexual intercourse that is meant to reduce the chance of pregnancy or infection.
condralgia	chondralgia Cartilaginous pain.
condritis	chondritis Cartilaginous inflammation.
condroma	chondroma Cartilaginous hyperplastic growth.
condromalacia	chondromalacia Excessive softening of the cartilages.
condromalacia rotuliana	chondromalacia of the patella Softening of the articular cartilage of the patella.
condrosarcoma	chondrosarcoma Cartilaginous tumor which exhibits rapid growth.
conducta de apetencia	feeding behavior
conducto	duct
conducto arterioso permeable	ductus arteriosus A fetal artery that communicates between the pulmonary artery and the descending aorta.
conducto arterioso permeable	patent ductus arteriosus A condition exhibited by failure of the ductus arteriosus (communication between the aorta the the pulmonary artery normally noted in a fetus) to close.
conducto cistico	cystic duct The duct connecting the gallbladder to the common bile duct.
conducto lactíferos	lactiferous duct A canal that carries milk.
conducto sacro	sacral canal The portion of the vertebral canal that progresses into the sacrum.
conducto semicircular	semicircular canal The anterior, posterior and lateral canals in the inner ear that assist in balance control.
conductos biliares	bile ducts The structures that are conduits for passage of bile from the liver and gallbladder to the duodenum.
confabulación	confabulation The fabrication of experiences to compensate for memory loss.
confiable	reliable
confianza	confidence
conflicto	conflict
conformidad	compliance The act of going along with a plan.
confusión	confusion
congelado	frozen
congestivo, congestiva	congestive
congénito, congénita	congenital A disease or anomaly present from birth.
conjunctivo coloración	color of conjunctiva A point of assessment to check for pallor.
conjuntiva	conjunctiva The membrane that lines the eyelid.
conjuntivitis	conjunctivitis Inflammation of the conjunctiva.
cono	cone
conocido	known
consado	tired
consanguinidad	consanguinity The relationship by blood.
consciente	conscious Being award and being able to respond to one's surroundings.
conservativo	conservative
consistente	consistent

Spanish	English
consolidación	consolidation An area of fixed secretions in the lung.
constipado	catch a cold
constricción	constriction
consumo	intake
consumo de oxígeno	oxygen consumption The body's utilization of oxygen per unit of time.
contacto	contact
contagioso, contagiosa	contagious Description of a disease that can be spread by direct or indirect contact.
contaminar	contaminate, to
contar	count, to
contenido	content
continuo	on going
contraceptivo	contraceptive A device or medication used to prevent pregnancy.
contractura de Dupuytren	Dupuytren's contracture A disease of the palmar fascia causing a flexion contracture of the fourth and fifth fingers.
contractura isquémica	ischemic contracture A muscle's resistance to passive stretch that is related to a decrease in arterial flow from any reason.
contradicción	contraindication
contradictorio	contradictory
control de la natalidad	birth control Any method of limiting contraception.
contusión	contusion An area of broken capillaries in the skin causing discoloration; commonly called a bruise.
conveniente	convenient
convexo, convexa	convex Having an exterior curved the outside of a sphere.
convulsión	convulsion An involuntary series of tonic and clonic movements.
convulsión	seizure An episode of tonic/clonic movement noted in epilepsy.
copofobia	kopophobia A morbid fear of fatigue.
copulación	copulation Sexual relations.
cor pulmonale	cor pulmonale Heart disease that is secondary to lung disease.
coracoides	coracoid A prominence on the scapula to which the biceps is attached.
corazón	heart
corcova	hunchback Synonym of kyphosis.
cordel	string
corditis	chorditis Inflammation of a vocal or spermatic cord.
cordón espermático	spermatic cord The structure containing the ductus deferens, testicular artery, and nerves that goes from the inguinal ring to the testis.
corea	chorea Involuntary, continuous rapid, jerking movements.
corea de Huntington	Huntington's chorea
corea de Sydenham	Sydenham chorea Historically known as Saint Vitus' dance, it is a childhood chorea associated with rheumatic fever.
coriza	coryza An acute condition exhibited by copious nasal discharge.
corneal	corneal Referring to the cornea.
cornete	concha A part of the body that is spiral shaped. Nasal concha are the small bones in the sides of the nasal cavity.
coroides	choroid Similar to the chorion (fertilized ovum or zygote)
coroiditis	choroiditis Inflammation of the choroid.
coroidocilitis	choroidocyclitis Inflammation of the ciliary processes and choroid.

Spanish	English
coronoide	coronoid Crown-shaped.
corpus luteum	corpus luteum A structure that is discharged from an ovary; it degenerates if it is not impregnated.
corpúsculo	corpuscle A red or white blood cell.
corriente	current
corriente	stream
corsé	brace; splint
cortada	cut
cortadura	nick
corteza suprarrenal	adrenal cortex The outer layer of the adrenal gland.
corteza, córtex	cortex An external layer.
cortical	cortical Referring to the cortex.
corticoesteroide	corticosteroid A hormone developed in the adrenal cortex.
corticotropina	corticotropin A hormone of the adrenal cortex.
cortisol	cortisol An adrenal cortical hormone, also called hydrocortisone.
cortisona	cortisone An adrenal cortical hormone responsible for carbohydrate regulation.
cosquilleo	tickle
costado	side
costilla	rib
costo	cost
costocondritis	costochondritis Inflammation of the rib and or its cartilage.
costra	crust
coxalgia	coxalgia Pain in the hip.
cóccix	coccyx The small bone formed by the natural fusion of rudimentary vertebrae.
cóclea	cochlea The essential organ of hearing which is in a spiral form.
cólera	cholera An infectious disease exhibited by vomiting and diarrhea and caused by Vibrio cholerae.
cólico	colic Acute abdominal pain.
cólico nefrítico	renal colic Pain caused by passage of a calculus through the ureter.
cóndilo	condyle A rounded protrusion of a bone.
córnea	cornea The transparent segment located at the anterior part of the eye.
craneal	cranial Referring to the skull.
craneoclasto	cranioclast An instrument used to crush a fetal skull.
craneofaringioma	craniopharyngioma A tumor that originates in the hypophyseal stalk.
craneosinostosis	craniosynostosis Closure of the sutures of the skull that occurs prematurely.
craneotabes	craniotabes Softening of the skull bones causing widened sutures; this occurs in rickets.
craneotomía	craniotomy Surgical creation of a hole in the skull.
craurosis vulvar Leucocraurosis.	kraurosis vulvae Dryness and shrinkage of the vulva.
cráneo	cranium The skeleton of the head.
creatina	creatine A compound involved with muscle contraction.
creatinina	creatinine A compound excreted in the urine that is produced by the metabolism of creatine.
crenoterapia	crenotherapy A form of treatment from mineral springs.
cresta acústica	acoustic crest A prominence on ampulla of the semicircular ducts.

Spanish	English
cresta ilíaca	iliac crest The upper border of the ilium.
cretinismo	cretinism A chronic condition caused by diminished thyroid hormone secretion.
cribiforme	cribriform Like a sieve; the olfactory nerves pass through the cribriform plate of the ethmoid bone.
cricoideo	cricoid The ring-shaped cartilage of the larynx
criestesia	cryesthesia Abnormal sensitivity to cold.
criocirugía	cryosurgery The application of extreme cold to destroy tissue.
crioterapia	cryotherapy The use of cold for therapeutic purposes.
criptorquismo	cryptorchism A condition characterized by the failure of the testes to descend into the scrotum.
criptosporidiosis	cryptosporidiosis A parasitic related diarrhea seen in AIDS.
cristaloide	crystalloid A substance that can pass through a semipermeable membrane; not a colloid.
cristaluria	crystalluria The presence of crystals in the urine.
Crohn, enfermedad de	Crohn's disease
cromatina	chromatin A desocyribose nucleic acid that carries the genes of inheritance.
cromosoma	chromosome A structure in the nucleus of living cells that carries genetic information.
crónico, crónica	chronic When referring to an illness, it means recurring or persistent.
cruciforme	cruciform Shaped like a cross.
crup	croup An acute laryngeal condition that is accompanied by a hoarse, barking cough.
crural	crural; femoral Referring to the femur or leg.
cruzamiento	decussation An area of intersection.
cuadriplejía	quadriplegia Paralysis of all four extremities.
cuadro clínico	clinical signs Physical assessment data.
cuarentena	quarantine A place of isolation for infectious persons until it can be certain it is safe to let them mingle.
cuarto	room; chamber
cuádriceps	quadriceps The anterior thigh muscle composed of four muscles.
cubitus	cubitus 1. The bend at the elbow. 2. Ulna.
cucaracha	cockroach
cucharada	spoonful
cucharada	tablespoon
cucharadita	teaspoon
cuello	neck
cuello del útero	cervix uteri The narrow end of the uterus.
cuello rígido	stiff-neck
cuenta	bill
cuerda	chorda A cord or sinew.
cuerdas vocales	vocal cords
cuero cabelludo	scalp
cuerpo calloso	corpus callosum A point of connection between the two cerebral hemispheres.
cuerpo celular	cell body
cuerpo ciliar	ciliary body The connection between the iris and the choroid.

185

Spanish	English
cuerpo geniculado	geniculate body Protrusions on the thalamus that relay visual and auditory signals to the brain.
cuerpos cuadrigéminos	quadrigeminal bodies The cranial and caudal colliculi.
cuerpos extraños	foreign bodies Term used to describe objects found in a body orifice that are not part of the body.
cuidado de heridas	wound care
cuidado intensivo	intensive care
cuidado prenatal	prenatal care Medical care received while one is pregnant.
culdoscopía	culdoscopy Examination of the female pelvic viscera with a scope inserted through the posterior vaginal fornix.
culebrilla	shingles Herpes zoster.
cultivo	culture The growth of bacteria in artificial medium.
cumplir	comply, to
cuna	cradle
cuneiforme	cuneiform The three bones between the navicular bone and the metatarsals.
curación	cure
curación	healing
curare	curare A toxic botanical substance used at one time in poison darts in South America. Curare derivatives have been used in general anesthesia.
curativo	curative A remedy capable of healing completely.
cureta	curette The instrument used during a curettage.
curetaje	curettage Removal of tissues from a cavity.
curso de la vida	lifetime
cutáneo, cutánea	cutaneous Referring to the skin.
cuticula	cuticle The dead skin at the base of the toenail or fingernail, also called the eponychium.
dacriadenitis	dacryoadenitis Inflammation of the lacrimal gland.
dacriocistitis	dacryocystitis Inflammation of a lacrimal sac.
dacriocistorrinostomía	dacryocystorhinostomy Surgical reaction of a communication between the lacrimal sac and nasal cavity.
dacriolito	dacryolith A stone in the lacrimal sac or duct.
dar	hit
dar a conocer	aquaint
dar a luz	bear, to To give birth to a child.
dar de alta	hospital discharge
de aquí	hence
de avanzada edad	elderly
de bacterium	bacteria Plural for any organism of the order Eubacteriales.
de larga acción	long acting
de larga duración	long-standing
de pie	standing
de tubos de sangre	blood tubing (used for infusion of blood)
debajo	under; infra Sometimes used when indicating a patient is "under treatment" for a condition (active treatment).
debido a	owing to
debilidad	debility Physical weakness.
debilidad	muscle weakness

Spanish	English
debilidad	weakness
decapitación	decapitation The physical separation of the head from the body.
decidua	decidua The mucous membrane lining the uterus during pregnancy.
decilbelio	decibel A unit used in the measurement of sound.
declaración	statement
declinación	decline
dedo	finger
dedo	digit Finger.
dedo del pie	toe
dedo en garra	hammer toe A condition characterized by extension of the proximal phalanx and flexion of the second and distal phalanges.
dedo en gatillo	trigger finger
dedo en maza	mallet finger Flexion contracture of the distal phalanx.
dedo en palillo de tambor	clubbing Increase in the mass of the soft tissue of the terminal phalanges.
dedo gordo del pie	hallux Referring to the first toe.
defecación	defecation The discharge of feces from the rectum.
defecto	defect
defecto del tabique ventricular	ventricular septal defect An abnormal communication between the right and left ventricles via a hole in the septum.
defecto septal atrial	atrial septal defect An abnormal communication between the atria of the heart.
defectuoso	impaired
defensa	guarding A symptom used to describe a patient resisting an examination because of severe pain; often seen in patients with peritonitis.
deficiencia	deficiency
deformidad	deformity
deglución	deglutition The process of swallowing.
deglutir	swallow, to
delantal	apron
delgado	thin
delirio	delusion A belief that is contradictory to rational thought.
delirium	delirium An acute mental state exhibited by altered thought processes and restlessness.
delirium tremens	delirium tremens A condition seen when alcohol is withdrawn which is exhibited by restlessness, hallucinations and tremors.
deltoideo, deltoidea	deltoid A term referring to "three". The deltoid muscle has its origin at three areas: clavicle, acromion, and spine of the scapula.
delusorio	delusional Referring to a delusion.
demarcación	demarcation Having a fixed boundary.
demencia	dementia A chronic brain disorder exhibited by memory loss, personality changes and faulty reasoning.
demografía	demography The study of the structure of human populations.
demulcente	demulcent Something that relieves irritation or inflammation.
dendrita	dendrite Impulses are transmitted along a dendrite to a nerve cell body.
dengue	dengue A mosquito-borne viral disease exhibited by fever and joint pain.
densidad	density The denseness of an object.
dentado	dentatum Also referred to as nucleus dentatus.

187

Spanish	English
dentadura	denture A frame that holds artificial teeth.
dental	dental Referring to teeth.
dentición	dentition The natural teeth.
dentición secundaria	permanent teeth
dentista	dentist A professional capable of treating diseases of the teeth and gums.
dentro de	inside
depilatorio	depilatory An agent used to remove hair.
depravación	deprivation The lack of a necessity.
depresión	depression A medical condition exhibited by profound despondency.
depresor de lengua	tongue depressor; tongue blade As the name implies, the stick pushes the tongue down so the posterior aspect of the mouth can be viewed more readily.
deprimido, deprimida	depressed
derecho	right
dermatitis	dermatitis Non-specific inflammation of the skin.
dermatografía	dermatography A description of the skin.
dermatología	dermatology The medical profession involving the treatment of skin conditions.
dermatoma	dermatome The area of sensation of the skin supplied by a single posterior spinal root.
dermatomicosis	dermatomycosis An infection of the skin by Trichophyton, Microsporum or Epidermophyton fungi.
dermatomiositis	dermatomyositis Inflammation of the skin, subcutaneous tissue and adjacent muscle.
dermatosis	dermatosis Any skin disease.
dermatosis actínico	actinic dermatosis A skin disease caused by exposure to radiation from the sun, ultraviolet waves or gamma radiation.
dermatófito	dermatophyte A fungal parasite living on the skin.
dermatólogo	dermatologist A physician specializing in dermatology.
dermis, piel	dermis The "true skin" that lies beneath the epidermis.
dermografía	dermographia A raised, pale line with hyperemic borders is elicited upon scratching the skin with a dull instrument, in this condition.
derrame pleural	pleural effusion
desaparecimiento	disappearance
desarreglo	disorder Impairment.
desarreglo emocional	behavior disorder An abnormal mental state.
desarrollo	growth
desarticulación	disarticulation The separation or amputation of a joint.
desbridamiento	debridement
descamación	desquamation The shedding of skin in flakes or sheets.
descanso	rest
descendencia	offspring
descendente	descending
descerebrado	decerebrate The removal of the brain.
descompensación	decompensation The inability of an organ to respond to functional overload.
descompresión	decompression The surgical procedure relieving pressure on a part.
desconocido	unknown
desecación	desiccation The act of drying up.

Spanish	English
desechar	ruling out
desensibilizar	desensitize, to To gradually expose a person to an offending agent to prevent an abnormal response upon a secondary exposure.
desequilibrio	disequilibrium The absence of stability.
desfibrilador	defibrillator A device used to convert an abnormal cardiac rhythm (ventricular fibrillation) into a normal rhythm with use of electrical stimulation.
desgarramiento	tear Referring to a vaginal tear after childbirth.
deshidratación	dehydration
desinfectante	disinfectant A substance that kills bacteria.
desmayo	blackout Common term for loss of consciousness.
desmayo	faint Weak and dizzy.
desmoide	desmoid A tumor typically found in the abdomen which contains. muscle and connective tissue.
desnervado	denervated To remove nerve supply.
desnudar	disrobe, to
desnutrición	malnutrition Lack of appropriate nutrition.
desorden	dysfunction
desorientación	disorientation Mental confusion.
despecho	despite
despedida	parting
despertamiento	awakening
desplazamiento	displacement Movement from normal position.
despuntado, despuntada	blunt
destoxificación	detoxification The process of removing toxins from the body.
desviación	deviation Away from the norm.
deterioración	deterioration
deterioro	impairment
determinación de grupos sanguineos	blood grouping Testing blood to determine which type should be used for transfusion.
determinación del grupo sanguíneo	ABO system The system using human blood antigens to determine blood type.
determinar	ascertain, to Synonym of "to determine".
detrito	detritus Particulate matter produced by the decomposition of an organic substance.
detrusor urinario	detrusor urinae Smooth muscle fibers that extend from the urinary bladder to the pubis.
deuteranomalía	deuteranomaly Abnormal color vision sometimes called "green weakness".
deviación precordiales	chest leads
dextráa	dextran A high glucose polymer used as a plasma substitute.
dextrocardía	dextrocardia Location of the heart in the right hemithorax.
débil	weak
década	decade
diabetes insípidia nefrógena	diabetes insipidus Caused by a deficiency in vasopressin, it is exhibited by great thirst and large volume urine output (and normal blood sugar).
diabetes mellitus	diabetes mellitus A disease exhibited by a deficiency of the pancreatic hormone insulin.
diabético, diabética	diabetic A person who has diabetes mellitus.

189

Spanish	English
diaforético	diaphoretic Exhibited by profuse perspiration.
diafragma	diaphragm The muscular separation between the thoracic and abdominal cavities.
diagnóstico	diagnostic A specific symptom or characteristic.
diagnóstico diferencial	differential diagnosis A list of possible alternative diagnoses for a patient who is ill.
diagnóstico doble	dual diagnosis Term used to describe the presence of alcohol/drug addicition associated with a psychiatric diagnosis such as depression.
diapasón	tuning fork A device used to distinguish between perceptive and conductive hearing loss.
diapédesis	diapedesis The outward passage of blood elements through an intact vessel wall.
diarrea	diarrhea Increase in frequency and a loose consistency of the stools.
diartrosis	diarthrosis An articulation allowing free movement.
diastasa	diastase Amylase.
diatermia	diathermy The use of heat produced from high-frequency electric currents to medically or surgically treat someone.
diáfisis	diaphysis The central part of a long bone.
diámetro conjugado del estrecho inferior de la pelvis	conjugate diameter A pelvic inlet measurement used to determine whether a woman is capable of delivering a fetus vaginally.
diástesis	diathesis A medical tendency to develop a specific condition.
diástole	diastole The period of dilatation of the heart; between the first and second heart sounds.
diente	tooth
diente molar	molar teeth The most posterior teeth bilaterally which includes 8 deciduous and usually 12 permanent teeth.
diestro	dexter; right; straight; erect
dieta, régimen	diet
dietista	dietitian A professional who works with diet and nutrition.
diferencial	differential A term used to refer to the various options for diagnoses.
difteria	diphtheria A contagious bacterial disease characterized by a grey membrane on the pharynx along with respiratory or cutaneous symptoms; caused by Corynebacterium diphtheriae.
digestión	digestion The process of enzymatic breakdown of food in the alimentary canal.
digitalis	digitalis Cardiac medication derived from the leaf of Digitalis purpurea.
dilatación	dilatation The process of becoming wider or larger.
dilatador	dilator An instrument that dilates.
dilución	dilution The process of making a weaker solution.
dimercaprol	dimercaprol A medication used as a binding agent for heavy metal poisoning.
diminuto	minute Something very small.
dioptría	dioptre Referring to refraction or transmitted and refracted light.
dióxido	dioxide A compound containing two oxygen atoms.
dióxido de carbono	carbon dioxide gas
diplejía	diplegia The paralysis of both arms or both legs.
diplococo	diplococcus A bacterium that occurs in pairs including pneumococcus and Neisseria gonorrhoeae and Neisseria meningitidis.
diploide	diploid A nucleus containing two complete sets of chromosomes.

190

Spanish	English
diplopía	diplopia Double vision.
dipsomanía	dipsomania Twins that are joined at some part of their bodies.
dirección de las manecillas del reloj	clockwise
disacárido	disaccharide A type of sugar that yields two monosaccharides upon hydrolysis.
disafia	dysaphia Altered sense of touch.
disartria	dysarthria Difficulty in articulation of speech.
disbarismo	dysbarism Condition caused by a change in pressure, noted most commonly among scuba divers.
discinesia	dyskinesia Abnormal movement.
disco óptico	optic disk The area of the retina where the optic nerve enters.
disco herniado	herniated disc Prolapse of the nucleus pulposus into the spinal cord.
discondroplasia	dyschondroplasia The formation of cartilaginous and bony tumors near the epiphyses.
discoria	dyscoria A discordance in pupillary reaction.
discrasia	dyscrasia An abnormal condition, mostly referring to the blood.
discreto	discrete
disdiadococinesia	dysdiadocokinesia The inability to arrest one motor response and substitute its opposite.
disección	dissection
diseminación	dissemination To be spread or dispersed widely.
disentería	dysentery A severe form of diarrhea with blood and mucous in the stool.
disestesia	dysesthesia 1. Impairment of the sense of touch. 2. The presence of persistent pain upon receiving a light touch.
disfagia	dysphagia Difficulty in swallowing.
disfasia	dysphasia Difficulty in speaking caused by cerebral dysfunction.
disgenesia gónada	gonadal dysgenesis The lack of complete development of the gonads.
dishidrosis	dyshidrosis Disregulation of sweating
dislalia	dyslalia The absence of comprehensible speech articulation.
dislexia	dyslexia Difficulty in learning or reading written language with no effect on intelligence.
dismenorrea	dysmenorrhea Pain during menstruation.
disminución	decrease
disnea	dyspnea Difficult breathing.
disnia por esfuerzo excesivo	exercise-induced dyspnea
disolución	dissolution Disintegration.
disostosis cleidocraneal	cleidocranial dysostosis A congenital condition exhibited by abnormal ossification of the cranial bones and absence of clavicles.
dispareunia	dyspareunia Pain during sexual intercourse.
dispepsia	dyspepsia Indigestion.
dispersión	scatter
displasia	dysplasia The increase in organ size due to an increase in the number of abnormal cell types.
disponibilidad	availability
disponible	available

Spanish	English
dispotivo intrauterino anticonceptivo (DIUA)	intrauterine contraceptive device (IUD) A device used to physically prevent the implantation of a fertilized ovum.
disquecia	dyschezia Pain experienced during defecation.
distal	distal Situated away from the center of the body.
distención	distension Swollen.
distender	strain As in a muscle strain.
distensión vesical	distended bladder
distiquia	distichiasis Presence of two rows of eyelashes on one eyelid which are turned inward toward the globe.
distocia	dystocia Difficult birth caused by fetal position, narrow pelvis or lack of opening of the cervix.
distribución	distribution
distrofia muscular	muscular dystrophy A hereditary condition exhibited by progressive muscular weakness and muscle atrophy.
disuria	dysuria Difficulty or pain upon urination.
diuresis	diuresis Increased excretion of urine.
diurético	diuretic Medication which causes an increased excretion of urine.
diurno, diurna	diurnal Occurring during the day.
diverticulitis	diverticulitis Inflammation of the diverticulum.
diverticulosis	diverticulosis Presence of diverticulum.
divertículo	diverticulum A sac or pouch created by herniation of a mucous membrane in the alimentary canal.
día de ingreso	date of admission
doble	double
doblez	duplication
dolor	pain
dolor de dientes	toothache
dolor de extremidad fantasma	phantom limb pain Pain sensed in an area where one has had an amputation as though the limb is still present.
dolor de oído	earache
dolor penetrante	stabbing pain
dolor referido	referred pain Pain felt in an area distinct from the original source.
doloroso	painful
dopamina	dopamine An intermediate product in the creation of norepinephrine.
dormido	asleep
dorsal	dorsal Referring to the back or back surface.
dorsiflexión	dorsiflexion Backward bending of the foot or hand.
dorso	dorsum The back part.
dos veces	two times
dosis	dosage The frequency and amount of a medication.
dosis	dose The quantity of a medication.
dosis excesiva	overdose An above normal dose of a medication.
dosis letal	lethal dose The amount of a drug required to cause death.
dotar	endow
dracunculiasis	guinea worm A parasitic nematode worm that lives under the skin, formally called Dracunculus medinensis.
droga	drug

Spanish	English
ducha	douche Cleansing of a canal; unless otherwise specified it refers to cleansing of the vaginal canal.
ducto hepático	hepatic duct The right and left hepatic ducts join the cystic duct to form the common bile duct.
duela	fluke Parasitic nematode worm; an example is Schistosoma.
duodenal	duodenal Referring to the duodenum.
duodenectomia	duodenectomy Excision of the duodenum.
duodeno	duodenum
duodnitis	duodenitis Inflammation of the duodenum.
duramadre	dura mater The outermost covering of the brain and spinal cord.
duro	hard
echar espuma por la boca	froth at the mouth, to
echarse a perder	spoiled (for food to go bad)
eclampsia	eclampsia A maternal condition characterized by convulsions and hypertension that can lead to maternal and fetal death.
ecmnesia	ecmnesia Memory loss for recent events but retained memory of remote events.
ecocardiografía	echocardiography The use of ultrasound waves to visualize the heart and its structures.
ecolalia	echolalia The meaningless repetition of the words spoken by another person.
ectasia	ectasia Expansion or distension.
ectodermo	ectoderm The outermost layer of the three layers of the embryo.
ectópico	ectopic Abnormal position.
ectrodactilia	ectrodactylia A congenital anomaly exhibited by absence of one digit or part of a digit.
ectropión	ectropion Eversion of the eyelid, usually the lower lid.
eczema	eczema A medical condition exhibited by pruritic, red, scaly patches on the scalp, cheeks and extensor surfaces.
eczema dishidrosis	dyshidrotic eczema A dermatitis characterized by vescicobullous lesions.
edad	age
edema	edema Extravascular fluid accumulation.
edema angioneurótico	angioneurotic edema A condition exhibited by sudden edema of skin and mucous membranes.
edema de fóveo	pitting edema Edema of the lower extremities characterized by an indentation being left when the examiner applies pressure with their thumb.
edema dependiente	ankle edema or dependent edema
edema por declive	lower extremity edema
edema pulmonar	pulmonary edema Characterized by abnormal fluid buildup in the lungs.
edematoso	edematous Referring to the presence of edema.
edentado	toothless Edentulous.
educación	education
efecto acmulativo	cumulative effect A consequence of successive additions.
efecto adverso	adverse effect In reference to medication use, it is an undesirable consequence of the drug.
efecto secundario	side effect
efector	effector An organ that responds to a stimulus.

Spanish	English
efedrina	ephedrine A chemical used to treat asthma because it expands bronchial passages and used to control spinal anesthesia associated shock because it constricts blood vessels.
efelis	ephelis Medical term for the common freckle.
eficaz	efficacious Effective.
efusión	effusion The accumulation of fluid in a body cavity.
egocéntrico	egocentric Thinking of self without considering the feelings or thoughts of others.
ejaculación	ejaculation The emission of semen at the moment of sexual climax in a male.
ejecución	implementation
el óptico	optician A person who makes eyeglasses.
elastina	elastin A connective tissue-based glycoprotein.
elección	choice
electivo	elective Non-urgent and not life-saving.
electrocardiograma	electrocardiogram Display of a person's heart beat that can be used in the diagnosis of cardiac disorders.
electrodo	electrode A device used to facilitate conduction of electricity to or from a body.
electroencefalograma	electroencephalogram (EEG) A display of brain waves used in the diagnosis of brain disorders, especially epilepsy.
electroforesis	electrophoresis The movement of charged particles in a fluid that is under the influence of an electric field. This is used in testing for various maladies in the form of serum protein electrophoresis.
electrolito	electrolyte The ionized constituents including potassium, sodium, chloride and others.
electromiografía	electromyography The display of the electrical activity f muscle.
elefantiasis	elephantiasis A condition caused by nematode parasites leading to lymphatic obstruction and limb or scrotal swelling.
eliminación	removal
elixir	elixir A medical solution.
embarazo	gestation; pregnancy
embarazo	pregnancy
embarazo a término	full-term A normal length pregnancy.
embarazo ectópico	ectopic pregnancy A pregnancy that is not intrauterine.
embarazo prolongado	post-term pregnancy A pregnancy that has gone beyond the expected length of time.
embolectomie	embolectomy The removal of an embolus.
embolia gaseosa	air embolism The blockage of an artery or vein by an air bubble.
embolia grasosa	fat embolism A deposit of fat that obstructs a vessel.
embolismo	embolus A blood clot, air bubble or fatty deposit that cause obstruction of a vessel.
embolismo pulmonar	pulmonary embolism A sudden blockage of a lung artery frequently eminating from a blood clot in one's leg.
embriología	embryology The study of the embryo.
embrión	embryo The term used to describe a fertilized ovum in the first 8 weeks of development.
emetropía	emmetropia The normal correlation between eye refraction and the axial length of the eyeball.
emético	emetic An agent that induces vomiting.

Spanish	English
eminencia hipotenar	hypothenar eminence The prominence on the palm at the base of the fingers adjacent to the ulna.
eminencia tenar	thenar eminence Formed by the bellies of the abductor pollicis brevis, flexor pollicis brevis and opponens pollicis.
emoción	emotion An intense feeling.
emoliente	emollient Having softening or soothing qualities.
empatía	empathy To be concerned for and share the feelings of another.
empeine	instep The medial aspect of the foot between the ankle and the ball of the foot.
empeorar	worsen, to
empiema	empyema A collection of purulent material in a body cavity, usually referring to a thoracic empyema.
emulsión	emulsion The dispersion of one liquid into another, but it is not dissolved.
enano	dwarf Abnormally small person.
enartrosis	enarthrosis The type of joint in which a spherical bone is set into the socket of another bone.
encefalinas	enkephalins Peptides found in the brain that have similar effects as the endorphins.
encefalitis	encephalitis Inflammation of the brain.
encefalocele	encephalocele The protrusion of the brain through a defect in the skull.
encefalograma	encephalography Roentgenography of the brain.
encefalomalacia	encephalomacia Abnormal softness of the brain.
encefalomielitis	encephalomyelitis Inflammation of the brain and spinal cord.
encefalopatía	encephalopathy Degeneration of cerebral function.
encefalopatía espongiforme bovina	mad cow disease Bovine spongiform encephalopathy, a disease that cause cerebral degeneration exhibited by ataxia.
encefálico	encephalic Referring to the brain.
encía	gum
enclavamiento	rabbeting The interlocking of two sections of a fractured bone.
enconarse	fester To become infected.
encondroma	enchondroma An abnormal increase in cartilage growth on the inside of bone or of other cartilage.
encopresis	encopresis Involuntary defecation.
encordamiento	chordee Downward bending of the penis.
endarteritis	endarteritis Tunica intima inflammation.
endémico	endemic When a disease is commonly found in a location or in a people group.
endocarditis	endocarditis Inflammation of the endocardium.
endocervicitis	endocervicitis Inflammation of the mucosal lining of the cervix.
endocrino	endocrine Referring to glands that secrete hormones and other chemicals into the blood.
endodermo	endoderm The innermost layer of the embryonic germ cell layers.
endometrio	endometrium The mucous membrane lining of the uterus.
endometrioma	endometrioma An isolated benign mass containing endometrial tissue.
endometriosis	endometriosis Presence of uterine mucosal tissue in the pelvis in abnormal locations.
endometritis	endometritis Inflammation of the endometrium.
endoneurio	endoneurium The tissue in a peripheral nerve that separates the individual nerve fibers.

195

Spanish	English
endorfinas	endorphins Hormones secreted that activate the body's opiate receptors and act as analgesics.
endoscopio	endoscope A device used to view the interior of a hollow organ (sigmoidoscope, gastroscope)
endotelioma	endothelioma A mass that propagates from the endothelium of blood vessels, lymphatics or serous cavities.
endotraqueal	endotracheal Within the trachea.
endógeno	endogenous Originating from within.
endrocrinología	endocrinology The study of endocrine glands and hormones.
enema	enema A procedure involving insertion of fluid into the rectum.
enema de bario	barium enema Administration of barium into the rectum followed by roentgenography to check for rectal or colon abnormalities.
enfermedad	disease
enfermedad	sickness
enfermedad cardíaca reumática	rheumatic heart disease A manifestation of rheumatic fever, frequently causing valvular dysfunction.
enfermedad causada por rasguño de gato	cat scratch fever An infectious disease characterized by local inflammation a the site of the scratch, local lymph adenopathy and fever.
enfermedad de Addison	Addison's disease A disease of the adrenal gland exhibited by anemia, hypotension and a bronze tone to the skin.
enfermedad de Alzheimer	Alzheimer's disease A dementia of unknown cause or pathogenesis.
enfermedad de Hansen	Hansen's disease Leprosy
enfermedad de Hodgkin	Hodgkin's disease
enfermedad de Köhler	Köhler's disease Malformation of the navicular bone.
enfermedad de la orina en jarabe de arce	maple syrup urine disease A condition characterized by an enzyme defect causing an increase in leucine in the urine.
enfermedad de Lobo, Lobomicosis	Lobo's disease A condition exhibited by small, red, hard papules in the sacral region caused by Lacazia loboi.
enfermedad de los cajones	caisson disease Decompression sickness.
enfermedad de los legionarios	legionnaires' disease The name was derived after an outbreak at a convention of the American Legion; it is manifested by fever, chills, dyspnea, and cough.
enfermedad de Milroy	Milroy's disease Hereditary disease exhibited by leg edema.
enfermedad de Peyronie	Peyronie's disease Curvature of the penis during an erection to to plaque.
enfermedad del movimiento	motion sickness Nausea associated with travel.
enfermedad del sueño	sleeping sickness Also called Trypanosomiasis, this disease is caused by a parasitic protozoa and transmitted by the tsetse fly.
enfermedad desmielinizante	demyelinating disease A condition characterized by the loss of myelin.
enfermedad maligna	terminal illness
enfermedad matinal Náuseas del embarazo.	morning sickness Nausea associated with pregnancy.
enfermedad mortífera	life-threatening
enfermedad peridontal	periodontal disease Present around to a tooth.
enfermedad pélvica inflamatoria	pelvic inflammatory disease Generally a bacterial infection affecting a woman with potential invovlement of the uterus, fallopian tubes, ovaries and cervix.

Spanish	English
enfermedad transmitida sexual	sexually transmitted disease (STD) A condition one obtains from another during sexual relations.
enfermedad venéreo	venereal disease A condition transmitted via sexual intercourse.
enfermera	nurse
enfermería	nursing care
enfisema	emphysema Abnormal enlargement of the airspaces distal to the terminal bronchioles.
enfriamiento	chill
enoftalmia	enophthalmos Posterior displacement of the eyeball in the orbit.
enorme	enormous Very large.
enostosis	enostosis The abnormal bony growth inside a bone or on the cortex.
enredado	involved
ensayo	assay A procedure for measuring the activity of a biological sample.
enterectomie	enterectomy Surgical resection of part of the intestine.
enteritis	enteritis Inflammation of the intestines.
enterobiasis	enterobiasis An infection caused by worms from the genus Enterobius.
enterococo	enterococcus A gram positive cocci that occurs naturally in the intestine but is pathogenic elsewhere in the body.
enterolito	enterolith A calculus of the intestine.
enteroptosis	enteroptosis Inferior displacement of the intestines in the abdomen.
enterotomía	enterotomy A surgical opening of the intestines.
entérico	enteric Referring to the intestines.
entérico intestino	enteral feeding Nutrition supplied via the alimentary canal.
entuertos	after-pains The pain experienced after childbirth caused by uterine contractions.
entumecimiento	numbness
enucleación	enucleation Surgical removal of a globe.
enuresis	enuresis Involuntary urination.
envejecimiento	aging
envenenamiento por plomo	lead poisoning The ingestion of lead, exhibited in severe cases by paralysis, encephalopathy, purple gingiva, and colic.
enzima	enzyme A compound that acts as a catalyst for reactions within cells as assists with digestion outside of cells.
eosinofilia	eosinophilia An increased number of eosinophils in the blood.
eosinófilo	eosinophil A cell with eosin stain used to designate a type of leukocyte that is elevated during allergic reactions.
ependimoma	ependymoma A tumor composed of cells that line the ventricles of the brain.
epéndimo	ependyma The glial lined covering of the cerebral ventricles and the central portion of the spinal cord.
epibléfaron	epiblepharon A condition exhibited by the eyelashes pressing against the eyeball.
epicardio	epicardium The serous membranous, innermost lining of the pericardium.
epicondilitis	epicondylitis Inflammation of the epicondyle.
epicóndilo	epicondyle A protrusion at the distal end of the humerus.
epicráneo	epicranium The skin, fibrous layer (aponeurosis), and muscles lining the scalp.
epidemia	epidemic Ubiquitous development of an infectious disease.
epidemiología	epidemiology The study of the incidence, development and control of disease.
epidermis	epidermis The skin cells overlying the dermis.

197

Spanish	English
epidermofitosis	epidermophytosis A fungal skin infection caused by an organism from the genus Epidermophyton.
epididimitis	epididymitis Inflammation of the duct that moves sperm from the testis to the vas deferens.
epididimoorquitis	epididymo-orchitis Inflammation of the epididymis and the testis.
epidural	epidural The space around the dura of the spinal cord.
epiescleritis	episcleritis Inflammation of the tissue lying above the sclera.
epifisitis	epiphysitis Inflammation of the end of a long bone that is separated from the shaft by a cartilaginous disc.
epigastrio	epigastrium The section of the abdomen that overlies the stomach.
epiglotis	epiglottis Tissue at the base of the tongue that covers the trachea when one swallows.
epilación	epilation Removal of hair and the roots.
epilepsia	epilepsy A condition associated with abnormal brain activity and exhibited by sudden, recurrent convulsions, sensory disturbances and loss of consciousness.
epileptiforme	epileptiform Being similar to epilepsy.
epileptogénico	epileptogenic That which induces seizures.
epinefrina	epinephrine A hormone secreted by the adrenal gland.
epiplón	omentum A fold of peritoneum fastening the stomach to other organs in the viscera.
episiotomía	episiotomy A surgical incision of the vagina used to aid childbirth.
epispadius	epispadias A congenital condition characterized by the urethral meatus being at the superior aspect of the penis
epistaxis	epistaxis Bleeding emanating from the nose.
epistaxis	nosebleed Epistaxis.
epitelial	epithelial Referring to the epithelium.
epitelio	epithelium The tissue lining the skin and the gastrointestinal tract that is derived from the embryonic ectoderm and endoderm..
epitelioma	epithelioma A malignant tumor composed of epithelial cells.
epitróclea	epitrochlea The medial condyle of the humerus.
epífisis cerebral	epiphysis cerebri A small structure situated on the mesencephalon between the two sections of the thalamus.
equilibrio	equilibrium When opposing forces are in balance.
equilibrio	steady state In equilibrium.
equilibrio ácido-base	acid-base balance The equilibrium of the electrolytes in the body.
equimosis	ecchymosis Skin discoloration caused by bleeding beneath the epidermis.
Equinococo	Echinococcus A tapeworm of the family Taeniidae that can cause hydatid cysts.
equipo	equipment
ERGE enfermedad del reflujo gastroesofágico	GERD gastroesophageal reflux disease
ergonomía	ergonomics The study of workplace design that focuses on reducing work-related injuries.
ergosterol	ergosterol A compound converted to vitamin D2 upon exposure to ultraviolet light.
ergómetro	ergometer A device that measures energy expenditure.
erguido	upright

Spanish	English
erisipelas	erysipelas An acute infection caused by Streptococcus pyogenes that causes fever along with swelling and inflammation. The infection frequently effects the face or one leg.
eritema de los pañales	diaper rash
eritema multiforme	erythema mutliforme A skin condition exhibited by purpuric lesions and bullae usually on the distal parts of extremities but can affect the face and trunk.
eritema nudoso	erythema nodosum The presence of red or purple nodules on the pretibial area.
eritroblasto	erythroblast A nucleus containing immature erythrocyte.
eritroblastosis	erythroblastosis fetalis A hemolytic disease of the newborn.
eritrocianosis	erythrocyanosis A condition exhibited by purple patches with asymmetric swelling, pruritis and burning.
eritrocito	erythrocyte Called a red blood cell, it transports oxygen and carbon dioxide to and from the tissues.
eritrocitosis	erythrocytosis A higher than normal level of erythrocytes in the blood stream.
eritropoyesis	erythropoiesis The production of red blood cells.
erliquiosis	ehrlichiosis A tickborne infectious disease.
erosión	erosion The gradual destruction of surface tissue.
error, falta	error
ertitrocitopenia	erythrocytopenia Low level of erythrocytes in the blood stream.
eructación	eructation A belch or burp.
erupción	rash
erupción	skin rash
erupción por drogas	drug eruption A diffuse rash caused by a medication.
es decir	i.e. A latin derived abbreviation for "that is to say"(In latin: id est)
escafocefalia	scaphocephaly A condition exhibited by a long narrow skull because of early closure of the sagittal sutures.
escafoide	scaphoid bone The most lateral of the carpal bones; it articulates with the radius.
escala de coma de Glasgow	Glasgow coma scale A scale used to grade one's level of consciousness with a score of 3 being totally unresponsive and a score of 15 being normal.
escalapo, bisturí	bistoury; scalpel A surgical knife.
escaldaura	scalding A burn injury from extremely hot water.
escalpelo	scalpel A knife used during surgery for incision of skin and tissue.
escama	squama A scale or platelike body.
escamoso	squamous Scaly.
escapulagia	scapulalgia Scapular pain.
escara	eschar Dry, hard, dead tissue commonly seen with a chronic pressure ulcer or anthrax.
escarificación	scarification Multiple small scratches of the skin, as is sometimes used for vaccine administration.
escápula	scapula Medical term for the shoulder blade.
escirro	scirrhus A cancer that is hard to palpation.
escíbalo	scybalum A hard, dry formation of stool in the bowel.
escleritis	scleritis Inflammation of the eyeball.
esclerodactilia	sclerodactylia Scleroderma of the digits.
esclerodermia	scleroderma A systemic disease of the connective tissues.

Spanish	English
esclerosis múltiple	multiple sclerosis A chronic neurologic disease exhibited by numbness, vision and speech problems, and motor incoordination.
esclerosis tuberosa	tuberous sclerosis An inherited neurocutaneous disorder exhibited by benign hamartomas of the brain, lung, kidney, skin and other organs.
esclerotomía	sclerotomy Surgical incision of the sclera.
escoliosis	scoliosis A lateral curvature of the spine.
escopofilia	scopophilia Sexual please attained by viewing sexual organs.
escorbuto	scurvy A disease of vitamin C deficiency exhibited by bleeding gums.
escotoma	scotoma A blind spot within an otherwise normal visual field.
escólex	scolex The front end of a tapeworm.
escrotal	scrotal Referring to the scrotum.
escroto	scrotum The sac which contains the testes.
escrófula	scrofula Cervical tuberculous lymphadenitis.
escrutinio	screening
escrutinio familiar	family history
escudo	shield
escútulo	scutulum A crust of tinea capitis.
esencial	essential
eserina	eserine Physostigmine.
esferocito	spherocyte An erythrocyte without the usual central pallor; it is noted in spherocytosis and some hemolytic anemias.
esferocitosis	spherocytosis The presence of spherocytes in the blood.
esferocitosis hereditario	hereditary spherocytosis A familial hemolytic disease exhibited by abnormally thick erythrocytes.
esfigmomanometría	sphygmomanometer Device for measuring blood pressure.
esfinterotomía	sphincterotomy Surgical incision of the anal sphincter.
esfínter	sphincter
esfuerzo	effort
esguince	sprain
esmegma	smegma A thick curdled secretion found around the clitoris and the prepuce.
esofagectomía	esophagectomy Surgical removal of the esophagus.
esofagitis	esophagitis Inflammation of the esophagus.
esofagoscopia	esophagoscopy Visual inspection the esophagus utilizing a scope.
esofágico	esophageal Referring to the esophagus.
esotropia	esotropia Medial deviation of the eye at primary gaze.
esófago	esophagus The muscular tube that connects the throat to the stomach.
espacio muerto	dead space The area in the respiratory tract where air is not exchanged.
espacio muerto anatómico	anatomical dead space
espacio muerto fisiológico	physiologic dead space
espasmo	spasm
espasmo carpopedal	carpopedal spasm A spasm of the carpus and the foot.
espasmo de torsión	torsion spasm Also called dystonia musculorum deformans, a genetic condition exhibited by twisting contortions sideways and forward while walking.
espasmo muscular	twitch

200

Spanish	English
espasmolítico	spasmolytic A substance that diminishes spasms.
espasticidad	spasticity Refers to continuous spastic movement.
espástico	spastic Stiff, awkward movement of the muscles.
específico	specific
espectrometría	spectrometry The use of a device to measure spectra.
espectroscopio	spectroscope A device for producing and recording spectra.
espejo	mirror
espejuelos	eyeglasses
esperar	expect, to
esperatogénesis	spermatogenesis The production of spermatozoa.
esperma	sperm
espermatocele	spermatocele A cyst in the epididymis containing spermatozoa.
espermatozoide	spermatozoon A mature male germ cell that is capable of fertilizing an ovum.
espermicida	spermicide A substance capable of killing sperm.
espesar	inspissate, to To thicken or congeal.
espéculo	speculum A device used to open a canal, like the vagina, for inspection.
espina	spine The spinal column or a thorny protrusion.
espinal	spinal Referring to the spine.
espinilla	shin
espirógrafo	spirograph A device used to record respiratory movements.
espirómetro	spirometer A device used to measure pulmonary capacity.
espícula	spicule A sharp, slender part.
esplenectomía	splenectomy Surgical excision of the spleen.
esplenomegalia	splenomegaly An abnormally enlarged spleen.
esplénico	splenic Referring to the spleen.
espolón calcáneo	calcaneal spur A bony protrusion on the calcaneus.
espondilitis	spondylitis Inflammation of the vertebrae.
espondilitis anquilosante	ankylosing spondylitis A type of arthritis found in the spine that is exhibited by bony fusion.
espondilolistesis	spondylolisthesis The overlapping of one vertebra over another.
espondilólisis	spondylolysis Dissolution of the vertebra.
espongiosis	spongiosis Edema of the spongy layer of the skin.
esponja	sponge
espontáneo	spontaneous
esporotricosis	sporotrichosis A Sporotrichum schenckii infection manifested by formation of lymphatic and subcutaneous nodules.
espuma	foam
espuma	froth
esputo	sputum A mixture of respiratory tract secretions and saliva.
esqueleto	skeleton
esquema	scheme
esquistocito	schistocyte Part of a red blood cell seen in hemolytic anemia.
esquistosomiasis	schistosomiasis A condition, sometimes known as bilharzia, which involves infestation with flukes of the genus Schistosoma.
esquizofrenia	schizophrenia A chronic mental condition exhibited by delusions, hallucinations, and faulty perception.
estadificación	staging Refers to a stratification of cancer for example.

Spanish	English
estado	state
estado	status
estado antecesor	prior status Referring to a person's previous state of health.
estado de condición	status of illness
estado nutrición	nutritional status
estafiloma	staphyloma Protrusion of the cornea due to inflammation.
estafilorrafia	staphylorrhaphy Surgical repair of a defect between the soft palate and uvula.
estapedectomía	stapedectomy Surgical excision of the stapes.
estapedio	stapedius muscle Located in the tympanic interior, it reduces stapedial movement.
estasis	stasis Lack of movement.
estático	static Not changing.
esteatorrea	steatorrhea Excrement with an abnormally high fat content.
esteatosis	steatosis Fatty degeneration; when referring to the liver it involves invasion of fat into hepatocytes.
estenosis	stenosis Narrowing of an orifice.
estenosis mitral	mitral stenosis Narrowing of the left atrioventricular orifice.
estenosis o estrechamiento	aortic stenosis Narrowing of the aortic orifice.
estenosis pulmonar	pulmonary stenosis A stricture between the pulmonary artery and the right ventricle.
estercobilina	stercobilin A substance created by the reduction of bilirubin and gives excrement the brown hue.
estereognosis	stereognosis The ability to identify an object by touch.
esterilización	acyesis Feminine sterility.
esterilización	sterilization A procedure done to prevent production of offspring.
esternal	sternal Referring to the sternum.
esternocleidomastoideo	sternocleidomastoid The pair of muscles that connect the sternum, clavicle and mastoid process.
esternón	sternum
esterol	sterol Unsaturated steroid alcohols such as cholesterol.
estetoscopia	stethoscope Device used to auscultate the heart, lungs and over arteries to assess for abnormalities.
estéril	sterile 1. Infertile 2. Refers to equipment that is free of contamination.
estilete	stylet A thin wire within a catheter that is removed after the catheter is in place.
estimulación artificial	cardiac pacing Electromechanical stimulation of the heart.
estomacalgia	stomach pain
estomatitis aftosa	aphthous stomatitis Grouped small lesions that occur on the tongue or in the mouth.
estornudar	sneeze, to
estómago	stomach
estrabismo	strabismus An anomaly of ocular movement.
estrabismo convergente	Esotropia or commonly "cross-eyed".
estrechez	stricture
estrellado	stellate ganglion Formed by the seventh cervical, eighth cervical and first thoracic ganglia.
estremecimiento	shiver

202

Spanish	English
estreñimiento	constipation A condition exhibited by difficulty in having a bowel movement due to hard stools.
estribo	stapes This auditory ossicle is the innermost of three ossicles and is shaped like a stirrup.
estribo	stirrup An attachment to an exam table where a woman puts her legs to assist examination of the genitalia.
estridor	stridor
estría	stria A narrow bandlike body.
estroma	stroma A term used to describe the framework of an organ.
estrógeno	estrogen A hormone involved with developing and maintaining female sexual characteristics.
estupor	stupor
etanol	ethanol Synonym for ethyl alcohol.
etmoides	ethmoid A bone at the root of the nose which has perforations for the olfactory nerves to transit.
etología	etiology
eunuco	eunuch A man who has been castrated.
eutanasia	euthanasia Killing someone painlessly who is thought to have a terminal condition.
evacuación	evacuation The emptying of an organ of fluids or gas.
evacuar	void
evaluación	assessment An evaluation.
evaluación	evaluation
evantración	eventration Protrusion of the intestines from the abdomen.
eversión	eversion To turn outward.
evidente	evident Obvious.
evisceratión	evisceration The removal of bowels from the body.
evitable	avoidable
evulsión	evulsion Forcible extraction.
ex-sanguinotransfusión	exchange transfusion Treatment of hyperbilirubinemia in neonates.
exacerbación	exacerbation Worsening of an existing problem.
examen	examination
examen fisico	physical exam
examen rectal digital	rectal digital examination Use of a gloved finger to assess the rectal vault.
examinar para	check for, to
exantema	exanthema A rash that accompanies a disease or fever.
excavació rectouternia	Douglas' pouch A recess in the peritoneum between the rectum and the uterus. Also called the rectouterine pouch.
excesivamente pesado	overweight
exceso	excess
excipiente	excipient An inactive substance used to deliver an active substance.
excitación	arousal Awaken an emotion.
excondroma	ecchondroma Hyperplastic growth of cartilage on the surface of other cartilage.
excoriación	excoriation Superficial loss of skin.
excreta	excreta Fecal material.
excretmento	excrement Feces.

Spanish	English
exfoliación	exfoliation The shedding of scales.
exhumación	exhumation The process of removing a dead body from a grave.
exigente	demanding
exomphalos	exomphalos Umbilical hernia.
exophthalmic goiter	Graves' disease A form of hyperthyroidism exhibited by a goiter and exophthalmos.
exotoxina	exotoxin A toxin released from a living cell.
exotropía	exotropia A type of strabismus that is characterized by the eyes turned outward.
exógeno	exogenous Referring to external factors.
exóstosis	exostosis A bony prominence growing from the surface of a bone.
expansión	expansion
expectativa de vida	life expectancy
expectoración	expectoration The presence of sputum that has been coughed out.
expectoración	spitting
expectorante	expectorant A substance that promotes the secretion of sputum.
expiratorio	expiratory Referring to exhalation of air from the lungs.
expulsión	expulsion Evacuation or elimination.
expulsión de la placenta	expulsion of placenta
extender	extend
extendido	widespread
extensión	extension Going from a bent to straight position.
extensor	extensor Referring to the extension of an extremity or part of an extremity.
extenteración	exenteration Complete surgical removal of an organ.
extenuación	emaciation Abnormally thin and weak.
exterior	external Outside of the body.
extirpar	extirpate To totally destroy.
extracapsular	extracapsular Situated outside a capsule.
extracelular	extracellular Outside the cell.
extracto	extract A substance in a concentrated form.
extraño	strange
extrasístole	extrasystole
extravasación	extravasation Referring to a situation in which blood or fluid goes out of a vessel it is normally flowing into.
extremidad	extremity
extremidad superior	upper limb
extrínseco	extrinsic Coming from outside or external sources.
exudado	exudate The fluid, cells, and debris found in the tissues or a cavity (like pleural space) during inflammation.
exudar	ooze To slowly leak.
éxito	success
faceta	facet A small flat surface of a bone.
facies	facies A facial expression that is typical for a particular disease.
factor antihemofílico	antihemophilic factor Also called factor VIII. A deficiency of the factor causes hemophilia.
factor antinuclear	antinuclear factor Also called antinucleic antibody (ANA); it is found in conditions such as lupus and rheumatoid arthritis.

Spanish	English
factor de liberación de la hormona de crecimiento	growth hormone-releasing factor
factor natriurético auricular	atrial natriuretic factor A chemical secreted by the right atrium that promotes sodium excretion in the urine.
fagocito	phagocyte A cell capable of surrounding and digesting microorganisms.
fagocitosis	phagocytosis The action of a phagocyte.
falange	phalanx
falciforme	falciform Referring to something that is curved. The falciform ligament attaches the liver to the diaphragm.
falta de aire	air hunger
falx cerebri	falx cerebri A fold in the dura that separates the two cerebral hemispheres.
familia	family
familiar	familial Referring to the family
famrmacocinética	pharmacokinetics The study of the distribution, absorption and excretion of drugs within the body.
faradismo	faradism The gradual increasing and decreasing of the amplitude of electricity.
faringe	pharynx The membranous cavity from the mouth to esophagus.
faringectomía	pharyngectomy Surgical excision of part of the pharynx.
faringitis	pharyngitis Inflammation of the pharynx.
faringitis	sore throat
faringolaringectomía	pharyngolaryngectomy Surgical removal of part of the pharynx and larynx.
faríngeo	pharyngeal Referring to the pharynx.
farmacéutico	pharmacist A professional who prepares and sells medicine through various systems, including governmental organizations like the Veterans Administration.
farmacia	pharmacy
farmacología	pharmacology The study of all aspects of medicines.
fascia	fascia The fibrous sheath enclosing a muscle or organ.
fasciculación	fasciculation Involuntary contraction of muscle fibers.
fascietomía	fasciotomy Incision into a fascia.
fascitis	fasciitis Inflammation of a fascia.
fascículo	fascicle A bundle of nerve or muscle fibers.
fascículo auriculoventricular	atrioventricular bundle Also called bundle of His.
fase terminal	end stage Terminal stage. End stage cancer means there is no cure possible and death is imminent.
fatal	fatal
favo	favus Tinea capitis caused by Trichopyton schoenleini.
febril	febrile Presence of an supraphysiologic temperature.
fecha	deadline
fecha de alta	discharge date
fecha de nacimiento	date of birth
fecha de vencimiento	expiration date
fecundidad	fecundity The capability of producing offspring quickly and frequently.
fenestración	fenestration Usually referring to a surgical window.
fenilcetonuria	phenylketonuria A hereditary condition in which a person cannot excrete phenylalanine; untreated it causes brain and spinal cord dysfunction.

205

Spanish	English
fenotipo	phenotype The visual expression exhibited by a person from the association of the genotype with the environment.
fertilidad	fertility The ability of a person to contribute to contraception.
fertilización	fertilization The melding of male and female gametes to form a zygote.
fetal	fetal Referring to the fetus.
fetichismo	fetichism The glorification of an inanimate object.
feto	fetus
fetor	fetor A foul odor.
fémur	femur The long bone in the thigh.
férula	splint A rigid support used to immobilize and extremity.
férula muñeca	cock-up splint A splint used to maintain the wrist in dorsiflexion; used for carpal tunnel syndrome.
fibra musgosas	mossy fiber Nerve fibers that surround the nerve cells of the cerebellar cortex.
fibrilación	fibrillation Uncoordinated, ineffective contraction as in atrial fibrillation.
fibrina	fibrin An insoluble protein formed when fibrinogen is acted upon by thrombin.
fibroadenoma	fibroadenoma A benign breast mass composed of fibrous and glandular tissue.
fibroblast	fibroblast A collagen producing cell in connective tissue.
fibrocondritis	fibrochondritis The inflammation of a structure composed of cartilage and fibrous tissue.
fibroelastosis	fibroelastosis The abnormal increase in growth of fibrous and elastic tissue.
fibroide	fibroid A benign mass, typically uterine, composed of fibrous and muscle tissue.
fibromatosis plantar	plantar fibromatosis Deep fascia nodules on the plantar aspect of the feet.
fibromioma	fibromyoma A mass containing fibrous and muscle tissue.
fibroscarcoma	fibrosarcoma A sarcoma composed primarily of malignant fibroblasts.
fibrosis cistica	cystic fibrosis A congenital disorder exhibited by abnormal thick mucous which leads to problems in the intestines, pancreas and lungs.
fibrosis cistica	fibrosis Connective tissue that is scarred and thickened after injury.
fibrositis	fibrositis Fibrous connective tissue that is inflammed.
fiebre	fever
fiebre aftosa	foot and mouth disease A contagious viral disease exhibited by oral and digital vesicles.
fiebre amarilla	yellow fever A viral, hemorrhagic fever transmitted by mosquitos.
fiebre ácaro	mite fever Synonym of typhus fever.
fiebre del agua negra	blackwater fever A term used to describe the fever associated with malaria when the urine is reddish-black.
fiebre del heno	hay fever An allergy exhibited by pruritis of the eyes and nose, rhinorrhea and excessive lacrimal secretion.
fiebre escarlatina	scarlet fever A condition caused by streptococci that is exhibited by fever and a bright red (scarlet) rash.
fiebre por flebótomos	sandfly fever A febrile illness transmitted by a sandfly, from the genus Phlebotomus, and found in the Mediterranean.
fiebre por garrapata	tick-borne fever A relapsing fever caused by a spirochete of the genus Borrelia.
fiebre por mordedura de rata	rat bite fever As the name implies, it is a condition exhibited by fever, nausea and skin erythema after one is bitten by a rat.
fiebre Q	Q fever A disease caused by rickettsiae from the ingestion of unpasteurized milk.

Spanish	English
fiebre recurrente	relapsing fever A recurrent bacterial infection, with fever, caused by Spirochetes.
fiebre reumática	rheumatic fever A febrile streptococcal disease causing pain and joint swelling.
fiebre terciana Fiebre de Paludismo vivax.	tertian fever A febrile syndrome caused by Plasmodium vivax which produces a fever spike every 48 hours.
fiebre tifoidea	typhoid fever A condition caused by ingestion of food or water containing salmonella typhi that is exhibited by fever and abdominal signs and symptoms.
fiebre tifus	typhus fever A rickettsiae infection exhibited by rash, fever, headache and myalgia.
fijación	fixation 1. An obsessive interest. 2. The securing of a body part.
filaria	filaria A parasitic nematode worm that is transmitted by flies and mosquitos causing filariasis.
filiforme	filiform Threadlike.
filum terminale	filum terminale The thin structure at the end of the conus medullaris which connects the spinal cord with the coccyx.
fimbria	fimbria A slender projection at the end of the fallopian tube near the ovary.
fimosis	phimosis Stricture of the prepuce preventing it from being pulled back over the glans penis.
firme, sólido	firm
fisiología	physiology A subspecialty of biology that studies the normal functioning of the body.
fisura	fissure A general term for a cleft or deep groove. An anal fissure, for example, is a small ulcer adjacent to the anus.
fíbula,peroné	fibula The smaller of two bones in the lower leg.
fístula	fistula An abnormal communication between two organs or an organ and the skin, as in rectovaginal fistula.
fístula anal	anal fistula
flagelación	flagellation 1. The protrusion found on flagella. 2. Massage administered by tapping a body part with fingers.
flagelo	flagellum A slender appendage that allows protozoa to swim.
flata de ortografía	misspelling
flato	flatus
flatunecia	flatulence The gas expulsed from the anus.
flácido	flaccid Limp. A term applied to an extremity one cannot move actively.
flebectomía	phlebectomy Surgical excision of a vein.
flebitis	phlebitis Inflammation of a vein.
flebotrombosis	phlebothrombosis Presence of a clot in a vein, without associated inflammation.
flegmasia	phlegmasia Inflammation or fever.
flemasia alba dolens	phlegmasia alba dolens Phlebitis of the femoral vein that can occur after pregnancy or typhoid fever.
flexor	flexor A muscle that bends an extremity or part of an extremity.
flexura	flexure The action of bending.
flexura esplénica	splenic flexure of the colon
flexura hepática	hepatic flexure of the colon
flexura sigmoidea	sigmoid flexure
flicentular	phlyctenular Related to the formation of small vesicles on the cornea or conjunctiva.

207

Spanish	English
fliujo aire	air flow
flojedad	laxity A description of a joint that is loose.
flotante	floating
fluido amniótico	amniotic fluid The fluid surrounding the fetus.
fluido intraocular	intraocular fluid
fluido sinovial	synovial fluid The fluid that surrounds, for example, the knee within a capsule.
flujo	flow
flujo espiratorio máximo	peak flow A measurement of lung function used in asthma.
flujo expiratorio forzado	forced expiratory flow rate Amount of air forcibly exhaled in liters per unit of time.
fluorescina	fluoresceine A fluorane dye used to check for corneal ulcers.
fluorización	fluoridation The addition of fluorine to something.
fluorocopía	fluoroscopy The continuous viewing of roentgenographic images with a fluorescent screen.
flúido endolinfático	endolymph The fluid collection the labyrinth of the ear.
flúor	fluorine A chemical that causes severe burns if exposed to the skin.
fobia	phobia An profound fear of something.
fogaje	hot flash A symptom of menopause manifested as a sudden sensation of fever.
folicular	follicular Referring to a small secretory gland.
foliculitis de la barba	barber's itch Ringworm that is transmitted by contaminated shaving equipment.
folículo piloso	hair follicle
fonación	phonation The vocalization of sounds.
fondo	fundus Referring to the upper part of the stomach or the part of the globe opposing the pupil.
fondo del ojo	eyeground The fundus that is visualized with an ophthalmoscope.
foniatría	phoniatrics The treatment of speech abnormalities.
fontanella	fontanelle or fontanel The space between the bones in the skull that are separate at birth.
foramen	foramen An opening in a bone.
foramen oval	foramen ovale A hole in the atrial septal wall in a fetus.
forense	forensic Referring to the scientific method of studying crime.
formulario	formulary A list of medicines that are permissible to prescribe.
fornix	fornix A vaulted structure.
fosa	fossa A shallow depression.
fosfatasa ácida	acid phosphatase A phosphate derived chemical that is optimally active in an acidic environment.
fosfaturia	phosphaturia Presence of phosphates in the urine.
fosfolípido	phospholipid A substance, such as lecithin, that when hydrolyzed produces fatty acids, glycerin, and a nitrogen compound.
fosfonecrosis	phosphonecrosis The breakdown of the mandible caused by excessive exposure to phosphorus.
fotofobia	photophobia Abnormal sensitivity to light.
fotosensibilización	photosensitization The process of reacting to sunlight by developing edema and dermatitis.
fotómetro de llama	flame photometer A device used to measure the intensity of light.
fórceps	forceps A surgical instrument, commonly called tweezers.

208

Spanish	English
fóvea	fovea The area on the retina where the visual acuity is optimal.
fracción por tensión	stress fracture A long bone fracture caused by repetitive mechanical stress.
fractura	break
fractura	fracture
fractura cerrada	fracture, closed
fractura communita	fracture, comminuted
fractura compuesta	compound fracture Open fracture.
fractura con hundimiento	fracture, depressed
fractura de sobrecarga	fracture, stress
fractura de tallo verde	fracture, greenstick
fractura expuesta	fracture, open
fractura patológica	fracture, pathologic
fractura por avulsión	fracture, avulsion
fragilitas ossium	fragilitas ossium A condition exhibited by excessively brittle bones. Also called osteogenesis imperfecta.
frambesia	yaws A tropical disease characterized by ulcers on the extremities, caused by Treponema pertenue.
frambesía	framboesia; yaws An endemic tropical disease caused by Treponema pertenue.
frecuencia	frequency
frecuencia cardíaca	heart rate
fremitus	fremitus A vibration that is appreciated with palpation.
freniconeurectomía	phrenicectomy Surgical excision of the phrenic nerve.
frenoplejía	phrenoplegia Paralysis of the diaphragm.
frente	forehead
frenulum	frenulum The tissue that connects the inferior portion of the tongue to the base of the mouth.
frénico	phrenic Referring to the diaphragm.
fricción	friction
frío	cold Having a sense of being cold.
frío	cool
frontal	frontal Referring to the anterior aspect, as in frontal lobe.
frotis	smear Used to refer to a specimen smeared on a slide.
fructosuria	fructosuria
fuerte	strong
fuerza	potency Strength or power.
fuerza	strength
fuerza compresiva	grip strength Quantitative measurement of the force of a hand grip.
fuga	leakage
fulminante	fulminant Sudden and severe.
fumar	smoke, to
función	function
fungi, hongo	fungus A spore-producing organism that feeds on organic matter.
fungicida	fungicide An agent that destroys fungus.
funiculitis	funiculitis Inflammation of the funiculi.
funículo	funiculi of the spinal cord The white matter of the spinal cord that is further defined by location.

Spanish	English
furunculosis	furunculosis The presence of multiple furuncles.
furúnculo	furuncle A painful erythematous nodule with a central core.
fusiforme	fusiform Spindle-shaped.
galactocele	galactocele A milk-filled cyst in the mammary gland.
galactorrea	galactorrhea Excessive production of milk.
galactosa	galactose A sugar that is a constituent of lactose.
galactosemia	galactosemie 1. Galactose in the blood. 2. A congenital condition exhibited by impaired carbohydrate metabolism.
galope	gallop An abnormal heart sound.
galvanismo	galvanism The use of electric currents for medical treatment.
galvanómetro	galvanometer A device used to measure small electric currents.
gameto	gamete A germ cell that is able to unite with another germ cell of the opposite gender to form a zygote.
gamma globulina	gamma globulin A blood serum protein with little electrophoretic mobility.
ganglio espinal	spinal ganglion The ganglion located on the dorsal root of each spinal nerve.
ganglio geniculado	geniculate ganglion The sensory ganglion of the facial nerve.
ganglio linfático	lymph node An area of organized lymphatic tissue.
ganglionectomía	ganglionectomy The removal of a benign swelling on a tendon sheath.
ganglios basales	basal ganglia Structures adjacent to the thalamus that are involved with coordination of movement.
gangrena	gangrene Tissue death from either impaired blood flow or an infection.
gangrena gaseosa	gas gangrene A life and limb threatening disorder caused associated with tissue death and caused by an anaerobic bacterium in the genus of Clostridium.
garganta	throat
gargarizar	gargle, to
gargolismo	gargoylism A congenital anomaly exhibited by mental retardation, bone deformities and an abnormally large head.
garra	talon The ball of the ankle joint.
garrapata de venado	deer tick
gasa	gauze A fabric used for dressing changes.
gastrectomía	gastrectomy Complete or partial surgical resection of the stomach.
gastrinas	gastrin Hormones that stimulates gastric secretions.
gastritis	gastritis Inflammation of the stomach.
gastrocele	gastrocele Protrusion of part of the stomach in the form of a hernia.
gastroenteritis	gastroenteritis A bacterial or viral infection that leads to vomiting and diarrhea.
gastroenterotomie	gastroenterostomy A surgical opening in the stomach or intestine.
gastronemio	gastrocnemius A large muscle in the lower leg, responsible for ankle plantar flexion, that is attached to the distal femur and achilles tendon.
gastropexia	gastropexy Securing the stomach to the abdominal wall.
gastroscopio	gastroscope A device used to directly visualize the stomach.
gastroscopía	gastrostomy A surgical creation of an opening in the stomach.
gastroyeyunostomía	gastrojejunostomy A surgical procedure that directly connects the stomach to the jejunum.
gatillo	trigger
gavaje	gavage The instillation of food into the stomach with use of a tube.
gástrico	gastric Referring to the stomach.

Spanish	English
gel	gel
gemelo monocigóticos	identical twins Twins from the same zygote.
gemelos	twins
gemelos dicigóticos	dizygotic twins Twins from two separate zygotes (non-identicle twins).
gemir	groan
gen	gene A unit of heredity that is passed on from parent to child.
general	general
genético	genetic Referring to genes or heredity.
geniculado	geniculate Bent at a sharp angle.
genitales	genitalia Genitals.
genitourinario	genitourinary
genoma	genome A full set of genetic information for an organism.
genu valgum	genu valgum A condition exhibited by the knees turning inward, commonly referred to as knock-knee.
genu varum	genu varum A condition exhibited by the knees turning outward, commonly referred to as bowleg.
geriatría	geriatrics The study of the health of old people.
germen	germ
gerontología	gerontology The study of old persons.
gestación	gestation The development of a fetus from conception until birth.
gestión	management
giardiasis	giardiasis A flagellate protozoa, Giardia lamblia, that causes diarrhea.
gigante	giant
gigantismo	gigantism Abnormally large size.
ginecología	gynecology The branch of medicine associated with the reproductive system of women.
ginecomastia	gynecomastia Enlargement of the breasts.
gingival	gingival Referring to the gums.
gingivitis	gingivitis Inflammation of the gums.
gínglimo	ginglymus A joint that allows movement in one direction only.
glabela	glabella The area of the forehead above and between the eyebrows.
glande	glans The distal aspect of the penis or clitoris.
glaucoma	glaucoma A condition characterized by increased intraocular pressure.
glándula apocrina	apocrine gland A gland that releases some of its cytoplasm in secretions; an example is axillary sweat glands.
glándula mamaria	mammary gland The mass of tissue posterior to the nipples which has the essential task of milk production.
glándula pineal	pineal gland A small body posterior to the third ventricle of the brain.
glándula pituitaria	pituitary gland
glándula sebácea	sebaceous gland A gland in the skin that secretes sebum.
glándula suprarrenal	adrenal gland A gland located on the superior aspect of both kidneys.
glándulas endocrinas	endocrine glands Glands that secrete hormones and other substances into the blood.
glándulas salivales	salivary gland The parotid, submandibular and sublingual glands that secrete saliva.
glenoideo	glenoid Referring to the fossa that is a shallow depression, such as the hollow of the scapula where the humeral head sets.

Spanish	English
glicerina	glycerin A byproduct in the manufacture of soap that is used as a laxative.
glicoproteína	glycoprotein A protein that has a carbohydrate attached to its polypeptide chain.
glicólisis	glycolysis The production of energy and pyruvic acid when glucose is broken down by enzymes.
glioma	glioma A neural malignant tumor of glial cells.
gliomioma	gliomyoma A mass with gliomatous and myomatous characteristics.
globo	glomus tumor A reddish-blue painful papule that occurs on the distal aspects of the digits.
globo pálido	globus pallidus A portion of the lentiform nucleus in the brain.
globulina antilimfocite	antilymphocyte globulin The gamma globulin portion of antilymphocyte serum.
glomerulonefritis	glomerulonephritis Inflammation of the renal glomeruli, usually from hemolytic streptococcus.
glomérulo	glomerulus A grouping of capillaries where waste is filtered from the blood.
glomo carotídeo	carotid body Carotid artery receptors that are sensitive to blood chemistry changes.
glosa, lengua	glossal Referring to the tongue.
glosectomía	glossectomy Surgical resection of the whole or part of the tongue.
glositis	glossitis Inflammation of the tongue.
glosodinia	glossodynia Tongue pain.
glosofaríngeo	glossopharyngeal The name for cranial nerve IX that supplies the tongue and pharynx.
glotis	glottis Essentially the vocal structure, including the true vocal cords and the opening between them.
glucagón	glucagon A pancreatic enzyme responsible for breakdown of glycogen to glucose.
glucemia	glycemia The amount of glucose in the blood.
glucogénesis	glycogenesis The production of glycogen from glucose.
glucosuria	glycosuria Presence of glucose in the urine.
glucógeno	glycogen A compound that stores glucose and when it undergoes hydrolysis forms glucose.
glúteo	gluteal Referring to the gluteus.
gnático	gnathic Referring to the jaws.
gnosia	gnosia Ability to recognize things and people.
goma	gumma A soft granulomatous tumor of the skin or cardiovascular system seen in tertiary syphilis.
gonadotropina	gonadotrophin Pituitary hormone that promotes gonadal activity.
gonococo	gonococcus A diploccocal bacteria that is the causative agent in gonorrhea, formally Neisseria gonorrhoeae.
gonorrea	gonorrhea A sexually transmitted disease that is exhibited by purulent discharge from the vagina or penis.
gordo, obeso	fat
gordura	fatness
gota	drop
gota	gout
gota a gota	drop by drop
gota por minuto	drops per minute

Spanish	English
gotas para los ojos	eye drops
goteo	dribble, to
goteo postnasal	post-nasal drip
gotero	dropper A device used to administer medicines one drop at a time.
gónada	gonad A testis or an ovary.
grado	grade
Graefe, signo de	Graefe's sign Also called lid lag, a sign characterized by the upper eyelid not closing over the globe. This is seen commonly in exophthalmic goiter.
gramo	gram
granulocito	granulocyte A white blood cell with cytoplasmic secretory granules.
granuloma	granuloma A mass of granulation tissue.
graso	fatty
gráfico anatómico (a)	anatomical chart A pictorial diagram of part of the anatomy.
grieta	crevice A narrow opening.
gripe de las aves	avian flu A viral disease found in birds and fowl that can be transmitted to humans; it is exhibited by respiratory and gastrointestinal symptoms but can lead to encephalitis.
gripe, influenza	influenza Viral infection causing fever, muscle aches and catarrh.
gritar	yell, to
grosero	rude
grueso	gross
gruñido	grunting A low guttural sound used to describe a person with profound respiratory difficulty.
grupo sanguíneo	blood type Determined and listed in the ABO system.
guante	glove
guardo cama	bed rest
guayaco	guaiac A substance derived from guaiacum trees used to test for trace amounts of blood, in stool for instance.
gubia	gouge A chisel with a concave blade used in surgery.
Guillan-Barré, síndrome de	Guillain-Barré syndrome An acute autoimmune disorder that causes nerve inflammation subsequently muscle weakness.
guía colorimétrica	color chart
gusano	worm
gusano látigo Trichuris trichiura.	whipworm A parasitic, intestinal nematode worm of the genus Trichuris.
gustativo	gustatory Referring to sense of taste.
gusto	taste
gutural	guttural
habla	speech
hacia adelante	forwards
halitosis	halitosis Foul odor eminating from the mouth.
hallus varus	hallux varus
hallux valgus	hallux valgus
hamartoma	hamartoma A nodule of superfluous tissue.
hambre	hunger
haploide	haploid Either a single set of chromosomes or a set of nonhomologous chromosomes.

Spanish	English
hapteno	hapten The molecular component that determines immunologic specificity.
hábito	habit
hebefrenia	hebephrenia A type of schizophrenia exhibited by hallucinations and inappropriate laughter.
heces	feces Excrement.
hedonismo	hedonism Devoting oneself to being happy.
helado	freezing (as in ambient temperature)
helio	helium An inert gas that is the lightest of the noble gases.
helioterapia	heliotherapy Treatment of disease with sunlight.
helmintiasis	helminthiasis Being infected by a helminth.
helminto	helminth A fluke, tapeworm or nematode.
hem	heme A constituent of hemoglobin that is an insoluble iron protoporphyrin.
hemangioma	hemangioma A benign tumor composed of blood vessels.
hemangioma cavernosa	cavernous hemangioma A tumor composed of connective tissue with blood filled areas.
hemartrosis	hemarthrosis Presence of intra-articular blood.
hematemesis	hematemesis Vomiting blood.
hematina	hematin The insoluble iron protoporphyrin component of hemoglobin.
hematocele	hematocele A mass or area of swelling caused by the accumulation of blood.
hematoma	hematoma A mass containing blood.
hematoma epidural	epidural hematoma Formation of a collection of blood outside the dural layer of the brain; usually caused by trauma.
hematoma subdural	subdural hematoma Formation of a blood clot between the dura mater and the arachnoid membrane.
hematomielia	hematomyelia Accumulation of blood in the spinal cord.
hematoporfirina	hematoporphyrin A derivative of heme that does not contain iron.
hematoquesia	hematochezia Presence of blood in the excrement.
hematosálpinx	hematosalpinx Presence of blood in the fallopian tube.
hematócrito	hematocrit The measurement of the volume of red blood cells compared to the total volume of blood; recorded in percent.
hematómetra	hematometra The accretion of blood in the uterus.
hematuria	hematuria The presence of blood in the urine.
hemático	hematinic A substance that increases hemoglobin in the blood.
hembra	female
hemeostasis	homeostasis The tendency of an organism to maintain a stable and uniform state.
hemeralopía	hemeralopia Night blindness.
hemianopia	hemianopsia Blindness over half the field of vision.
hemianopsia bitemporal	bitemporal hemianopsia A visual defect seen commonly in pituitary tumors in which the visual defect is in the temporal portion of each eye.
hemibalismo	hemiballismus Severe motor restlessness unilaterally, usually from a subthalamic lesion.
hemicigoto	hemizygote A cell with only one set of genes.
hemicolectomía	hemicolectomy Surgical removal of part of the colon.
hemicrania	hemicrania 1. Pain on one side of the head. 2. Incomplete anencephaly.
hemiparesis	hemiparesis Unilateral muscle weakness (half the body).
hemiplejía	hemiplegia Paralysis of one side of the body.

214

Spanish	English
hemisferio	hemisphere Referring to either the right or left portion of the cerebrum.
hemoaglutinación	hemagglutinin An antibody that facilitates the agglutination of blood.
hemocitómetro	hemocytometer A device used for counting cells from a blood sample.
hemoconcentración	hemoconcentration Decrease in the total fluid content of the blood, leading at times to a falsely elevated hematocrit.
hemocromatosis	hemochromatosis A hereditary condition exhibited by iron deposition in the tissue and leading to liver disease, bronze discoloration of the skin and diabetes.
hemodiálisis	hemodialysis The process of filtering blood outside the body to remove toxins normally excreted by functioning kidneys.
hemofilia	hemophilia A hereditary bleeding disorder characterized by hemarthroses and deep tissue bleeding as a result of absence of a coagulation factor such as factor VIII.
hemofílico	hemophiliac A person with hemophilia.
hemoftalmía	hemophthalmia Bleeding within the eye.
hemoglobina	hemoglobin An iron containing protein used for the transport of oxygen in blood.
hemoglobinuria	hemoglobinuria Presence of free hemoglobin in the urine.
hemolítico	hemolytic Something that causes hemolysis.
hemoneumotórax	hemopneumothorax Accumulation of blood and air in the pleural space.
hemopericardio	hemopericardium Abnormal presence of blood in the pericardium.
hemoperitoneo	hemoperitoneum Abnormal presence of blood in the peritoneum.
hemopoyesis, hematopoyesis	hemopoiesis The production of blood cells from stem cells.
hemopoyetina	hemopoietin A hormone secreted by the kidneys that stimulates the bone marrow to produce erythrocytes.
hemoptisis	hemoptysis Expectoration of blood.
hemorragia	hemorrhage Bleeding from a damaged blood vessel.
hemorroide	hemorrhoids Engorgement of the veins in the anus or rectum.
hemorroidectomía	hemorrhoidectomy Surgical excision of a hemorrhoid.
hemostasis	hemostasis The control of bleeding.
hemotórax	hemothrorax The abnormal presence of blood in the pleural cavity.
hemólisis	hemolysis Breakdown of hemoglobin.
hendidura vulvar	vulval cleft The area between the labia majora where the vagina and urethra rest.
heparina	heparin A polysaccharide that occurs naturally in the liver and is used as a medication to induce a hypocoagulable state.
hepatectomía	hepatectomy Partial or complete surgical resection of the liver.
hepatitis	hepatitis Inflammation of the liver.
hepatitis colestática	cholestatis hepatitis
hepatocito	hepatocyte A liver cell.
hepatoma	hepatoma A tumor of the liver.
hepatomegalia	hepatomegaly Enlargement of the liver.
hepatosplenomegalia	hepatosplenomegaly Enlargement of the spleen and the liver.
hepático	hepatic Referring to the liver.
hereditario	hereditary That which is transmitted genetically
herida	wound
herida de arma blanca	stab wound

Spanish	English
herida de bala	gunshot wound
hermafrodita	hermaphrodite A person possessing gonadal characteristics of both sexes.
hermano	sibling
hernia cerebral	brainstem herniation Movement of the brainstem into the incisura because of increased intracranial pressure.
hernia diafragmática	diaphragmatic hernia Protrusion of visceral contents through the diaphragm.
hernia femoral	hernia, femoral
hernia hiatal	hiatus hernia Protrusion of part of the stomach through the esophageal hiatus of the diaphragm.
hernia incarcerada	hernia, incarcerated
hernia inguinal	hernia, inguinal
hernia lumba	hernia, lumbar
hernia umbilical	hernia, umbilical
herniorrafía	herniorrhaphy The surgical repair of a hernia.
heroína	heroin A morphine derivative that is highly addictive.
herpangina	herpangina An infectious disease caused by Coxsackie virus exhibited by vesicular lesion on the soft palate.
herpes	herpes A skin condition exhibited by formation of clustered vesicular lesions; herpes simplex is at times referred to, albeit incompletely, as herpes.
herpes genital	genital herpes
herpes zóster	herpes zoster; shingles A unilateral vesicular rash along one dermatome and caused by inflammation of a posterior nerve root by "the chicken pox virus".
herpetiforme	herpetiform Something that is characteristic of herpes.
herpético	herpetic Referring to herpes.
heterocigótico	heterozygous Having different alleles concerning a certain trait.
heterocromía del iris	heterochromia iridis or syndrome of Eric Congenital anomaly in which the iris of each eye is of a different color.
heterogéneo	heterogenous That which originates outside the organism.
heterotopía	heterotropia Synonym of strabismus.
hialino	hyaline Having a glassy, transparent appearance.
hialoide	hyaloid Transparent.
hidatidiforme	hydatiform Referring to a hydatid cyst.
hidradenitis	hidradenitis Inflammation of a sweat gland. When there is purulent discharge it is called hidradenitis suppurativa.
hidrartrosis	hydrarthrosis An accumulation of water-like fluid in a joint cavity.
hidratación	hydration Used to describe fluid balance.
hidrocele	hydrocele The accumulation of fluid in a body sac.
hidrocele escrotal	scrotal hydrocele A benign collection of fluid in the scrotum.
hidrocéfalo	hydrocephalus The excessive accumulation of cerebral spinal fluid in the brain causing enlargement of the head.
hidrocortisona	hydrocortisone A natural steroid hormone secreted by the adrenal cortex and used in a synthetic formulation for treatment of various medical conditions.
hidrofobia	hydrophobia Abnormal fear of water.
hidroma	hygroma A cyst or bursa filled with fluid.
hidronefrosis	hydronephrosis Enlargement of a kidney due to interruption of outflow of urine from that kidney.
hidroneumotórax	hydropneumothorax Abnormal accumulation of fluid and air in the pleural space.

Spanish	English
hidropesía	hydrops The abnormal collection of fluid in a cavity.
hidropesía fetal	hydrops fetalis The total body accumulation of fluid in a fetus; the result of a hemolytic reaction in a Rh neg mother.
hidrosálpinx	hydrosalpinx Collection of fluid in a fallopian tube.
hidrosis	hidrosis The production and secretion of sweat.
hidrotórax	hydrothorax Accumulation of fluid within the thoracic cavity.
hidrólisis	hydrolysis A reaction with water causing a compound to breakdown.
hierro	iron An element found in hemoglobin.
hifema	hyphema A blood collection in the front of the eye.
higiene bucal	oral hygiene
higroscópico	hygroscopic The tendancy to absorb moisture from the air.
hija	daughter
hiliar	hilar Referring to a hilus.
hilio	hilum or hilus A depression where blood vessels and nerve fibers enter an organ.
himen	hymen A membrane in the vagina.
himenotomía	hymenotomy Surgically creating an opening in the hymen.
hinchazón	puffiness
hioides	hyoid bone
hiperacidez	hyperacidity An abnormally high acid level.
hiperactividad	hyperactivity Abnormal increase in activity.
hiperalgesia	hyperalgesia Greater than normal sensitivity to pain.
hiperbárico	hyperbaric Use of gas at a higher than normal pressure.
hiperbilirrubinemia	hyperbilirubinemia Higher than normal level of bilirubin in the blood.
hipercalcemia	hypercalcemia Higher than normal level of calcium in the blood.
hipercalemia	hyperkalemia Higher than normal level of potassium in the blood stream.
hipercapnia	hypercapnia Higher than normal level of carbon dioxide in the blood stream.
hipercinesia	hyperkinesis Excessive activity and inability to concentrate.
hipercromía	hyperchromia An excessive level of hemoglobin in erythrocytes.
hiperemia	hyperemia An increase in blood for the area of concern.
hiperesplenismo	hypersplenism Excessive splenic activity resulting in decreased peripheral blood elements and sometimes splenomegaly.
hiperestesia	hyperesthesia Higher than normal skin sensitivity.
hiperextensión	hyperextension Extension of an articulation beyond the normal range.
hiperfagia	hyperphagia Excessive food ingestion.
hiperflexión	hyperflexion Flexion of an articulation beyond the normal range.
hiperforia	hyperphoria Upward deviation of the visual axis of the eye.
hiperglucemia	hyperglycemia Higher than normal level of glucose in the blood.
hipergonadismo	hypergonadism A condition of excessive gonadal activity and subsequently precocious sexual development.
hiperhidrosis	hyperhidrosis Excessive perspiration.
hiperlipidemia	hyperlipidemia Higher than normal level of lipids in the blood stream.
hipermenorrea	menorrhagia Abnormally large amount of menstrual blood.
hipermetropía	hypermetropia Farsightedness.
hipermiotonía	hypermyotonia Excessive muscle tone.
hipermnesia	hypermnesia Unusually good memory.
hipernatremia	hypernatremia Elevated level of sodium in the blood.

Spanish	English
hipernefroma	hypernephroma A renal tumor that mimic adrenal cortical tissue.
hiperoniquia	hyperonychia Hypertrophic nails.
hiperopia	hyperopia
hiperopía. Presbicia.	longsighted Synonym of hyperopia.
hiperosmia	hyperosmia
hiperparatiroidismo	hyperparathyroidism Excessive level of parathyroid hormones in the blood stream causing weak bones and hypocalcemia.
hiperpirexia	hyperpyrexia Fever.
hiperplasia	hyperplasia Excessive growth of normal cells.
hiperpnea	hyperpnea Abnormal increase in rate and depth of respiration.
hiperqueratosis	hyperkeratosis Excessive thickening of the outer layer of skin.
hiperreflxia	hyperreflexia
hipersensibilidad	hypersensitivity Abnormal increase in sensitivity.
hipertensión	hypertension Higher than normal blood pressure.
hipertensión maligno	malignant hypertension Sudden, severe hypertension associated with neuroretinitis.
hipertermia	hyperthermia Fever.
hipertiroidismo	hyperthyroidism Increased thyroid activity resulting in exophthalmos and increased metabolic rate.
hipertituitarismo	hyperpituitarism Excessive eosinophilic hormone resulting in acromegaly or excessive basophilic hormone resulting in pituitary compression and ultimately hypopituitarism.
hipertonía	hypertonia Excessive tone or tension.
hipertónica	hypertonic Increased osmotic pressure.
hipertricosis	hypertrichosis Excessive hair growth.
hipertropia	hypertrophy Pathologic organ enlargement.
hiperuricemia	hyperuricemia Elevated level of uric acid in the blood.
hiperventilación	hyperventilation Rapid and deep respirations.
hipervolimia	hypervolemia Abnormally large amount of fluid in the blood stream.
hipnótico	hypnotic Sleep inducing agent.
hipo	hiccup
hipocalcemia	hypocalcemia Lower than normal level of calcium in the blood.
hipocalemia	hypokalemia Diminished level of potassium in the blood stream.
hipocampo	hippocampus The area at the base of the cerebral ventricles thought to be the center of memory and emotion.
hipocapnia	hypocapnia A decreased level of carbon dioxide in the blood.
hipocloridria	hypochlorhydria A state of decreased secretion of hydrochloric acid in the stomach.
hipocondriasis	hypochondriasis Abnormal increase in concern about one's own health.
hipocondrio	hypochondrium The upper abdomen lateral to the epigastrium.
hipocondríaco	hypochondriac A person suffering from hypochondriasis.
hipocromía	hypochromic Referring to the abnormal decrease in hemoglobin content of erythrocytes.
hipoestesia	hypoesthesia Abnormally decreased skin sensitivity.
hipofibrinogenemia	hypofibrinogenemia Diminished blood fibrinogen level.
hipofisectomía	hypophysectomy Surgical removal of the pituitary gland.
hipoforia	hypophoria Downward deviation of the visual axis of the eye.

Spanish	English
hipofosfatasia	hypophosphatasia A genetic defect of diminished alkaline phosphatase in the cells leading to bone demineralization.
hipogastrio	hypogastrium The area of the central abdomen located below the stomach.
hipogástrico	hypogastric Referring to the hypogastrium.
hipoglicémico	hypoglycemia Abnormally low blood sugar.
hipogonadismo	hypogonadism Abnormal decrease in gonadal function with associated diminished growth and sexual development.
hipomanía	hypomania A moderate form of mania.
hiponatremia	hyponatremia Diminished level of sodium in the blood stream.
hipoparatiroidismo	hypoparathyroidism Abnormal decrease in parathyroid function.
hipopión	hypopyon The presence of purulent fluid in the anterior chamber of the eye.
hipopituitarismo	hypopituitarism Diminished pituitary activity exhibited by obesity and persistence of adolescent characteristics.
hipoplasia	hypoplasia Incomplete development.
hiposalivación	hyposalivation Secretion of saliva below the normal rate.
hipospadias	hypospadias Congenital condition exhibited by development of the urethral meatus on the inferior aspect of the penis.
hipostasis	hypostasis The formation of a deposit.
hipotálamo	hypothalamus Located inferior to the thalamus it controls visceral activities, water balance, temperature and sleep.
hipotensión	hypotension Abnormally low blood pressure.
hipotensión postural	postural hypotension
hipotermia	hypothermia Lower than normal temperature.
hipotiroidismo	hypothyroidism Reduced functioning of the thyroid.
hipotonía	hypotonia Reduced tone or activity.
hipoxia	hypoxia Diminished oxygen content.
hipófisis	hypophysis Pituitary gland.
hirsutismo	hirsutism Abnormal growth on hair on a person's face and body.
hisopo	swab
histamina	histamine A chemical responsible for the reaction exhibited when a person has an allergic reaction.
histerectomía	hysterectomy Surgical removal of the uterus.
histeria	hysteria A psychological condition exhibited by uncontrolled emotion or exaggerated manifestations.
histerografía	hysterography 1. Recording of uterine contractions. 2. Roentgenography of the uterus after administration of contrast media.
histeromiomectomía	hysteromyomectomy Surgical removal of a uterine myoma.
histeropexia	hysteropexy Surgical fixation of the uterus by shortening of the round ligaments or by other means.
histerosalpingografíe	hysterosalpingography Roentgenography of the uterus and fallopian tubes after instillation of contrast media.
histerotomía	hysterotomy Surgical opening of the uterus.
histidina	histidine An amino acid precursor to histamine.
histiocito	histiocyte A phagocytic cell found in connective tissue.
histología	histology The study of the structure and composition of minute structures.
histoplasmosis	histoplasmosis A fungal pulmonary infection from bat and bird excrement.
histoquímica	histochemistry
historia	story

Spanish	English
historia clínica previa	past history Prior medical problems experienced by a patient.
hito	milestone An event indicative of a certain stage of development.
híbrido	hybrid An animal or plant produced from two different species.
hígado	liver A large glandular organ in the right upper quadrant that functions in digestive processes, as well as, neutralizing toxins.
hoja clínica	clinical record
hombre	man
hombro	shoulder
hombro congelado	frozen shoulder Common term for adhesive capsulitis.
homeopatía	homeopathy A treatment of disease by use of minute doses of toxic substances that would normally be harmful.
homicidio	homicide When one person kills another.
homocigótico	homozygous Having identical alleles for a particular trait.
homoinjerto	homograft A graft of tissue from the same species as the recipient.
homolateral	homolateral Ipsilateral.
homosexual	homosexual A person sexually attracted to someone of the same gender.
homólogo	homologous Referring to something derived from the same species but different genotype.
hormigueo	tingling
hormona	hormone A substance produced in the body that effects a specific organ.
hormona estimulante	releasing hormone Hormones that come from one gland such as the thalamus that cause release of hormones from another gland such as the pituitary.
hormona foliculoestimulante	follicle stimulating hormone (FSH) An anterior pituitary gland hormone responsible for production of sperm or ova.
hormona luteinizante	luteinizing hormone (LH) A pituitary hormone that stimulates ovulation in females and androgen in males.
hormona tiroideoestimulante	thyroid stimulating hormone (TSH) A thyroid secreted by the pituitary that regulates the thyroid.
horquilla	fourchette The fork shaped fold of skin where the labia minora meet superior to the perineum.
hospital	hospital
hueco	hollow
huesecillo	ossicle A small bone. The stapes is an auditory ossicle.
hueso	bone
hueso cancellus	cancellous bone Describing the cancellous interior of bone.
hueso ganchoso	hamate bone; uncinate bone The medial bone in the distal row of carpal bones adjacent to the fifth metacarpal.
hueso lunar	lunate bone A carpal bone that articulates with the wrist.
hueso navicular de la mano	navicular bone The most lateral bone in the proximal row of carpal bones.
huesos cornete	turbinate bones The three curved shelves in the nasal cavity.
huevo	egg
humano	human
humor	mood
humor acuoso (a)	aqueous humor The fluid between the cornea and lens, anterior to the globe.
humor acuoso (a)	humor, aqueous
humor vítreo	humor, vitreus

Spanish	English
huso acromático	achromatic spindle The threads between the poles of the spindle in karyokinesis.
húmedo	moist
húmero	humerus The long bone in the upper arm.
iatrogénico	iatrogenic A problem caused by medical treatment.
ictericia	jaundice Yellowing of the sclerae and skin because of excessive bilirubin in the blood.
icterus	icterus Yellowing of the skin and sclerae because of excess bilirubin.
ictiosis	ichthyosis A congenital anomaly exhibited by excessively dry, thick skin.
idiopático	idiopathic Relating to a disease with an unknown cause.
igual	equal
ileítis	ileitis Inflammation of the ileum.
ileocolitis	ileocolitis Inflammation of the ileum and cecum.
ileocolostomía	ileocolostomy Creating a surgical opening between the ileum and colon.
ileoproctostomía	ileoproctostomy Creating a surgical opening between the ileum and the rectum.
ileostomía	ileostomy Surgical creation of an opening in the ileum that is placed at the skin surface.
iliococcígeo	iliococcygeal Referring to the ilium and coccyx.
ilium	ilium The large bone at the superior aspect of the pelvis which is present bilaterally.
imágenes por resonancia magnética	magnetic resonance imaging (MRI) Images are produced by evaluating the response of body tissue. nuclei to radio waves in a magnetic field.
imán	magnet
impacción dental	impacted tooth A tooth that does not erupt because adjacent teeth prevent it.
impacción fecal	fecal impaction The presence of hard excrement in the rectum that requires manual removal.
impenetrable	impervious Not affected by.
imperforado	imperforate Lack of an opening. An infant with an imperforate anus has a congenital defect with no anal opening.
implante	implant
impotencia	impotence Absence of power. A term used to describe erectile dysfunction.
impulso nervio	nerve impulse A signal transmitted along a nerve fiber.
inadaptación	maladjustment
inanición	inanition Generalized weakness from lack of nutrition.
inanición	starvation
inarticulado	inarticulate Indistinct speech.
incapacidad	disability
incapacidad para distinguir colores	color blindness The inability to distinguish colors.
incesto	incest Sexual relations between related people.
incipiente	incipient Starting to happen.
incisión	incision
incisivo	incisor Sharp-edged tooth; humans have four incisors.
incisura	incisura A notch or indentation usually on the edge of a bone.
incisura	incisure A notch or incision.
incisura supraesternal	jugular notch The notch on the upper border of the sternum.

221

Spanish	English
inclusión celulares	inclusion body Variably shaped bodies in the nuclei of cells found in infections such as rabies and herpes.
incoherente	incoherent Absence of intelligible speech.
incomodidad	discomfort
incompetencia del cuello uterino	Cervical insufficiency (formerly incompetent cervix) Painless changes in the cervix that result in recurrent second semester pregnancy loss.
inconsciencia	unconsciousness Unable to respond to sensory stimuli.
incontinencia	incontinence Inability to control urination.
incoordinación	incoordination Absence of smooth, efficient body movement.
incremento	increment
incubadora	incubator A warming device for infants.
incus	incus The middle ear bone between the stapes and malleus.
indice de sedimentación de eritrocito	blood sedimentation rate (ESR) The settling time of erythrocytes in a prepared sample. This is a measure of the abnormal concentration of substances that are associated with pathological states.
indigestión	indigestion Inadequate digestion for various reasons.
individual	single
indígena	indigenous Naturally occurring.
indolente	indolent 1. Causing little pain. 2. Slow healing ulcer.
inducir	induce, to Facilitated. When referring to labor, it means medication was given to assist in delivery of the fetus.
induración	induration An area that is abnormally hard.
inebriación	inebriation Intoxication with drugs or alcohol.
ineficaz	ineffective
inercia	inertia The tendency to remain unchanged.
inervación	innervation The presence of a nerve supply.
inesperado	unexpected
inevitable	inevitable Not preventable.
infancia	childhood
infancia	infancy
infantil	infantile Referring to babies or young children.
infarto	infarct Referring to dead tissue.
infarto	infarction Dead tissue, for example, myocardial infarction.
infarto miocardio	myocardial infarction The death of myocardial tissue as a result of an interruption in flow to the region supplied by a coronary vessel.
infecciones de los oídos	ear infections
infeccioso	infectious
infección cruzada	cross-infection Transfer of infection between individuals, each with a different organism.
inferior	inferior
infestación	infestation The presence of large numbers, as in lice infestation.
inflamación	inflammation Localized redness, excessive warmth and swelling.
infraespinoso	infraspinous Below the scapular spine.
infundíbulo	infundibulum The connection between the hypothalamus and the posterior pituitary gland.
infusión	infusion The injection of fluid into tissue or a vein.
infusión intravenoso	intravenous infusion Administration of fluid into a vein.

Spanish	English
ingestion alimento	food intake
ingestion fluido	fluid intake The amount of oral consumption plus the amount of intravenous fluids administered.
ingestión	ingestion The intake of food or liquid orally.
ingle	groin The genital region.
inguinal	inguinal Referring to the groin.
inhalación	inhalation The act of breathing in.
inhibidor de monoaminooxidasa	monoamine oxidase inhibitor (MAOI) A drug used to treat depression that allows accumulation of serotonin and norepinephrine.
inicio	onset
injerto	graft
injerto óseo	bone graft The transfer of bone to aid in the healing of a complex fracture.
inmune	immune Being resistant to an infection.
inmunización	immunization A medication given to provide immunity.
inmunodeficiencia	immunodeficiency An inadequate immune response.
inmunoelectroforesis	immunoelectrophoresis A means of differentiating proteins and other compounds by comparing their mobility and antigenic specificities.
inmunoglobulina	immunoglobulin Serum and cellular proteins of the immune system.
inmunoquímica	immunochemistry The study of immune response and biochemistry.
inmunosupresión	immunosuppression The inhibition of the immune response.
innominado	innominate Referring to the innominate artery.
inoculación	inoculation Injection with a vaccine to provide immunity.
inofensivo	harmless
inorgánico	inorganic Not coming from natural growth.
inquietar	worry, to
insania	insanity Referring to a serious mental illness.
insano	insane A term not used in formal medical evaluations that when used by a layperson means a serious mental illness.
insensible	insensible Unable to perceive a stimulus.
inserción	insertion
inserción tubo nasogástrico	nasogastric tube placement
insidioso	insidious A slow, gradual and harmful advancement.
insolación calor	heat stroke A condition caused by excessive exposure to high ambient temperature; it is exhibited by dry skin, thirst, vertigo, muscle cramps and nausea. The three forms are heat exhaustion, heat cramps and sunstroke.
insomnio	insomnia Sleeplessness.
inspiración	inspiration Drawing in a breath.
insuficiencia aórtico (a)	aortic insufficiency A dysfunction of the aortic valve allowing backflow of blood into the heart.
insuficiencia cardíaca	cardiac failure Decreased cardiac output of the heart.
insuficiencia cardíaca congestiva	congestive heart failure A diminished cardiac output leading to passive engorgement.
insuficiencia coronaria	ischemic heart disease Inadequate blood supply to the heart.
insuficiencia renal	renal failure Diminution of kidney function.
insuficiencia vertebrobasilar	vertebrobasilar insufficiency Diminished flow to the vertebral and basilar arteries causing posterior fossa symptoms.

223

Spanish	English
insulina	insulin A hormone produced by the pancreas and synthetically to control blood glucose levels.
insulinoma	insulinoma An islet cell tumor that causes abnormally high insulin secretion and thus hypoglycemia.
integumento	integument Outer protective layer.
intensivo	intensive
interarticular	interarticular Between the articular surfaces of a joint.
intercelular	intercellular Between cells.
intermitente	intermittent
interno	internal
interóseo	interosseous Referring to something between bones, like the interosseous muscles of the hand.
intersticial	interstitial Referring to the interstices of tissue.
intertrigo	intertrigo Irritation present because adjacent surfaces rub together.
intertrocantéreo	intertrochanteric Referring to the space within the trochanter.
intervalo	interval
intervalo medicina	dosing interval The number of times per unit a medication is given.
interventricular	interventricular Between the ventricles.
intestinal	intestinal Referring to the intestines.
intestino	intestine A general term used for the section of bowel from the stomach to the anus.
intolerencia a la lactosa	lactose intolerance
intoxicación alimenticia	food poisoning
intraabdominal	intraabdominal Within the abdominal cavity.
intraarticular	intraarticular Within a joint space.
intracelular	intracellular Within a cell.
intracerebral	intracerebral Within the cerebrum.
intracraneal	intracranial Within the cranial vault.
intradérmico	intradermal Within the dermis.
intradural	intradural Within the dural space.
intramedular	intramedullary 1. Within the medulla oblongata. 2. Within the bone marrow.
intramuscular	intramuscular Within a muscle.
intraóseo	intraosseous Within a bone.
intraperitoneal	intraperitoneal Within the peritoneal cavity.
intratecal	intrathecal Technically means within a sheath but this term is used when medication is instilled in the dura mater spinalis.
intrauterino	intrauterine Within the uterus.
intravenoso	intravenous Within a vein.
intubación (intubación endotraqueal)	intubation Placement of a tube; commonly used to refer to endotracheal intubation.
intususcepción	intussusception The inversion of one portion of the bowel into another.
inulina	inulin A polysaccharide used in the testing of renal function.
inunción	inunction The application of lotion with friction.
involucrum	involucrum A wrap or covering (referring to a sequestrum).
involutivo	involutional The shrinkage of an organ when it is not in use, as in the uterus after childbirth.
inyección	injection The act of a needle being inserted into a body.

Spanish	English
ipsilateral	ipsilateral On the same side.
ira	rage
iridectomía	iridectomy Surgical removal of part of the iris.
iridocilitis	iridocyclitis Inflammation of the ciliary body and the iris.
iridoplejía	iridoplegia Paralysis of part of the iris with subsequent lack of contraction or dilation of the pupil.
iridotomía	iridotomy A surgical opening of the iris.
iris	iris The colored membrane posterior to the cornea.
irradiación	irradiation The process of being irradiated.
irrelevante	irrelevant Not pertinent.
irrigar	flush, to
islote	islet Tissue that is structurally separate from adjacent tissues.
isoanticuerpo	isoantibody A situation in which an antibody of person A reacts with an antigen of person B.
isquemia	ischemia Inadequate blood supply to a part of the body.
isquión	ischium The inferoposterior portion of the pelvis.
istmo	isthmus A narrow piece of tissue connecting two larger body parts.
izquierda	left
íleo	ileus A temporary obstruction in the intestine.
íleon	ileum The portion of the small bowel from the jejunum to the cecum.
jabón	soap
jarabe	syrup
jején de búfalo	black fly From the family Simuliidae, a gnat that can cause disease in humans; also called buffalo fly.
jeringa	syringe
jeringa gastrogavaje	gavage syringe
jeringa hipodérmico	hypodermic needle
joven	young
jugo gástrico	gastric secretions
juramento hipocrático	Hippocratic oath An vow taken by doctors, indicating they will treat people properly.
juventud	youth
kala azar Leishmaniasis visceral.	kala-azar A disease caused by Leishmania donovani that is exhibited by weight loss, fever, anemia and hepatosplenomegaly.
kernicterus	kernicterus A condition associated with high bilirubin levels that causes yellow staining of cerebral tissues and subsequent neurologic dysfunction.
kra-kra	craw-craw A pruritic papular skin eruption sometimes caused by Onchocerca.
kubisagari Vértigo epidémico.	kubisagari Vestibular neuronitis.
kwashiorkor	kwashiorkor A form of malnutrition from inadequate protein intake.
laberintitis	labyrinthitis Inflammation of the labyrinth.
laberinto	labyrinth Inner ear structure concerned with balance.
labial	labial Referring to the lip.
labio inferior	lip, lower Labium inferius oris.
labio leporino	cleft lip
labio pudendo mayor	labium majus (plural= labia majora) The folds of skin forming the lateral borders of the pudendal cleft.

Spanish	English
labio pudendo menor	labium minus (plural=labia minora) The folds of skin posterior to the labia majora.
labio superior de la boca	lip, upper Labium superius oris.
labium	labium Referring to any lip shaped structure.
laboratorio	laboratory
labrum	labrum An edge or lip. The labrum acetabular is the fibrocartilagous rim attached to the acetabulum.
laceración	laceration An injury that produced a cut in the skin or tissue such as a tear during childbirth.
laceración de cuero cabelludo	scalp laceration
lactación	lactation The secretion of milk from mammary glands.
lactalbúmina	lactalbumin Proteins found in milk.
lactancia materna	breast feeding
lactante	infant
lactante de término	infant, term
lactante postérmino	infant, post-term
lactante pretérmino	infant, pre-term
lactasa	lactase An enzyme that facilitates the breakdown of lactose to glucose and galactose.
lactosa	lactose A disaccharide present in milk.
ladilla	crab louse Phthirus pubis is formal name for a louse that infests pubic hair and causes intense itching.
lagoftalmos	lagophthalmos Characterized by the inability to close the eyelid completely over the eye.
lagrimal	lacrimal Referring to the secretion of tears.
lagrimeo	lacrimation The secretion of tears.
laguna	lacuna A small cavity or depression.
lalofobia	laliophobia Abnormal fear of speaking or stuttering.
laloquecia	lalochezia Relief of stress by uttering obsenities.
laminectomía	laminectomy The surgical removal of part of a vertebrae.
laminilla	lamella A thin layer of bone.
lanceta	fingerstick device A device used to project a lancet into the skin so a drop of blood can be obtained for analysis.
lanceta	lancet A small sharp instrument used to obtain a drop of blood for testing.
lanzar un chorro	squirt, to
laparoscopia	laparoscopy A procedure utilizing a laparoscope.
laparoscopio	laparoscope A fiber-optic instrument used to visualize the peritoneal contents.
laparotomía	laparotomy A surgical incision of the abdomen.
laringe	larynx A hollow muscular structure that contains the vocal cords.
laringectomía	laryngectomy Surgical removal of the larynx.
laringismo	laryngismus stridulus Sudden, severe laryngeal spasm.
laringitis	laryngitis Inflammation of the larynx.
laringoespasmo	laryngospasm Sudden, involuntary muscle contraction of the larynx.
laringoestenosis	laryngostenosis Abnormal narrowing of the larynx.
laringofaringe	laryngopharynx The pharyngeal space between the superior aspect of the glottis and the opening of the larynx.

226

Spanish	English
laringología	laryngology The study of the larynx and related diseases.
laringotomía	laryngotomy Surgical creation of an opening in the larynx.
laríngeo	laryngeal Referring to the larynx.
las gafas de buceo	goggles
lateral	lateral Referring to the side of the body.
laterodesviación	laterodeviation
latido cimiento fetal	fetal heart tone
latido, pulsación	beat As in heart beat.
latido, pulsación	heart beat
latir	throb, to
latirismo Lupinosis.	lathyrism A disease characterized by tremors, spastic paralysis and paresthesias caused by Lathyrus sativus.
lavado gástrico	gastric lavage Instillation and removal of large quantities of saline into the stomach in order to treat poisoning.
lábil	labile Easily altered; emotionally unstable.
láctico	lactic Referring to milk.
lágrima	tear As in, to shed a tear.
lámina del techo del mesencéfalo	tectum mesencephali The posterior portion of the mesencephalon including the sup. and inf. colliculi and tectal lamina.
LCR líquido cefalorraquídeo	CSF Abbreviation for cerebrospinal fluid.
leche de vaca	cow's milk
lecitina	lecithin A compound widely used by tissues, derived from egg yolks and it consists of phospholipids linked to choline.
leishmaniasis	leishmaniasis A condition caused by a flagellate protozoan parasite that is exhibited by visceral or dermatologic manifestations.
leishmaniasis cutánea	oriental sore A stigmata of cutaneous leishmaniasis caused by a bite from a sand fly.
lejía	bleach
lengua	tongue
lengua nigra	lingua nigra A condition characterized by a dark fur-like covering on the dorsum of the tongue.
lengua vellosa	hairy tongue
lens	lens The transparent chamber between the posterior chamber and the vitreous body.
lentes de contacto	contact lenses
lenticular	lenticular Referring to the lens of the eye.
lento	slow
leontiasis ósea Enfermedad de Virchow.	leontiasis ossea Bilateral hypertrophy of the bones of the face and cranium.
lepra	leprosy A contagious disease caused by Mycobacterium leprae that causes insensate papules and disfiguration.
leproma	leproma A superficial granulatomous papule that is seen in leprosy.
leptomeningitis	leptomeningitis A general term used to describe meningitis of the pia and arachnoid of the brain.
leptospirosis	leptospirosis A zoonosis caused by the spirochete Leptospira interrogans transmitted by rats and contaminated water.
lesbiana	lesbian

227

Spanish	English
lesionar	injure, to
lesión	injury
lesión céfalica cerrada	injury, closed head
lesión de hiperextensión-hiperflexión	injury, hyperextension-hyperflexion
lesión encontragolpe del cerebro	injury, contrecoup of brain
lesión piel	skin lesion
lesión por desguantamiento o desguante	injury, degloving
letal	lethal
letargia	lethargy Absence of energy.
leucemia	leukemia A malignant disease causing an increase in the number of abnormal and immature leukocytes.
leucemia linfocítica	lymphocytic leukemia Chronic accumulation of functionally incompetent lymphocytes.
leucina	leukine (or leucine) An amino acid obtained from hydrolysis of some proteins.
leucinosis	leucinosis; maple syrup urine disease A condition characterized by an enzyme defect causing an increase in leucine in the urine.
leucocitemia	leukocythemia Synonym of leukemia.
leucocito	leukocyte A white blood cell.
leucocitosis	leukocytosis An increase in the number of leukocytes.
leucocitólisis	leukocytolysis Destruction of white blood cells.
leucodermia	leukodermia A localized loss of skin pigment.
leuconiquia	leukonychia A whitish discoloration of the fingernails and toenails.
leucopenia	leukopenia A decreased number of leukocytes in the blood.
leucopoyesis	leukopoiesis Production of white blood cells.
leucorrea	leukorrhea Thick white vaginal discharge.
levadura	yeast
levantar	lift, to
levantar	raise, to
levator	levator A muscle that raises part of the body; the levator labii superioris raised the upper lip.
levulosa Fructosa	levulose Synonym for fructose.
léntigo	lentigo A benign condition exhibited by flat brown patches on the skin.
libertad	freedom
libido	libido Sexual desire.
libre	free
libre de	free of
ligadura	ligature A thread used to tie a vessel.
ligamento	ligament
ligamento ancho del útero	broad ligament of uterus Supports the uterus on both sides.
ligamento bifurcado	bifurcate ligament A ligament on the dorsum of the foot that includes the calcaneonavicular and calcaneocuboid ligaments.

228

Spanish	English
ligamento pectíneo	pectineal ligament A continuation of the lacunar ligament along the pectineal line in the pubis.
ligamento redondo del útero	round ligament The supporting structure of the uterus.
lima	file Patient record or folder.
liminal	liminal Referring to a threshold.
linctura	lincture A medicine mixed with a sweet substance.
linfa	lymph A transparent and sometimes opalescent fluid that flows in the lymph channels.
linfadenitis	lymphadenitis Inflammation of a lymph node.
linfangiectasia	lymphangiectasis Distention of the lymph channels.
linfangioma	lymphangioma A mass composed of newly formed lymph tissue.
linfangitis	lymphangitis Inflammation of the lymph vessels.
linfático	lymphatic Referring to the lymph system.
linfocitemia	lymphocythemia Abnormally high number of lymphocytes in the blood.
linfocito	lymphocyte A white blood cell produced by the lymph tissue.
linfocitopenia	lymphocytopenia Decrease in the usual number of lymphocytes in the blood.
linfocitosis	lymphocytosis The organization of cysts containing lymph.
linfoide	lymphoid Similar to lymph.
linfoma	lymphoma A malignant disease of the lymph system, Hodgkin's lymphoma for example.
linfosarcoma	lymphosarcoma A malignant disease of the lymph system that does not include Hodgkin's lymphoma.
lipasa	lipase A pancreatic enzyme that facilitates the breakdown of fats.
lipemia	lipemia Abnormally high fat content in the blood.
lipoatrofía	lipoatrophy Fatty tissue atrophy.
lipocito	lipocyte A fat cell.
lipocondrodistrofia	lipochondrodystrophy A congenital condition exhibited by short stature, kyphosis, mental deficiency and short fingers.
lipodistrofia	lipodystrophy Abnormal fat metabolism.
lipoide	lipoid Referring to fat.
lipoidosis	lipoidosis Abnormal lipid metabolism.
lipoma	lipoma A benign tumor consisting of fat cells.
lipoproteína	lipoprotein A soluble protein used to transport fat or lipids.
liquen	lichen A term used to describe a variety of papular skin diseases. Lichen planus is a shiny, flat, violaceous eruption of the mucous membranes, skin and genitalia.
liquido cerebroespinal	cerebrospinal fluid (CSF) The fluid between the pia mater and arachnoid membrane.
lisiado, lisiada	cripple
lisina	lysine An amino acid found in most proteins.
lisis	lysis The rupture of a cell wall or membrane.
lisosoma	lysosome An organelle contained in the cytoplasm of eukaryotic cells.
lisozima	lysozyme An enzyme in tears that facilitates destruction of certain bacterial cell walls.
litagogo	lithagogue A treatment of a calculus.
litolapaxia	litholapaxy The crushing and then removal of a calculus.
litotomía	lithotomy Surgical removal of a calculus.

Spanish	English
litotrito	lithotritor An instrument used to crush a calculus.
litro	liter
límbico	limbus The margin of a structure, for example, of the cornea and sclera.
límite terapéutico	therapeutic range
línea de Hunter	linea alba The tendinous portion of the anterior abdomen between the two rectus muscles.
línea media del cuerpo	midline
lípido	lipid A compound that is a fatty acid which is insoluble in water but soluble in organic solvents.
lítico	lytic Referring to lysis.
llevar a cabo, realizar	achieve
lo largo de	throughout
loasis	loiasis A disease caused by the filarial nematode Loa loa.
lobar	lobar Referring to a lobe.
lobectomía	lobectomy Surgical removal of a lobe (generally lung or liver).
lobotomía	lobotomy Surgical incision into the prefrontal lobe; historically a treatment of mental illness.
lobulillo	lobule A small lobe.
localización	localization Establishment of a site of a disease process.
localizado	localized Toward one point or area.
loculado	loculated Divided into small cavities.
locura	madness
longevidad	longevitiy
longitud	length
loquios	lochia Vaginal secretions noted within two weeks of childbirth.
lordosis	lordosis An abnormal depth of the inward curvature of the spine.
lóbulo	lobe A body part divided by a fissure.
lubricante	lubricant
lumbago	low back pain
lumbago	lumbago Pain in the region of the lumbar spine.
lumbalgia	back pain
lumbar	lumbar Referring to the spinal region inferior to the thoracic spine.
lumen	lumen A hollow cavity.
lupus eritematoso	lupus erythematosous An autoimmune inflammatory disease exhibited by a butterfly shaped rash on the face along with visceral and connective tissue abnormalities.
luteotrófico	luteotropic Synonym of prolactin.
luto	mourning A period of grieving.
luxación, dislocación	dislocation The displacement of a bone when referring to an articulation.
luz	light
lúnula	lunula The pale area at the base of a fingernail.
macrocito	macrocyte A large red blood cell.
macrocitosis	macrocytosis Referring to the status of an increased number of large erythrocytes as seen in Vitamin B12 deficiency.
macrodactilia	macrodactyly Abnormally large digits.
macroencefalia	macroencephaly Having an abnormally large head.

Spanish	English
macroglobulinemia	macroglobulinemia A condition exhibited by an increase number of macroglobulins in the blood.
macroglosia	macroglossia Abnormally large tongue.
macromastia	macromastia Abnormally large breasts.
macromelia	macromelia Abnormally large head or extremity.
macroqueilia	macrocheilia Abnormally large lips.
macrostomía	macrostomia Abnormal increase in the width of the mouth.
macrófago	macrophage A phagocytic cell that originates in the tissues.
macula	macula 1. The area of the eye of greatest visual acuity that surrounds the fovea. 2. A small flat discoloration of the skin (synonym for macule).
maculopápula	maculopapule A skin lesion that is similar to both a macule and a papule.
magnético	magnetic
magnum foramen	foramen magnum The hole in the skull that the spinal cord passes through.
malacia	malacia The abnormal softening of a body part or tissue.
malalineación	malalignment (dental) Displacement of the teeth from their normal position.
malaunión	malunion The union of a fracture in a faulty position.
malestar	malaise
maléolo	malleolus A bony protrusion on medial and lateral aspect of each ankle.
maléolo interno	malleolus, medial
maléolo lateral	malleolus, lateral
maligno	malignant
malleus	malleus Small bone in the inner ear that articulates with the incus.
malpraxis	malpractice Negligent professional activity.
maltosa	maltose A disaccharide hydrolyzed by amylase.
mamario	mammary Referring to the breast.
mamilar	mammillary Referring to a nipple.
mamografía	mammography Roentgenography of the breasts, used as a screening test for cancer.
mamoplastia	mammaplasty Plastic surgery of the breast.
mancha de Koplik	Koplik's spots Red buccal macules with a blue center; seen in measles.
manchas	blemishes
mandíbula	jaw
mandíbula	mandible The lower jaw.
manera de caminar	gait The way one walks.
manguito rotatotio del hombro	rotator cuff The structure around the capsule of the shoulder joint formed by the infraspinatus, supraspinatus, teres minor and subscapularis muscles.
maniobra de Adson	Adson maneuver A test used to screen for thoracic outlet syndrome.
maniobra de Bill	Bill maneuver During childbirth, use of forceps at midpelvis to help extract the head.
maniobra de Bracht	Bracht maneuver Delivery of a fetus in a breech position.
maniobra de Buzzard	Buzzard maneuver Testing of the patellar reflex while the client firmly touches the floor with their toes in a sitting position.
maniobra de Credé	Credé's maneuver Manual pressure over the bladder to assist in expression of urine in an atonic bladder.
maniobra de Hampton	Hampton maneuver Rolling a patient during gastrointestinal fluoroscopy in order to obtain an air contrast of the antrum and duodenum.
maniobra de Heimlich	Heimlich maneuver A forceful upward thrust to the diaphragm to dislodge an airway obstruction.

231

Spanish	English
maniobra de Hillis-Müller	Hillis-Müller maneuver A procedure to determine the descent of the head during active labor.
maniobra de Hueter	Hueter's maneuver The application of downward and forward pressure on the tongue while passing an gastric tube.
maniobra de Jendrassik	Jendrassik's maneuver A method of distracting a patient while checking the patellar reflex.
maniobra de Leopold	Leopold's maneuver Used to determine fetal position.
maniobra de Mcdonald	Mcdonald's maneuver A measurement of the uterus in centimeters that corresponds to gestational age in weeks.
maniobra de Ritgen	Ritgen's maneuver A procedure that controls the rate of delivery of the infant's head during childbirth.
maniobra de Valsalva	Valsalva's maneuver A technique in which one attempts to exhale with the mouth and nose closed; this equalizes pressure in the ears.
manía	mania A mental disorder exhibited by hyperexcitability, delusions and euphoria.
mano	hand
mano en garra	clawhand A hand deformity caused by ulnar nerve palsy exhibited by the hyperextension of the metacarpophalangeal joints and flexion of the interphalangeal articulations.
mano péndula	wrist drop
manojo de His	bundle of His The atrial contraction rhythm is facilitated by this bundle to the ventricles.
manómetro	manometer Device used for pressure monitoring.
mantenimiento	maintenance
manubrio del esternón	manubrium sterni The superior segment of the sternum which articulates with the clavicle and first rib.
mapeo	mapping
marasmo	marasmus Progressive weight loss and emaciation.
marca en vino de Oporto. Nevus flammeus	port-wine mark Also called nevus flammeus, it is a vascular anomaly characterized by purplish skin discoloration.
marcapaso	pacemaker An electrical device used to stimulate the heart used for bradyarrhythmias.
marcha festinante	festinating gait Walking with increased speed involuntarily; often seen in Parkinson's disease.
marcha pie caído	drop foot gait A gait characterized by dragging the foot, as there is no ankle dorsiflexion.
mareo	dizziness Sensation of losing one's balance.
marijuana o marihuana	marijuana Cannabis.
mariscos	shellfish
marsupialización	marsupialization Creation of a surgical pouch.
masa	mass Tumor.
mascullar	mumble, to
mastectomía	mastectomy Surgical resection of one or both breasts.
masticación	mastication Chewing.
masticar	chew, to
mastitis	mastitis Inflammation of the breast.
mastodinia	mastodynia Breast pain.
mastoidectomía	mastoidectomy Surgical removal of the mastoid.

Spanish	English
mastoideo	mastoid Referring to the mastoid process.
mastoiditis	mastoiditis Inflammation of the mastoid process.
materia gris periacueducto	periaqueductal gray matter Refers to the brain gray matter adjacent to the periaqueductal.
maxilar	maxilla The upper jaw that also forms the inferior portion of the orbit and part of the nose.
maxilofacial	maxillofacial
mazamorra	mazamorra Dermatitis caused by hookworm larvae indigenous to Peurto Rico.
máquina corazón-pulmón	heart lung machine Device used during cardiac surgery to replace the function of the heart and lungs while surgery is performed.
más allá de	beyond
más viejo	older
máscara de Hutchinson	Hutchington's mask The sensation the face is covered in cobwebs, associated with tabes dorsalis.
máscara respiratoria única o de sentido único	non-rebreather mask
meato	meatus Opening to the body, such as urethral meatus.
meato auditivo externo	external ear canal, auditory canal
mecha	wick; drain
meconio	meconium The first newborn feces which are green. Presence of meconium on the newborn is a sign there was fetal distress in utero.
medial	medial Situated toward the midline.
mediastino	mediastinum The thoracic area between the lungs.
mediastinoscopia	medianoscopy Visual inspection of the mediastinum with a scope.
medicación	medication
medicina	medicine
medicina nuclear	nuclear medicine The branch of medicine associated with the use of radioactive material in the evaluation and treatment of disease.
medicoquirúrgico	medicosurgical Referring to medicine and surgery.
medio de cultivo	culture broth A medium used to grow bacteria.
medio sordo	hard of hearing
mediodía	noon
medula óseo	bone marrow The soft material filling the cavity of bones.
medular	medullary 1. The inner part of an organ. 2. Referring to the medulla oblongata.
meduloblastoma	medulloblastoma A malignant tumor of the cerebellum found mostly in children.
megacariocito	megakaryocyte A cell found in the bone marrow that is a source of platelet production.
megacefalia	megacephaly Having a larger than normal cranial capacity.
megacolon	megacolon
megaloblasto	megaloblast A large red blood cell noted primarily in pernicious anemia.
megalomanía	megalomania A mental disorder characterized by abnormal feelings of self-importance.
meiosis	meiosis Cell division creating two daughter cells each with half the number of cells as the parent cell.
mejilla	cheek
mejor	best
mejorar	ameliorate

233

Spanish	English
melancolía	melancholia Profound sadness.
melanina	melanin A dark pigment found on the skin, hair or iris.
melanoma	melanoma Malignant cancer, typically found in the skin.
melanoma de ojo	ocular melanoma. An aggressive cancer that, when involving the eye, is located in the choroid layer.
melena	black stools Common term for melena.
melena	melena The passage of black, tarry stools indicative of upper gastrointestinal bleeding.
melisofobia	melissophobia Also called apiphobia, a fear of bees.
melitis Inflamación de la mejilla.	melitis Inflammation of the cheek.
membrana celular	cell membrane The semipermeable structure surrounding the cytoplasm of a cell.
membrana timpánica	tympanic membrane The membrane between the external and middle ear.
memoria	memory
menarca	menarche The time of the initial menstrual period.
mencionar	mention, to
meningioma	meningioma A tumor of the meningeal tissue; generally benign.
meningismo	meningism Signs and symptoms of meningitis without infection of the meninges.
meningitis	meningitis Inflammation of the meninges exhibited by fever, photophobia, nuchal rigidity and in severe cases coma and convulsions.
meningocele	meningocele A congenital defect exhibited by protrusion of the meninges through a defect in the spinal column.
meningococemia	meningococcemia
meniscectomía	meniscectomy Surgical excision of a meniscus.
menisco	meniscus A thin cartilage between joint surfaces.
menitgitis criptocóccica	cryptococcal meningitis A meningeal infection associated with AIDS.
meníngeo	meningeal Referring to the dura mater, arachnoid and the pia mater.
menopausia	menopause The time when menstruation ceases.
menos	less
menstruación	menstruation
menstruo	menses The blood and other material expelled from the uterus during menstruation.
mental	mental
mentón	chin
mesarteritis	mesarteritis Inflammation of the middle layer of an artery.
mesencéfalo	mesencephalon Midbrain.
mesentario del apéndice	mesoappendix The portion of the mesentery vermiform appendix.
mesenterio	mesentery The fold of peritoneum that connects the small bowel, pancrease and spleen to the posterior portion of the abdominal wall.
mesénquima	mesenchyme Organized mesodermal cells that produce connective tissue, lymphatics and bone.
mesocolon	mesocolon The mesentery connecting the colon to the posterior abdominal wall.
mesodermo	mesoderm The middle germ layer in an embryo that is the source of bone, muscle and skin.

Spanish	English
mesonefroma	mesonephroma Usually a tumor of the female genital tract that is thought to stem from the mesonephros.
mesoovario	mesovarium The portion of the mesentery connecting the ovary with the abdominal wall.
mesosálpinx	mesosalpinx A portion of the broad ligament supporting the fallopian tubes.
mesotelioma	mesothelioma A tumor that stems from mesothelial tissue; a known cause is asbestos exposure.
metabólico	metabolic Referring to the physical and chemical reactions involved with keeping an organism functioning.
metacarpiano	metacarpal The name for any of the five hand bones.
metacarpofalángico	metacarpophalangeal Referring to the metacarpus and the phalanges.
metahemoglobina	methemoglobin A substance formed with the oxidation of hemoglobin.
metaplasia	metaplasia Abnormal change in the nature or character of tissue.
metatarsalgia	metatarsalgia Foot pain.
metatarsiano	metatarsal Any of the bones of the foot.
metáfisis	metaphysis The region between the diaphysis and the epiphysis.
metionina	methionine A sulfur-containing amino acid used in the biosynthesis of cysteine.
metro	meter
metrorragia	metrorrhagia Uterine bleeding in normal amounts but at irregular intervals.
médico	physician
médico forense	coroner A person who investigates sudden or suspicious deaths.
médula espinal	spinal cord The bundle of nerves that with the brain comprise the central nervous system.
médula oblongata	medulla oblongata The inferior portion of the brainstem.
médula suprarrenal	adrenal medulla The innermost part of the adrenal gland.
método de tratamient	treatment regimen
mialgia	myalgia Muscle pain.
miastenia grave	myasthenia gravis An autoimmune disease characterized by fluctuating weakness of the ocular, limb and respiratory muscles.
micciones nocturnas	nocturnal emission Involuntary emission of semen at night.
micetoma	mycetoma Persistent inflammation of the tissues caused by an infection.
micosis	mycosis A disease caused by a fungal infection.
micotoxinas	mycotoxin A substance toxic to fungus.
microbio	microbe A microorganism.
microbiología	microbiology The study of microorganisms.
microcefálico	microcephalic A congenital deformity exhibited by an abnormally small head.
microcito	microcyte An unusually small erythrocyte associated with anemias, such as iron deficiency anemia.
microftalmo	microphthalmos A congenital condition characterized by smallness of the eyes.
micrognatia	micrognathia Abnormally small maxilla or mandible.
microgramo	microgram One millionth of one gram.
microorganismo	microorganism An organism only seen with a microscope.
microscopio	microscope
microscopio electrópio	electron microscope A device that uses electron beams and lenses to give high magnification.
micrómetro	micrometer One millionth of one meter.

Spanish	English
micturición	micturition Synonym of urination.
midriasis	mydriasis Pupillary dilation.
mielina	myelin The substance that forms a sheath around some nerve fibers.
mielitis	myelitis Inflammation of the spinal cord.
mielocele	myelocele Protrusion of the spinal cord through a defect in the bony structure.
mieloide	myeloid Referring to the bone marrow or spinal cord.
mieloma	myeloma Malignant tumor of the bone marrow.
mielomatosis	myelomatosis A leukemic disease in which there is an abnormally high amount of myeloblasts in the blood.
mielomeningocele	myelomeningocele A protrusion of the spinal cord and its meninges through a defect in the vertebral canal.
mielopatía	myelopathy A condition of the spinal cord.
miembro	member Referring to an extremity (arm or leg).
migraña	migraine An episodic, unilateral headache accompanied by nausea.
miliar	miliary Referring to a disease that is exhibited by small seed-like lesions (millet), such as miliary tuberculosis.
miligramo	milligram
mililitro	milliliter
mililitro cúbico	cubic millimeter A unit of volume.
milímetro	millimeter
mimar	pamper, to
minuto	minute A unit of time.
miocardio	myocardium The middle layer of the heart wall.
miocarditis	myocarditis An inflammation of the heart.
miocárdico	myocardial Referring to the muscular tissue of the heart.
mioclono	myoclonus Contraction or spasm of a group of muscles.
mioclono palatino	palatal myoclonus An involuntary, persistent, rapid regular tremor of the soft palate and face.
mioglobina	myoglobin
mioma	myoma
miomas uterinos Tumores no cancerosos que aparecen en el útero.	uterine fibroids Benign tumors made up of muscular and fibrous tissue in the uterus.
miomectomía	myomectomy Surgical resection of a myoma.
miometrio	myometrium The smooth muscle layer of the uterus.
miopatía	myopathy Muscle disease.
miope	myope A person who is nearsighted.
miopía	myopia Nearsightedness.
miosarcoma	myosarcoma A mass with myoma and sarcoma characteristics.
miosina	myosin A protein that when coupled with actin form the contractile complex of a muscle cells.
miosis	myosis Profound pupillary constriction.
miositis	myositis Inflammation of muscle tissue.
miositis osificante	myositis ossificans Inflammation of muscle tissue with presence of bony deposits.
miotásico	myotic Referring to miosis.
miotonía	myotomy The surgical removal of muscle tissue.

Spanish	English
miotonía distrófica	myotonia dystrophica; Steinert's disease A condition exhibited initially by hypertonic muscles followed by atrophy of the facial and neck muscles.
mirada	gaze
mirada	glance
miriaquita	miryachit A disease of Siberia characterized by an exaggerated startle response.
miringitis	myringitis Inflammation of the tympanic membrane.
miringoplastia	myringoplasty Surgical repair of tympanic membrane defects.
miringotomíe	myringotomy Surgical opening of the tympanic membrane.
misantropía	misanthropy A severe dislike of homo sapiens.
misofobia	mysophobia Severe fear of dirt or contamination from common objects.
mitad	half
mitocondria	mitochondria Organelle found in cells responsible for energy production.
mitosis	mitosis Cell division in which two daughter cells are formed that have the same number of chromosomes as the parent cell.
mitral	mitral Referring to the mitral valve.
mixedema	myxedema Diffuse edema with a wax-like appearance of the skin; this condition is associated with hypothyroidism.
mixoma	myxoma A tumor composed of mucous tissue.
mixosaroma	myxosarcoma A sarcoma that also has mucous tissue.
moco	mucus A substance secreted by mucous membranes.
moderado	mild
mojado	wet
molalidad	molality The number of moles of a solution per kilogram of pure solvent.
molde para andar	walking cast A cast used for simple fractures of the lower leg.
molécula	molecule A combination of at least two atoms.
monitor de Holter para 24 horas	ambulatory electrocardiographic monitoring A continuous recording of the electrocardiogram used to detect occult dysrhythmias.
monitoreo	monitoring
monitorización fetal	fetal monitoring
monocito	monocyte A leukocyte with an oval nucleus and grey cytoplasm.
monocitosis	monocytosis An abnormal increase in the number of monocytes in the blood.
monoclonal	monoclonal Asexual formation of a clone from a single cell.
monodiplopía	monodiplopia Double vision in only one eye.
monomanía	monomania A psychotic obsession about a single subject.
mononeurapatía del III par craneal	cranial mononeuropathy III Dysfunction of the third cranial nerve causes double vision and eyelid drooping.
mononeuritis	mononeuritis Inflammation of a single nerve.
mononeuropatía del VI par craneal	cranial mononeuropathy VI A disorder of the sixth cranial nerve causes double vision.
mononuclear	mononuclear A cell having only one nucleus.
mononucleosis	mononucleosis An infectious disease exhibited by malaise and lymphadenopathy.
monoplejía	monoplegia Paralysis of a single limb.
mons pubis	mons pubis The fleshy protuberance over the symphysis pubis.
morfea	morphea A condition exhibited by an elevated or depressed patch of pink skin with a purple border.
morfina	morphine An opioid analgesic.

237

Spanish	English
morfología	morphology The study of living organisms and the correlation between their structure.
morgue	morgue
moribundo	moribund Near death.
morir	die, to
mosca tsetse	tsetse fly An insect that transmits the protozoa trypanosoma and can cause sleeping sickness.
mosquitero	mosquito net
moteado	mottling An irregular arrangement of patches of color.
motor, motora	motor
movimiento ocular rápido	Rapid Eye Movement The movement of a person's eyes during this period of sleep.
movimiento ocular rápido (MOR)	REM (rapid eye movement) sleep This period of sleep is associated with irregular respirations and heart rate, involuntary movements and dreaming.
mórbido	morbid
mórula	morula A solid mass created by the splitting of an ovum.
mucho	lots of
mucho tiempo	long time
mucina	mucin A glycoprotein that is the primary constituent in mucous.
mucílago	mucilage 1. A viscous bodily fluid. 2. A polysaccharide used in medicines and glue.
mucocele	mucocele An accumulation of mucous in a dilated cavity.
mucoide	mucoid Referring to mucous.
mucolítico	mucolytic A substance that breaks down mucous.
mucopurulento	mucopurulent That which contains both mucous and pus.
mucosa	mucosa A mucous membrane like the buccal mucosa.
mudo	mute
muerte	death
muerte cerebral	brain death Cessation of cerebral functioning.
muerto, muerta	dead
muestra	specimen
muestra de orina limpia	clean catch urine specimen
muestra de orina limpia	midstream urine A specimen of urine that is collected after the initial stream of urine is initiated and before one finishes urinating.
muestreo	sampling
muguet	thrush Candida albicans
mujer embarazada	gravida Pregnant.
muleta antebrazo	forearm crutch A long stick with a place for a hand-grip to aid in ambulation when there is lower extremity weakness.
muletas	crutches
multigrávida	multigravida A woman who has been pregnant more than once.
multilocular	multilocular The presence of more than one cells within a cavity.
multípara	multipara A woman with more than one live births.
mummular	nummulated Formed as round, flat discs.
muscular	muscular
muslo	thigh
mutación	mutation A gene alteration that can be passed to the next generation.

Spanish	English
mutismo	mutism Inability to speak.
músculo	muscle
músculo abductor corto del pulgar	abductor pollicis brevis Abducts the thumb.
músculo abductor largo del pulgar	abductor pollicis longus Abducts and flexes the thumb.
músculo aductor	adductor A muscle that brings a part to the midline.
músculo buccinador	buccinator muscle Pulls the mouth posteriorly.
músculo glúteo	gluteal or gluteus muscle A paired set of three muscles, the gluteus maximus, medius and minimus, that all have origins in the ilium and insertions in the femur. (buttocks)
músculo occipitofrontal	occipitofrontal muscle Raises the eyebrows.
músculo recto del abdomen	rectus abdominis muscle The pair of long, flat muscles that connect the sternum with the pubis.
muñeca	wrist
muñón	stump Term used to designate what remains of an amputated extremity.
myelograma	myelogram CT scan or roentgenography of the spinal canal after injection of contrast media.
nacido muerto	stillborn Refers to a newborn that died in utero.
nacido, nacida	born
nacimiento	birth
nalgas	buttocks
narcisismo	narcissism Abnormally excessive self-interest.
narcolepsia	narcolepsy A condition exhibited by a strong desire to sleep and by sudden onset of sleep at increased intervals.
narcosis	narcosis A reversible medication-induced condition of excessive drowsiness or unconsciousness.
narcótico	narcotic A medication that produces narcosis.
naris	nostril
nariz	nose
nasal	nasal Referring to the nose.
nasofaringe	nasopharynx The part of the pharynx which lies superior to the soft palate.
nasofaríngeo	nasopharyngeal Referring to the nose and pharynx.
nasolagrimal	nasolacrimal Referring to the nose and tear apparatus.
natalidad	birth rate The number of live births per 1000 of a given population per year.
navicular	navicular 1. boat shaped 2. Referring to the navicular bone of the hand or foot.
náusea	nausea
nebulizador	nebulizer A device used for transforming a liquid into a fine mist for inhalation as in nebulized albuterol for an acute exacerbation of asthma.
necesitar	need
necroscopia	necropsy Synonym of autopsy.
necrosis	necrosis The death of most of the cells of the affected part.
necrosis avascular	avascular necrosis
necrótico	necrotic Referring to necrosis.
nefrectomía	nephrectomy Surgical removal of a kidney.
nefritis	nephritis A general term meaning inflammation of a kidney that is further categorized depending on the associated pathology.
nefroblastoma	nephroblastoma Congenital tumor of the kidney, also called Wilms' tumor.

Spanish	English
nefrocalcinosis	nephrocalcinosis A condition exhibited by calcium phosphate deposition in the renal tubules; a cause of renal insufficiency.
nefrolitiasis	nephrolithiasis A calculus in the kidney.
nefrolitotomía	nephrolithotomy Surgical removal of a renal calculus.
nefroma	nephroma A renal tumor.
nefrona	nephron A functional unit of the kidney that consists of the glomerulus, the proximal and distal convoluted tubules, the loop of Henle and the collecting tubule.
nefropatía	nephropathy Renal disease.
nefropexia	nephropexy The surgical fixation of a kidney that was previously floating.
nefroptosis	nephroptosis Inferior displacement of the kidney.
nefrosclerosis	nephrosclerosis Hardening of the kidney.
nefrosis	nephrosis A kidney disease exhibited by edema and proteinuria; also called nephrotic syndrome.
nefrostomía	nephrostomy Surgical creation of an opening between the renal pelvis and an opening in the skin.
nefrotomía	nephrotomy Surgical incision of the kidney.
nefrótico	nephrotic Referring to nephrosis.
negación	negation
negar	deny, to
negro	black
nematodo	nematode An endoparasite belonging to the class of the Nemathelminthes including roundworms and threadworms.
neonatal	neonatal Referring to the first four weeks after birth.
neonato	neonate The term for a newborn infant for the first four weeks.
neoplasma	neoplasm A new and abnormal growth.
nervi motot ocular común	oculomotor nerve Referring to cranial nerve III which is one of the nerves responsible for extraocular movements.
nervio	nerve
nervio abducens	abducens nerve A motor nerve (6th cranial nerve) that controls the lateral rectus muscle of the eye.)
nervio accesorio	accessory nerve (XI) Supplies motor innervation to the sternocleidomastoid and trapezius.
nervio circunflejo	circumflex nerve The axillary nerve that has an origin in the posterior branch of the brachial plexus.
nervio esplánico	splanchnic nerves The nerves supplying the abdominal viscera and blood vessels.
nervio facial	facial nerve Cranial nerve VII that supplies the face and tongue.
nervio femoral	femoral nerve Supplies the motor function of the quadriceps and the sensation over the anterior and medial thigh.
nervio hipogloso	hypoglossal nerve Twelfth cranial nerve pair.
nervio neumogástrico	vagus nerve The tenth cranial nerve that supplies the heart, lungs visceral organs; its function is tested by assessment of elevation of the uvula.
nervio sensitivo	sensory nerve A nerve that receives input from various receptors.
nervio trigémino	trigeminal nerve The fifth cranial nerve which supplies the motor function of mastication and has three sensory branches, the ophthalmic, maxillary and mandibular.
nervio troclear	trochlear nerve The fourth cranial nerve that supplies the superior oblique muscle of the eyeball.

Spanish	English
nervios espinales	spinal nerve The term for each of the thirty pairs of nerves that originate in the spine and traverse between the vertebrae. There are eight cervical, twelve thoracic, five lumbar, five sacral and one coccygeal nerve pairs.
neumatocele	pneumatocele 1. A hernia-like protrusion of lung tissue. 2. A collection of gas in a sac such as the scrotum.
neumaturia	pneumaturia Presence of air or gas in the urine.
neumococo	pneumococcus A bacterium causing pneumonia and meningitis. A common type is Streptococcus pneumoniae.
neumoconiosis	pneumoconiosis Fibrosis of the lung due to dust inhalation.
neumonectomía	pneumonectomy Surgical excision of all or part of a lung.
neumonía	pneumonia Inflammation of the lung due to an infection caused by a virus or bacterium.
neumonía por pneumocystis jiroveci	pneumocystis jiroveci pneumonia. A pulmonary infection associated with AIDS. Formerly called pneumocystis carinii pneumonia.
neumoperitoneo	pneumoperitoneum Abnormal or induced presence of air or gas in the peritoneum.
neumotórax	pneumothorax Abnormal presence of air between the lung and chest wall.
neural	neural Referring to a nerve or nerve impulse.
neuralgia	neuralgia Severe pain along the course of a nerve.
neuralgia del trigémino	trigeminal neuralgia Pain in the region of one or more branches of the fifth cranial nerve sensory branches.
neurapraxia	neurapraxia Paralysis from nerve injury but no degeneration of the nerve.
neurectomía	neurectomy Excision of a section of a nerve.
neurilema	neurilemma The membrane covering a myelinated nerve fiber or the axon of an unmyelinated nerve fiber.
neuritis	neuritis Inflammation of a nerve.
neuritis retrobulbar	retrobulbar optic neuritis An inflammatory, demyelinating condition in the retrobulbar region.
neuroastenia	neurasthenia A psychoneurosis exhibited by severe fatigue.
neuroblastoma	neuroblastoma A nervous system malignant tumor composed of neuroblasts.
neurocirugía	neurosurgery Surgery of the brain or spinal cord.
neurodermatitis	neurodermatitis A pruritic, thickened eruption in the axillary and inguinal thought to be exacerbated by emotions.
neuroepitelio	neuroepithelium Cells specialized to serve as sensory cells such as cells of the cochlea and tongue.
neurofibroma	neurofibroma A tumor formed by excessive growth of perineurium and endoneurium.
neurofibromatosis; Enfermedad de von Recklinghausen.	neurofibromatosis A hereditary condition exhibited by formation of multiple soft tumors scattered throughout the skin surface. Also known as von Recklinghausen disease.
neuroglia	neuroglia A type of connective tissue of the nervous system.
neuroléptico	neuroleptic A drug that causes neurologic symptoms.
neurología	neurology The study of the nervous system.
neuroma	neuroma A mass composed of nerve cells and fibers.
neuroma acústica	acoustic neuroma A nonmalignant tumor that can cause deafness, tinnitus and vertigo.
neurona	neuron A nerve cell.
neuropatía	neuropathy Structural of pathologic changes of the peripheral nervous system.

Spanish	English
neuropatía de atrapamiento	entrapment neuropathy Weakness or numbness caused by compression of a peripheral nerve.
neuropatía del plexo braquial	brachial plexus neuropathy
neuropatía diabética	diabetic neuropathy
neuropatía en bulbo de cebolla	onion bulb neuropathy Also known as hypertrophic interstitial neuropathy which is a sensorimotor polyneuropathy.
neuropatía óptica isquémica	ischemic optic neuropathy
neuropatía por vitamina B12	vitamin B12 neuropathy
neuropático	neuropathic Referring to neuropathy.
neurosis	neurosis A mental disorder.
neurosis de ansiedad	anxiety neurosis Abnormal presence of anxiety.
neurosífilis	neurosyphilis Infection of the central nervous system with Treponema pallidum.
neurotmesis	neurotmesis The severing of a nerve.
neurotomía	neurotomy Surgical incision into a nerve.
neurotransmisor	neurotransmitter A substance released at the end of a nerve fiber that facilitates transmission of an impulse.
neurólgo	neurologist A physician who specializes in the study of the nervous system.
neutropenia	neutropenia Diminished number of neutrophils in the blood.
neutrófilo	neutrophil A polymorphonuclear leukocyte.
nevo	nevus A benign, well-circumscribed growth of tissue of congenital origin.
nevo araña	spider nevus A papule with telangiectases radiating from the center.
nevo capilar	capillary nevus A growth of skin that involves the capillaries.
nébula	nebula An opaque spot on the cornea causing impaired vision.
nigua	chigger A parasitic mite of the genus Trombicula.
niño	child
nistagmo	nystagmus Rapid involuntary movement of the eyes; it can be horizontal, vertical or rotary.
nitrato de plata	silver nitrate stick A medical device used to treat hypergranulation tissue.
nitrógeno	nitrogen A colorless, odorless gas used as a coolant in the liquid form.
nixis	nyxis Paracentesis or a puncture.
nocivo	noxious Harmful or poisonous.
nocturia	nocturia Urination at night.
nocturno	nocturnal Referring to events that happen at night.
noicomicosis	onychomycosis Fungal disease of the toenails or fingernails.
nombre	name
norepinefrina	norepinephrine A hormone secreted by the adrenal medulla and a synthetic drug used as a pressor agent.
normoblasto	normoblast A precursor cell for erythrocytes.
normocito	normocyte A normal erythrocyte.
nosocomial	nosocomial infection An infection occurring after admission to a hospital.
nosofobia	nosophobia Unwarranted, excessive fear of any disease.
nosología	nosology The medical science of disease classification.
nódulo	nodule

Spanish	English
nódulo de la hermana Joseph	Sister Mary Joseph nodule A nodule at the umbilicus associated with metastatic abdominal cancer.
nódulo de Caplan	Caplan nodules These are pulmonary nodules noted in people with rheumatoid arthritis who were exposed to coal dust.
nódulo de Schmorl	schmorl's nodule Protrusion of the nucleus pulposus through the vertebral body endplast into the adjacent vertebra.
nódulos de Heberden	Heberden's node Hard nodules formed at the distal interphalangeal joints in osteoarthritis.
NR no resucitar	DNR Do not resuscitate.
nuclear	nuclear Referring to a nucleus.
nucleoproteína	nucleoprotein A substance composed of a nucleic acid and a protein.
nudillo	knuckle
nudo	knot
nudo	node A swelling or prominence.
nudo sinctitial	syncytial knot Aggregation of syncytiotrophoblastic nuclei in the villi of the placenta during early pregnancy.
nudo sinoauricular	sinoatrial node A mass of cardiac tissue that acts as the pacemaker.
nuez de Adán	Adam's apple A prominence on the anterior neck caused by the thyroid cartilage of the larynx.
nuligrávida	nulligravida A woman who has never been pregnant.
nulípara	nullipara A woman who has never given birth.
nutación	nutation Referring to nodding of the head.
nutrición	nutrition
nutriente	nutrient
núcleo arqueados	arcuate nucleus Small masses of gray matter found on the medulla oblongata.
núcleo rojo	red nucleus A collection of gray matter near the subthalamus that receives data from the superior cerebellar peduncle.
obesidad	corpulence Fatness.
obesidad	obesity
obilgatorio	mandatory
obsesión	obsession A pathologic preoccupation.
obsoleto	obsolete
obstetra	obstetrician A physician who specializes in the management of pregnancy, labor and the peuperium.
obstétrico	obstetric Referring to The management of pregnancy, labor and the peuperium.
obstrucción	obstructed To be blocked or halted.
obstrucción intestinal	intestinal obstruction Blockage of the intestine by mass or volvulus.
obturador	obturator A device used to close an artificial or natural opening.
obtuso	obtuse Rather insensitive or hard to understand.
occipital	occipital Referring to the back part of the head.
ocena	ozena Various nasal conditions, all of which include fetid discharge.
oclusión	occlusion
oclusión coronaria	coronary occlusion A blockage in a coronary artery.
ocular	ocular Referring to the eye.
oculógiro	oculogyric Referring to movement of the eye around the anteroposterior axis.
odinofagia	odynophagia Pain associated with swallowing.
odinofonía	odynophonia Pain associated with speaking.

243

Spanish	English
odontalgia	odontalgia Tooth pain.
odontoide	odontoid A prominence on the second cervical vertebra on which the first cervical vertebra pivots.
odontología	odontology Synonym of dentistry.
odor	odor
odorífero	odiferous
ofrecer	volunteer
oftalmía	ophthalmia Profound inflammation of the eye or its structures.
oftalmía gonorreica	gonorrheal ophthalmia
oftalmolgía	ophthalmology The study of diseases of the eye.
oftalmoplejía	ophthalmoplegia Paralysis of the eye muscles.
oftalmoplejía supranuclear	supranuclear ophthalmoplegia A disorder that effects the extraocular movements especially limiting the upward movement of the eyes.
oftalmoscopio	ophthalmoscope A device used to visually inspect the interior eye.
oftalmólogo	ophthalmologist A physician specializing in diseases of the eye.
oftálmico	ophthalmic Referring to the eye.
oído	ear
olécranon	olecranon The bony protrusion at the proximal ulna at the elbow.
olfatología	olfactory Referring to the sense of smell.
oligodactilia	oligodactyly Presence of fewer than 5 digits on a hand or foot.
oligodendroglia	oligodendroglia The ectodermal cells forming part of the central nervous system.
oligohidramnios	oligohydramnios Inadequate amount of amniotic fluid.
oligomenorrea	oligomenorrhea Infrequent menstruation or low volume menstrual flow.
oligoptialismo	oligoptyalism Insufficient secretion of saliva.
oligospermia	oligospermia Abnormally low sperm count.
oligotrofia	oligotrophia Inadequate nutritional state.
oliguria	oliguria Abnormally low urine output.
ombrofobia	ombrophobia An abnormal fear of rain.
omentocele	omentocele A herniated protrusion of omentum.
omentopexia	omentopexy Surgically fastening the omentum to an adjacent tissue it was not previously attached to.
oncología	oncology
oncólogo	oncologist
onda alfa	alpha wave Electroencephalographic waves with a frequency of 8-13 per second.
onfalitis	omphalitis Inflammation of the umbilicus.
onfalocele	omphalocele A large congenital, umbilical hernia with only a thin membranous covering.
ONG oído nariz y garganta	ENT Abbreviation for ears, nose and throat.
onicocriptosis	onychocryptosis Ingrown toenail.
onicofagia	onychophagia Habitually chewing on one's fingernails.
onicogrifosis	onychogryphosis A deformed nail that is incurved or hooked.
oniquia	onychia Inflammation of the toenail or fingernail matrix.
oniquia seca	onychia sicca Brittle fingernails or toenails.

244

Spanish	English
oocito	oocyte An ovarian cell that needs to undergo meiotic division to become an ovum.
ooforectomía	oophorectomy Surgical removal of an ovary.
ooforitis	oophoritis Inflammation of an ovary.
ooforosalpingectomía	oophorosalpingectomy Surgical removal of an ovary and fallopian tube.
oogénesis	oogenesis The initiation and development of an ovum.
oóforo	oophoron Synonym for ovary.
opiáceo	opiate Referring to opium.
opio	opium An addictive drug derived from opium poppy; synthetic versions are used as analgesics.
opioide	opioid A substance similar to opium that binds to at least one of the opium receptors in the body.
opistótonos	opisthotonos A profound spasm in which the head/neck is hyperextended, the feet are touching the bed and with the patient supine the body arched upward.
opometrista	optometrist
oponente	opponens Synonym for opponent muscle.
oposonina	opsonin An antibody used to facilitate phagocytosis of a bacterium.
optometría	optometry The profession of examination of the eyes for disease (not a medical doctor).
oral	oral
oralmente	orally
orbicular	orbicular Rounded or circular.
orbitario	orbital Referring to the orbit.
oreja interno	inner ear
Organizació Mundial de la Salud	World Health Organization (WHO)
organomegalia	organomegaly
orificio	orifice Synonym of foramen.
orina residual	residual urine The amount of urine remaining in the bladder after a person voids.
ornitosis	ornithosis A viral infection transmitted by birds that is manifested by chills, headache, photophobia, fever, nausea and vomiting.
oro	gold
orofaringe	oropharynx The portion of the pharynx between the soft palate and the superior aspect of the epiglottis.
orquialgia	orchialgia Testicular pain.
orquidectomía	orchidectomy Synonym of orchiectomy; removal of one or both testes.
orquiepididimitis	orchiepididymitis Inflammation of the testis and epididymis.
orquiopexia	orchidopexy Surgical repair of an undescended testis.
orquitis	orchitis Inflammation of one or both testes.
ortodoncia	orthodontics A subspecialty of dentistry concerned with treatment of dental irregularities and malocclusion, including the use of braces.
ortopédico	orthopedics A surgical specialty concerned with treatment of skeletal problems.
ortopnea	orthopnea The inability to breath comfortably except in the upright position.
ortosis	orthosis Straightening of a malaligned part with the use of braces and other supportive devices.

Spanish	English
ortostático	orthostatic Referring to the standing position. Orthostatic hypotension is low blood pressure in the standing position.
orzuelo	hordeolum Inflammation of the sebaceous gland of the eye.
oscilliopsia	oscillating nystagmus Abnormal movement of the eyes in a wave-like pattern.
osificación	ossification The formation of bone.
osmol	osmole The recognized unit of osmotic pressure.
osmolaidad	osmolality The concentration expressed in total number of solute particles per kilogram.
osmótico	osmotic Referring to osmosis.
osteítis	osteitis Inflammation of the bone.
ostensiblemente	ostensibly Synonym of apparently and seemingly.
osteoartritis	osteoarthritis A long term, progressive degenerative joint disease.
osteoartrosis	osteoarthrosis Arthritis without inflammation.
osteoblasto	osteoblast A cell that matures from a fibroblast and produces bone.
osteocito	osteocyte An osteoblast within the bone matrix.
osteoclasia	osteoclasis The surgical fracture of a bone usually in order to restore proper alignment.
osteoclasto	osteoclast A large bone cell that is associated with bone reabsorption and removal.
osteoclastoma	osteoclastoma A tumor composed of giant cells or osteoclasts.
osteocondral	osteochondral Referring to bone and cartilage.
osteocondritis	osteochondritis Inflammation of bone and cartilage.
osteocondroma	osteochondroma A tumor with bony and cartilaginous characteristics.
osteodistrofia	osteodystrophy Abnormal bone formation.
osteofonía	osteophony The sound conduction of bone.
osteogénesis	osteogenesis Development of new bones.
osteogénesis imperfecta	ostogenesis imperfecta
osteolítico	osteolytic Referring to the removal or loss of calcium from the bone.
osteomalacia	osteomalacia Softening of the bones because of a deficiency of vitamin D, calcium or phosphorus.
osteomielitis	osteomyelitis Inflammation of the bone or bone marrow because of a microorganism.
osteopatía	osteopathy 1. Any disease of the bone. 2. Medical practice concerning treatment of disease by manipulation and massage of bones, joints, and muscles.
osteopetrosis	osteopetrosis Increased bone density with no change in modeling.
osteoporosis	osteoporosis Loss of bone substance because the osteoblasts fail to produce bone matrix.
osteosarcoma	osteosarcoma A tumor composed of a sarcoma and osseous material.
osteosclerosis	osteosclerosis Abnormal hardening of bone.
osteotomía	osteotomy Creation of a surgical opening in bone.
osteófito	osteophyte Abnormal growth of a bone protuberance.
ostium	ostium A vessel or body cavity opening.
otalgia	otalgia Ear pain.
otalgia geniculada	geniculate neuralgia Severe intermittent pain in the external ear and deep in the ear.
otitis	otitis Inflammation of the ear. (otitis media or otitis externa)

Spanish	English
otolaringólogo	otolaryngologist Surgical specialist concerned with organs of the ears, nose and throat.
otolito	otolith A calcium based calculus in the inner ear.
otología	otology Study of conditions and anatomy of the ear.
otomicosis	otomycosis Fungal infection of the ear.
otosclerosis	otosclerosis A hereditary condition exhibited by progressive hearing loss because of bone overgrowth in the inner ear.
otoscopio	otoscope A device used for inspection of the tympanic membrane.
ototóxico	ototoxic A substance harmful to the ear or its nerve supply.
ovaritis	ovaritis Synonym for oophoritis.
oviducto	oviduct The channel which an ovum passes from the ovary.
ovulación	ovulation The release of an ova from the ovary.
oxaluria	oxaluria Existence of oxalates in the urine.
oxicefalia	oxycephaly The deformation of the skull so that it appears pointed.
oxidación	oxidation The process of a chemical combining with oxygen.
oxigenación	oxygenation Saturated with oxygen.
oxihemoglobina	oxyhemoglobin The combination of oxygen and hemoglobin using a covalent bond.
oxitocina	oxytocin A natural hormone released by the pituitary or a synthetic hormone that facilitates uterine contraction.
oxitócico	oxytocic Referring to rapid parturition.
oxiuro	pinworm Common term for Enterobius verminicularis; a nematode worm that is a parasite.
oxígeno	oxygen
oxímetro	oximeter A medical device used to measure the percent of oxygen that is saturated in the blood (oxygen saturation).
ozono	ozone A toxic chemical that has profound oxidizing properties. It has three atoms in its molecule compared with oxygen which has two.
óptico	optic Referring to the eye.
órbita	orbit The bony structure enclosing the eyeball.
órgano	organ
órgano terminal	end organ The encapsulated end of a sensory nerve.
óseo	osseous Possessing the quality of bone.
ósmosis	osmosis The movement of a solvent from a solution of greater concentration to one of lower concentration through a semi-permeable membrane until the two solutions have equal concentration.
óvulo	ovule An immature ovum.
óxido nitroso	nitrous oxide An inhalant gas used as an anesthetic agent.
paciente	patient
padrastro	hangnail
pagofagia	pagophagia Compulsive need to eat ice which is usually associated with iron deficiency anemia.
paladar	palate The roof of the mouth.
paladar hendido	cleft palate A congenital abnormal opening in the palate.
palangana	basin
palatoplejía	palatoplegia Paralysis of the palate.
paliativo	palliative A treatment used to reduce pain when cure is not possible.
palidectomía	pallidectomy Surgical resection of all or part of the palate.

Spanish	English
palidez	pallor Unusually pale appearance.
palma	palm The anterior aspect of the hand.
palmar	palmar Referring to the palm.
palpación	palpation The assessment of the body with the use of one's hands.
palpebra, palpebrae	palpebra, palpebrae Eyelid, eyelids.
palpitación	palpitation Sensation of a forceful, rapid, irregular heartbeat present after exercise or with anxiety.
paludismo	malaria A condition caused by a protozoan of the genus Plasmodium. It is transmitted by mosquitos and is exhibited by fever, chills, headache. In the severe form it can lead to convulsions, increased ICP and death.
paludismo	paludism Synonym of malaria.
paludismo cerebral	cerebral malaria
panadizo	whitlow An abscess occurring on the palmar surface of the fingertips.
panadizo melanótico Melanoma subungular.	melanotic whitlow
panartritis	panarthritis Inflammation of the joints.
pancarditis	pancarditis Inflammation of pericardium, myocardium and endocardium.
pancreatectomía	pancreatectomy Surgical excision of part or all of the pancreas.
pancreatitis	pancreatitis Inflammation of the pancreas.
pancreocimina	pancreozymin A duodenal mucosal enzyme that facilitates the secretion of amylase and other enzymes from the pancreas.
pandémico	pandemic When a disease is present over an entire region.
panhipopituitarismo	panhypopituitarism Insufficiency of the anterior pituitary.
paniculitis	panniculitis Inflammation of a section of subcutaneous tissue containing large amounts of fat.
panoftalmía	panophthalmia Inflammation of the eye and all its structures.
panotitis	panotitis Inflammation of each part of a bone.
pantalla fluorescente	fluorescent screen A screen used to view x-rays.
pantorrilla	calf
pañal	diaper
paño higiénico	sanitary napkin
paperas	mumps A contagious viral disease that is exhibited by parotid swelling and puts males at risk for sterility.
papiledema	papilledema Swelling of the optic disc.
papilitis	papillitits Swelling of a papilla.
papiloma	papilloma A benign, lobulated tumor coming from epithelium.
paquidermia	pachydermia An abnormally thick skin.
paquimeningitis	pachymeningitis Inflammation of the dura mater.
para tratar los síntomas de la migraña	antimigraine Medication used to treat headaches.
paracentesis	paracentesis A procedure involving aspiration of fluid from the abdominal cavity.
paracusia	paracusia Any abnormality in the sense of hearing.
parafimosis	paraphimosis A condition in which the foreskin is retracted but cannot be replace because of a restricted foreskin.
paralítico	paralytic 1. Referring to paralysis. 2. A person who is paralyzed.
paramediano	paramedian Situated toward the middle of the body.

248

Spanish	English
parametrio	parametrium The connective tissue and smooth muscle between the broad ligament serous layers.
parametritis	parametritis Inflammation of the parametrium.
paramédico	paramedical Hospital support staff excluding physicians.
paramnesia	paramnesia A condition exhibited by a person's belief they have memory for an event that never happened.
paranasal	paranasal Situated next to the nose.
paranoia	paranoia A mental condition exhibited by delusions of persecution.
paranoide	paranoid A person who has paranoia.
paraplejía	paraplegia Paralysis of the lower extremities.
parapraxia	parapraxis 1. Unable to perform purposeful movements. 1. Irrational behavior.
pararectal	pararectal Adjacent to the rectum.
parasimpático	parasympathetic Part of the autonomic nervous system that opposes sympathetic stimulation.
parathormona	parathormone Synonym for parathyroid hormone.
paratiroides	parathyroid Positioned adjacent to the thyroid.
paravertebral	paravertebral Positioned adjacent to the vertebra.
parálisis	palsy
parálisis agitante	paralysis agitans Synonym of Parkinson's disease.
parálisis bulbar progresiva	bulbar palsy Paralysis due to changes in the motor center of the medulla oblongata.
parálisis cerebral	cerebral palsy A condition exhibited by motor incoordination and speech changes that is the result of brain injury occurring ante-, intra- or post- partum.
parálisis de Bell	Bell's palsy Unilateral facial paralysis related to dysfunction of the seventh cranial nerve
parálisis facial	facial paralysis Lack of movement or sensation in the distribution of the facial nerve.
parálisis periódica hipocaliémica	hypokalemic periodic paralysis An inherited disorder that leads to muscle weakness related to a low serum potassium level.
parálisis periódica tirotóxica	thyrotoxic periodic paralysis Weakness associated with an elevated TSH.
parálisis seudobulbar	pseudobulbar palsy Sudden outbursts of laughter or tearfulness sometimes seen in amyotrophic lateral sclerosis.
parásito	parasite An organism that lives on or within another organism without benefit to the latter.
parco	sparing
pared celular	cell wall
pared torácica	chest wall
parenquimal	parenchyma The functional elements of an organ.
parenteral	parenteral Other than the alimentary canal.
paresia	paresis Incomplete paralysis.
parestesia	paresthesia An abnormal sensation usually described as pins and needles.
pariente	relation 1. A person who has a blood or marriage connection.
parietal	parietal Referring to the wall of a part or cavity.
parihuela	stretcher A device used to carry a patient in the supine position.
parkinsonismo Enfermedad de Parkinson.	Parkinson's disease A progressive neuromuscular disease exhibited by masklike facial expression, resting tremor, cogwheel rigidity and abnormal gait.

Spanish	English
paro cardíaco	cardiac arrest Cessation of function of the heart.
paroniquia	paronychia Inflammation of the tissue bordering a fingernail
parosmia	parosmia An alteration in the sense of smell.
parotiditis	parotiditis Inflammation of the parotid gland.
paroxístico	paroxysmal Occurring in sudden attacks.
parótida	parotid A gland near the ear.
parpadeo	blinking
partear	deliver, to (as in, to give birth)
partenogénesis	parthenogenesis Reproduction that occurs without an egg being fertilized by sperm.
partera	midwife A person trained to assist in childbirth.
partería	midwifery The occupation of assisting in childbirth.
parto	childbirth
parturición	parturition The process of giving birth.
pasado	last
paseo	ambulation A walk.
pasivo	passive Not achieved through active effort.
paso	pace
pasta	paste
patizambo Genu valgum.	knock knees Common term for genu valgum.
pato o garra de mono	monkey-paw An appearance due to median nerve palsy causing atrophy of the thenar eminence with adduction and elevation of the thumb, resembling that of a simian.
patogénesis	pathogenesis The course of a disease.
patogénico	pathogenic Referring to an organism that can cause disease.
patognomónico	pathognomonic Characteristic of something.
patología	pathology 1. The branch of medicine dealing with the study of tissues and the forensic application. 2. Referring to a condition that is abnormal.
patológico	pathological Referring to pathology.
pavor nocturno	night terror Sensation of profound fear upon wakening.
páncreas	pancreas A gland that secretes digestive enzymes into the duodenum and insulin and glucagon into the blood.
pápula	papule A small, well-circumscribed elevation of the skin.
párpado	eyelid Palpebra.
peca	macula solaris Formal medical term describing a freckle.
pecho, seno	breast
pectoral	pectoral Referring to the pectoral muscle.
pectoriloquia	pectoriloquy The examiner's voice is clearly audible when the patient speaks as when the examiner listens to an area of consolidation in the lungs of the speaker.
pediatra	pediatrician Physician who is a specialist in pediatrics.
pediatría	pediatrics Medical specialty concerned with the treatment and prevention of childhood disease.
pediculado	pediculate Referring to pedicle.
pediculosis	pediculosis Lice infestation.
pedícle	pedicle Part of a skin/tissue graft temporarily left connected to the original site.

Spanish	English
pedúnculo	peduncle 1. A stalk-like protrusion. 2. A bundle of nerve fibers connecting two parts of the brain.
peenash	peenash Clear rhinitis induced by larvae presence in the nasal passages.
pegamento	glue
peine	comb
pelagra	pellagra A deficiency in nicotinic acid exhibited by diarrhea and dermatitis.
peloteo	ballottement Presence of movement of a floating object by palpation.
peludo	hairy
pelvimetría	pelvimetry Measurement of the dimensions of the pelvis to determine whether a patient is capable of natural childbirth.
pelvis	pelvis The bony structure at the base of the spine.
pelvis androide	android pelvis A pelvis shaped like a man's.
pelvis renal	renal pelvis The kidney collecting system.
pene	penis Male genital organ used for the transfer of sperm and elimination of urine.
penetración	penetration
penfigoide ampollar	bullous pemphigoid A benign disease of the aged characterized by large bullae forming on the torso and extremities.
penicilina	penicillin A synthetic antibiotic originally produced from blue mold.
pentosuria	pentosuria The presence of pentose in the urine (a monosaccharide with five carbon atoms in the molecule).
pepsina	pepsin A proteolytic gastric enzyme.
pequeño	slight
percusión	percussion A manual procedure involving tapping a body part to determine the size or density (liquid or air) of a part.
perforación	perforation Presence of a hole.
periartritis	periarthritis Inflammation of the tissues around a joint.
pericardio	pericardium The structure enclosing the heart which contains a fibrous outer layer and serous inner layer.
pericarditis	pericarditis Inflammation of the pericardium.
pericardíco	pericardial Referring to around the heart.
pericolitis	pericolitis Inflammation of the membrane covering the colon.
pericondrio	perichondrium The membrane that encloses a cartilage.
pericondritis	perichondritis Inflammation of the perichondrium.
periférico	peripheral Referring to an outward part or surface.
perilinfa	perilymph The fluid separating the membranous and osseous labyrinth.
perinatología	perinatology The study of disease in the period just before and right after birth.
perineal	perineal Referring to the perineum.
perineo	perineum The area between the anus and scrotum or anus and vulva.
perineorrafia	perineorrhaphy Surgical repair of the perineum.
perinéfrico	perinephric Around the kidney.
periostio	periosteum A layer of connective tissue covering the bones.
periostitis	periostitis Inflammation of the periosteum.
perióstico	periosteal Referring to the periosteum.
periproctitis	periproctitis Inflammation of the tissue encircling the anus and rectum.
peristalismo	peristalsis The contraction of the longitudinal and circular muscle fibers of the alimentary canal so food is propelled.

Spanish	English
peritomía	peritomy Surgically creating an opening of the periosteum.
peritoneal	peritoneal Referring to the peritoneum.
peritoneo	peritoneum The serous membrane covering the abdominal organs and lining the abdominal walls.
peritonitis	peritonitis Inflammation of the peritoneum.
periuretral	periurethral Surrounding the urethra.
perjudicial	detrimental Harmful.
permanencia dela sensación del gusto	after-taste
pernicioso	pernicious 1. Having a detrimental effect. 2. Pernicious anemia is a reduced red blood cell count due to Vitamin B12 deficiency.
perno	pin; wire
peroneo	peroneal Referring to the fibula or the outer part of the leg.
perotonsilitis	peritonsillar Surrounding the tonsils.
persona contribuyente	donor Referring to a person who donates tissue or an organ.
personalidad	personality
perspiración	perspiration
pertussis	pertussis Synonym for whooping cough.
pes cavus	pes cavus Excessive height of the longitudinal arch of the foot.
pes valgus	pes valgus Abnormal longitudinal arch- it is flat.
pesadilla	nightmare
pesado	heavy
pesar	grief
pesar	sorrow
pesario	pessary A supportive device placed in the rectum or vagina.
pescado	fish
peso corporal	body weight
pestaña	eyelash
peste bubónica	bubonic plague A form of plague exhibited by the formation of buboes.
petequia	petechia A small red or purple macule on the skin caused by bleeding.
pezón	nipple
pélvico	pelvic Referring to the pelvis.
pénfigo	pemphigus A skin disorder with large bullous lesions.
péptico	peptic Referring to pepsin or concerning digestion.
péptido	peptide A compound with low molecular weight and containing two or more amino acids.
pérdida de un ser querido	bereavement The sorrow one feels with the loss of a loved one.
pérdido el conocimiento	loss of consciousness Unresponsive to verbal and tactile stimuli.
pérdido el seguimiento	lost to follow-up This describes a situation in which a patient has a chronic medical problem but has not been seen regularly.
pétreo	petrous Possessing a density of a stone.
pétrissage	petrissage Massage using a kneading action.
piamadre	pia mater The first layer of three covering the brain and spinal cord.
pica	pica A desire for unusual substances as occurs in pregnancy and some psychological conditions.
picadura	sting

Spanish	English
picadura de garrapata	tick bite
picdura de abeja	bee sting
picnosis	pyknosis The degeneration of a cell with the nucleus shrinking.
pie	foot
pie caído	drop foot The symptom in a person with a nerve injury causing impaired ankle dorsiflexion.
pie caído	foot drop
pie de atleta	athlete's foot Common term for tinea pedis.
pie plano	flat foot
piel	skin
pielitis	pyelitis Renal pelvis inflammation.
pielografía	pyelography Roentgenography of the renal pelvis and ureters after administration of contrast media.
pielolitotomía	pyelolithotomy Surgical excision of a calculus from the renal pelvis.
pielonefritis	pyelonephritis Inflammation of the renal parenchyma usually due to bacterial infection.
pielonefrosis	pyelonephrosis Term, rarely used anymore,used to describe disease of the renal pelvis.
piemia	pyemia Sepsis characterized by the presence of secondary abscesses.
pierna	leg
pigmentos biliares	bile pigments The golden brown or green-yellow color associated with bile.
pildora anticonceptiva	oral contraceptive Tablet taken by mouth to prevent pregnancy.
pilorplastia	pyloroplasty Surgical enlargement of a pylorus that previously was stenotic.
pilórico	pyloric Referring to the pylorus.
pinguécula	pinguecula The yellow tissue on the bulbar conjunctiva adjacent to the sclerocorneal junction.
pinocitosis	pinocytosis The absorption of fluid into a cell by the formation of vesicles on the cell membrane.
pioderma	pyoderma A purulent skin infection.
piogénico	pyogenic Referring to the formation of pus.
piojo	lice Plural for louse, a small parasite that lives on the skin. Pediculus humanus capitis is a head louse.
pionefrosis	pyonephrosis Injury to the renal parenchyma due to pus.
piorrea	pyorrhea Emission of pus.
piosálpinx	pyosalpinx Purulent material in the oviduct.
pipeta	pipet A slender tube with a bulb used for transferring liquids.
piramidal	pyramidal A term that is used to describe various spinal tracts that originate in the cerebral cortex.
pirexia	pyrexia Fever.
pirodoxina	pyridoxine Synonym for vitamin B6.
pirosis	pyrosis Synonym for heartburn.
pirógen	pyrogen A fever producing substance released by bacteria.
pitiriasis rosea	pityriasis rosea A skin disease characterized by dry pink oval papulosquamous eruptions.
piuria	pyuria Presence of purulent material in the urine.
pícnico	pyknic Possessing a short, stocky physique.
píldora	pill
píloro	pylorus The opening at the distal stomach that opens into the duodenum.

Spanish	English
placa terminal motora	motor end plate The expansions on a motor nerve where the branches terminate on muscle fiber.
placenta	placenta The vascular tissue that nourishes a fetus through an umbilical cord.
placenta previa	placenta praevia A condition in which the placenta covers the cervical os.
placentario	placental Referring to the placenta.
plagiocefalia	plagiocephaly A condition characterized by an asymmetric skull because the cranial sutures do not close normally.
planificación familiar	family planning Birth control.
planta de pie	sole of foot
plantar	plantar Referring to the bottom of the foot.
plaqueta	platelet An oval cell without a nucleus used in coagulation; also called a thrombocyte.
plasmacitosis	plasmacytosis The existence of plasma cells in the blood.
plasmaféresis	plasmapheresis A method of removing blood and reinfusing it after the elimination of antibodies.
plata	silver
platelminto	flatworm A class of worms that includes parasitic flukes and tapeworms.
pledget	pledget A small plug of cotton or other synthetic material inserted into a wound.
pleomorfísmo	pleomorphism The ability of an organism or substance to attain distinct forms.
pletismógrafo	plethysmograph A device used to measure the amount of blood flowing through a body part; impedance plethysmography is used to check for deep venous thrombosis.
pleura	pleura The serous membrane lining each lung.
pleursía	pleurisy Inflammation of the pleura.
plexo braquial	brachial plexus A cluster of nerves coming off the last four cervical and first thoracic spinal nerves form the nerve supply the the chest and arms.
plexo solar	solar plexus A cluster of ganglia and nerves, located at the base of the sternum, that surround the celiac trunk.
plétora	plethora An excess of something.
plica	plica A fold, as in a fold in the peritoneum.
pliegue glúteo	gluteal fold
pliegue piel	skin fold
plomo	lead An element with an atomic number of 82.
poder con	cope with, to
poiquilocitosis	poikilocytosis The presence of abnormally shaped erythrocytes.
poiquilotermia	poikilothermy A condition of cold-blooded animals in which their temperature varies based on the ambient temperature.
poliarteritis nodusa	polyarteritis nodosa A systemic necrotizing vasculitis that effects medium sized arteries.
policitemia	polycythemia Excess in the number of erythrocytes in the blood.
policitemia vera (o rubra)	polycythemia vera Condition characterized by increase in erythrocytes, thrombocytes and leukocytes, as well as, splenomegaly.
policondritis	polychondritis Inflammation of the cartilage at more than one site.
polidactilia	polydactyly Congenital anomaly exhibited by more than 5 digits on the hands and/or feet.
polidipsia	polydipsia Profound thirst.
polimenorrea	polymenorrhea Increase in the frequency of menstruation.

254

Spanish	English
polimiositis	polymyositis Inflammation of several muscle groups at once.
polineuritis	polyneuritis Inflammation of more than one nerve.
polineuropatía	polyneuropathy A condition involving more than one nerve.
polioencefalitis	polioencephalitis Polio infection of the brain.
poliomielitis	poliomyelitis An infectious viral disease exhibited by constitutional symptoms that can lead to quadriplegia.
poliopía	polyopia A condition in which one object is seen abnormally as two or more.
poliposis	polyposis The formation of multiple polyps.
poliquístico	polycystic Possessing more than one cyst.
polisacárido	polysaccharide A carbohydrate that upon hydrolysis forms more than ten monosaccharides.
poliscelia	polysialia Abnormal increase in saliva.
poliuria	polyuria Abnormal increase in volume of urine excreted.
polvo	dust
polvo	powder
polypus	polypus Synonym of polyp (a prominent growth from a mucous membrane).
ponfólix Dishidrosis.	pompholyx A condition exhibited by interdigital vesicles of the hands and feet.
pons	pons The part of the brainstem that connects the medulla oblongata with the thalamus.
pontino	pontine Referring to the pons.
poplíteo	popliteal Referring to the posterior knee.
por todo el cuerpo	all over the body
porfiria	porphyria A hereditary condition currently classified based on the specific enzyme deficiency. The most common form is porphyria cutanea tarda that causes blistering lesions.
porfirina	porphyrin A class of pigments that contain a flat ring of four heterocyclic groups.
portaagujas	needle holder A surgical instrument used to grasp a needle during suturing.
portal	portal Referring to an entrance such as porta hepatis.
portaobjeto	slide A thin, rectangular piece of glass used for viewing specimen under a microscope.
poscarga	after-load Referring to the amount of pressure the heart needs to pump against. If one has left heart failure it is beneficial to reduce after-load.
posición fetal	fetal position
posición rodilla-codo	knee elbow position Knees and elbows are on the table and the chest is in the air.
posictal	postictal
positivo	positive
posponer	postpone
postemilla	gumboil Swelling noted on the gingiva over a dental abscess.
posterior	posterior
postmadurado	postmaturity Generally referring to a pregnancy that goes beyond the due date.
postración	collapse
postrado en cama	bedridden
postural	postural Referring to position or posture.
potasio	potassium A chemical of the alkali metal group.

Spanish	English
potencial de acción	action potential The alteration in electrical potential associated with the movement along a nerve cell.
potential evocada	evoked potential Electrical impulses that can be noted after stimulation of sensory organs.
pox	pox A general term for fluid filled papules that upon rupturing leave pockmarks.
practicante de enfermera	nurse practitioner
preauricular	preauricular Anterior to the ear.
precanceroso	precancerous Referring to an early stage in cancer development.
precipitina	precipitin An antibody-antigen reaction producing a precipitate.
precordialgia	precordialgia Pain in the precordium.
precordio	precordium The area occupying the epigastrum and lower sternum.
preeclampsia	preeclampsia Hypertension with proteinuria and/or edema in the setting of pregnancy.
prematuro	premature Occurring earlier than expected.
premenstrual	premenstrual Occurring prior to the onset of menstruation.
premolar	premolar The teeth anterior to the molars.
prenatal	prenatal Referring to the time prior to birth.
prepucio	foreskin Also called prepuce, the skin that naturally covers the glans but can be rolled back.
presbiacusia	presbyacusia An age related, progressive hearing loss.
presbiopía	presbyopia Farsightedness associated with aging.
presentación de cara	face presentation Referring to the part of the body coming out of the cervix first during childbirth.
presentación de nalgas	breech birth
presentación frontal del feto	brow presentation The term used to describe which part of the body (forehead) is being delivered first in childbirth.
presístole	presystole The time just before systole.
presión alta	high blood pressure
presión arterial	blood pressure Written as the measurement in mmHg at the time of systole of the left ventricle over the time of diastole.
prevenir	prevent, to
priapismo	priapism A painful and abnormally prolonged erection.
primera dentición	deciduous teeth The first teeth.
primeros auxilios	first aid
primípara	primipara A woman giving birth for the first time.
probabilidad	likelihood
problema	problem
proctalgia	proctalgia A chronic high, dull rectal pain worse with sitting position.
proctitis	proctitis Inflammation of the rectum.
proctocele	proctocele A hernia-type protrusion of the rectum into the vagina.
proctoscopia	proctoscopy Inspection of the rectum with a scope.
profiláctico	prophylaxis That which is done to prevent disease.
profundo, profunda	deep
progeria	progeria A childhood disorder exhibited by signs of aging including gray hair, wrinkled skin and short height.
progesterona	progesterone A steroid hormone that prepares the uterus for pregnancy.

Spanish	English
proglotis	proglottis Any segment of a tapeworm.
prognatismo	prognathism Protrusion of the mandible which can cause malocclusion.
progresivo	progressive
prolactina	prolactin A pituitary hormone that facilitates milk production.
prolapso	prolapse The slipping downward of a body part, such as rectal prolapse.
prolapso del útero	uterine prolapse
prolapso del cordón umbilical	prolapse of the umbilical cord
promonocito	promonocyte An intermediate cell stage between monocyte and monoblast.
promontorio	promontory A protruding eminence.
pronación	pronation Turning posteriorly. When the hand is pronated, it is turned medially until the palm is facing posteriorly (when the body was initially in the anatomic position).
prono	prone Lying with the abdomen and face downward.
pronóstico	prognosis
propicio	benign Not harmful.
propioceptor	proprioceptor A receptor that responds to sensory input including position sense.
proptosis	proptosis oculi Synonym of exophthalmos; bulging of the eye.
prosencéfalo	forebrain The part of the brain that includes the thalamus, hypothalamus and cerebral hemispheres.
prostaciclina	prostacyclin A prostaglandin that functions as an anticoagulant and vasodilator.
prostaglandina	prostaglandin A compound first found in semen (thus "prosta" in the name from prostate) with many effects including uterine contraction.
prostatectomía	prostatectomy Surgical excision of the prostate.
prostración	prostration Profound exhaustion.
protectomía	proctectomy Surgical excision of the rectum.
proteinuria	proteinuria The presence of protein in the urine.
proteína	protein A class of nitrogenous organic compound.
proteólisis	proteolysis Enzyme action on proteins to form amino acids.
protoplasma	protoplasm The cytoplasm, organelles and nucleus of a living cell.
protozoario	protozoa A single celled microscopic organism including amoebas among others.
protrombina	prothrombin A compound converted to thrombin during coagulation of blood.
protuberancia	bulging
protuberancia	lump
provisiones	supplies
provocar	provoke, to
proximal	proximal Situated closer to the center of the body (opposed to that which is farther away, as in distal).
próstata	prostate A gland found in men that surrounds the neck of the urethra and bladder.
prótesis	prosthesis An artificial body part.
próximo	next
prueba alérgica	patch test A test used to determine which substances provoke an allergic response in a patient.

257

Spanish	English
prueba controlada por placebo	placebo controlled When a study is placebo controlled it means part of the group received an inactive treatment while the other group received active therapy.
prueba de absorción de anticuerpo treponémico fluorescente	FTA test Fluorescent treponemal antibody test for syphilis.
prueba de antiglobinemia	antiglobulin test (Coombs' test) Test used to detect erythroblastosis fetalis.
prueba de capilar fragilidad	capillary fragility test Application of a blood pressure cuff high enough to restrict venous return and after five minutes count the number or petechiae produced.
prueba de fijación del complemento	complement fixation test A laboratory test for the presence of an antibody in the serum that involves inactivation of the complement in the serum.
prueba de Finkelstein.	Finkelstein test Pain elicited with thumb flexion and wrist flexion is indicitive of De Quervain tenosynovitis.
prueba de la nariz y el dedo	finger nose test
prueba de tolerancia a la glucosa	glucose tolerance test The oral administration of a carbohydrate load and then evaluation of the blood sugar at timed intervals.
prueba intradérmica de Casoni	Casoni's test Hydatid fluid is injected intradermally; subsequent formation of a larger papule indicates hydatid disease.
pruebas sanguíneas cruzadas	cross-matching (blood) Evaluation of blood to determine compatibility between the donor and recipient prior to transfusion.
prurigo	prurigo A chronic, pruritic papular skin eruption.
prurito	itch
prurito	pruritis A general term for conditions exhibited by itching.
prurito azoico	azo itch A pruritis noted in people who use azo dyes.
prurito de avicultor	poultryman's itch Pruritis associated with the mite Dermanyssus gallinae.
prurito de escarcha Dermatitis hiemalis.	frost itch A pruritis noted when exposed to cold weather.
prurito de Malabar. Tiña imbricata.	Malabar itch. Pruritis associated with tinea imbricata which is characterized by overlapping rings of papulosquamous patches. It is also known as oriental ringworm.
prurito de Noruega	Norway itch A severe pruritis caused by scabies and is associated with immune disorders such as AIDS.
prurito de paja	straw itch Pruritis associated with exposure to straw that is infested with the mite Pyemotes ventricosus. Also referred to as dermatitis pediculoides ventricosus.
prurito de San Ignacio. Pelagra.	Saint Ignatius' itch Pruritis noted with a cluster of symptoms related to niacin deficiency. Generally referred to as pellagra.
prurito de verano o prurito estival.	summer itch Pruritis noted upon exposure to hot weather, also known as pruritis aestivalis.
prurito del nadador	swimmer's itch Pruritis caused by exposure to schistosomes.
prurito del suelo	ground itch Marked pruritis caused by a hookworm larvae, known otherwise as cutaneous larva migrans.
prurito dhobie Tiña cruris	dhobie itch So called because the contact dermatitis is caused by the soap used by laundry workers in India who are called "dhobie".
prurito inguinal	jock itch Pruritis caused by tinea cruris.
prurito por copra	copra itch A pruritis noted in people working with copra (dried kernel from a coconut).
psicastenia	psychasthenia Essentially any non-hysterical neuroses.

258

Spanish	English
psicología	psychology The study of the human mind and emotions.
psiconeurosis	psychoneurosis A mental disorder that could include depression or anxiety but does not include hallucinations.
psicopatología	psychopathology Scientific examination of mental disease.
psicosis	psychosis A profound mental disorder that can include delusions and hallucinations.
psicosis del postpartum	postpartum psychosis A serious mental condition that occurs following pregnancy.
psicosis maniacodepresiva	manic-depressive psychosis A mental disorder exhibited by alternating periods of depression and mania.
psicosomático	psychosomatic Physical ailments arising from mental disease.
psicoterapia	psychotherapy Treatment of mental disease with cognitive-behavioral approaches.
psicólogo	psychologist A professional specializing in psychology.
psiquiatría	psychiatry A branch of medicine specializing in the treatment of mental disorders.
psitacosis	psittacosis A chlamydial pneumonia that is transmitted by birds.
psoriasis	psoriasis A chronic papulosquamous dermatosis characterized by silver plaques.
pterigión	pterygium A membrane in the interpalpebral fissure present from the conjunctiva to the cornea.
ptialina	ptyalin An enzyme found in saliva.
ptosis	ptosis Drooping of the upper eyelid usually due to paralysis of the third cranial nerve.
pubertad	puberty The time when adolescents become capable of sexual reproduction.
pubis	pubis The anterior inferior part of the hip bone on each side that articulates at the pubic symphysis.
pudendo	pudendal Referring to the female genitalia
puente nasal bajo	low nasal bridge A flattening of the top part of the nose.
pueperio	puerperium The six week period after childbirth.
puérpera	puerpera A woman who just gave birth.
pujar	bearing down As in during labor.
pulga	flea
pulgar	thumb
pulmonar	pulmonary Referring to the lungs.
pulmón	lung
pulmón de granjero	farmer's lung Coined because farmers are susceptible to this disease by inhaling fungi from hay; also called Aspergillosis.
pulpa	pulp The tissue filling the root canals of a tooth.
pulpitis	pulpitis Dental pulp inflammation.
pulsación	pulsation
pulsátil	pulsatile
pulso	pulse The rhythmic throbbing of arteries felt at major vessels.
pulso alternante	pulsus alternans A regular alternation of weak and strong beats of the pulse.
punción	tap
punción cisternal	cisternal puncture A trans-occipitoatlantoid ligament puncture of the cisterna magna so CSF can be obtained.

Spanish	English
punción lumbar	lumbar puncture Insertion of a needle into the spinal canal in the region of L3-4 to obtain a sample of CSF.
punta del dedo	fingertip
punteado	stippling
punto ciego	blind spot An area of insensitivity to light located at the point of entry of the optic nerve on the retina.
punto terminal	end point The last stage of a process.
puña	fist
pupila	pupil The opening at the center of the iris.
pupila de Adie	Adie's pupil Characterized by a weak light reaction and a strong but slow near response
pupilo amaurótica	amaurotic pupil A pupil that will not respond to light when directly exposed but will respond when the other eye is exposed to light.
pupilo de Bumke	Bumke's pupil Dilation of the pupil in response to anxiety.
pupilo de Hutchinson	Hutchinson's pupil Dilation of a pupil related to third nerve palsy on the side of the lesion as seen in herniation.
pupilo de ojo de gato	cat's eye pupil A pupil in the shape of an oval.
pupilo paradójica	paradoxical pupil Constriction of the pupil when exposed to darkness.
purulento	purulent Referring to pus.
pus	pus
putrefacción	putrefaction The rotting or decaying of organic matter.
púrpura	purpura The presence of patches of ecchymosis or petechiae.
púrpura de Henoch-Schönlein	Henoch purpura Exhibited by vomiting, diarrhea, abdominal pain and hematuria; a non-thrombocytopenic purpura.
queilitis	chelilitis Inflammation of the lip.
queja	complaint
quejarse continuamente	querulousness Whining or complaining.
queloide	keloid Hypertrophic scar tissue that forms after a minor cut or surgical procedure.
quemadura	burn
quemadura por frío	frostbite
quemosis	chemosis Swelling of conjunctival tissue adjacent to the cornea.
queratectasia	keratectasia Obtrusion of the cornea.
queratectomía	keratectomy Excision of a portion of the cornea.
queratina	keratin A protein found in the skin, hair, nails and enamel of the teeth.
queratoma	keratoma A protuberance of horny tissue.
queratomalacia	keratomalacia Softening of the cornea.
queratosis	keratosis A growth of keratin such as a wart or callosity.
querático	keratic Referring to the cornea.
quiasma	chiasma The optic chiasma is the area inferior to the hypothalamus where the optic nerves cross.
quiescente	quiescent A time of inactivity.
quilo	chyle A combination of lymph fluid and fat that enters the blood via the thoracic duct.
quilomicrón	chylomicron A one micron particle of emulsified fat.
quiloso, quilosa	chylous Referring to chyle.
quimera	chimera A mixture of genetically distinct tissues.
quimiorreceptora	chemoreceptor A sense organ that responds to stimuli.

Spanish	English
quimiotaxis	chemotaxis The response of an organism to chemical agents.
quimioterapia	chemotherapy Use of medication (chemical agents) in the treatment of disease. This term is commonly used to refer to the treatment of cancer patients with medication.
quimo	chyme The gruel produced by gastric digestion.
quinsy	quinsy Peritonsillar inflammation or abscess.
quinta enfermedad o eritema infeccioso	Fifth disease or erythema infectiosum is a viral disease caused by parovirus B19.
quiropodista	chiropodist A doctor trained in the treatment of feet.
quiropráctica	chiropractic Referring to the medical practice of adjusting malaligned joints.
quiropráctico	chiropractor A medical practitioner who is involved with the treatment of disease by manipulating malaligned joints.
quirúrgico	surgical Referring to surgery.
quiste tirogloso	thyroglossal cyst A common congenital growth in the thyroglossal duct.
quiste de Baker	Baker cyst A synovial fluid collection in the popliteal fossa.
quiste de Meibomio. Chalazión.	meibomian cyst An enclosed fluid collection along a sebaceous gland of the eyelid.
quiste de secuestración	dermoid cyst An abnormal growth containing hair follicles, skin and sebaceous glands.
quiste hidatídico	hydatid cyst A cyst produced by and containing tapeworm larvae.
quiste pilonidal	pilonidal cyst A small cone-shaped cluster of tissue situated posterior to the third ventricle of the brain.
quiste sebáceo	steatoma A sebaceous cyst or lipoma.
quistes ováricos	ovarian cysts
rabdomiólisis	rhabdomyolysis
rabia	rabies An infectious viral disease transmitted through the bite of a mammal. Symptoms include hydrophobia, pharyngeal spasms and hyperactivity.
racemoso	racemose A gland having the form of a cluster.
radiación	radiation 1. The emission of energy in the form of electromagnetic waves. 2. Divergence from a common point.
radiación ionizante	ionizing radiation High energy radiation that produces ion pairs in matter.
radiactivo	radioactive Referring to the emission of ionizing particles or radiation.
radial	radial Referring to the radius.
radiculitis	radiculitis Inflammation of a spinal nerve root.
radiobiología	radiobiology The study of the effects of radiation on organisms.
radioepitelitis	radioepithelitis The injury to epithelial cells due to effects of radiation.
radiografía	radiography The department where images are produced on sensitive film by x-rays.
radioisótopo	radioactive isotope An isotope with an unstable nucleus that is used in diagnostic imaging.
radiología	radiology The branch of medicine concerned with roentgenography and other high-energy radiation.
radionúclido	radionuclide A radioactive nuclide.
radiosensibilidad	radiosensitivity The susceptibility of the skin to radiation.
radioterapia	radiotherapy Treatment of cancer with radiation.
radiólogo	radiologist A physician specializing in radiology.
radón 219	actinon A radioactive element, radon-219.
raíz	root

Spanish	English
raíz anterior	anterior root A motor nerve root that is in the anterior part of the spinal cord between the anterior and lateral funiculi.
raíz cuadrada	square root
raíz dorsal	dorsal root A description of the site of ganglion found on the dorsal root of each spinal nerve.
rales	rale An abnormal lung sound noted during auscultation.
ramus	ramus A branch; a term used to describe a smaller vessel branching off from a larger one.
rana	frog
raquitismo	rickets A condition exhibited by softening and bowing of the long bones; caused by Vitamin D deficiency.
rasguño	scratch
raspadera	rugine A surgical instrument that resembles a rasp.
raspadura	scrape
rayos gamma	gamma rays A type of electromagnetic radiation.
rayos ultravioletas	ultraviolet rays Electromagnetic radiation with wavelength longer than x rays.
rayos X de pecho	chest x-ray
rágade	rhagade Fissures in the skin, particularly adjacent to body orifices.
ránula	ranula A retention cyst formed because of obstruction of a salivary gland in the floor of the mouth.
rápido, rápida	brisk
reacción	reaction
reacción dopa	dopa reaction A dopa-oxidase reaction, changing dopa into melanin.
reacción por drogas	drug reaction
reactivo	reactive
rebanada	slice
rebote	rebound A term used to describe a type of tenderness found with peritonitis.
receptor	receptor A cell or organ that accepts stimuli and transmits data to a sensory nerve.
recesivo	recessive This refers to genetic controlled traits that are only inherited when code from both parents is the same.
receta	prescription
recidiva	relapse
rectal	rectal Referring to the rectum.
rectocele	rectocele A herniation of the wall between the rectum and vagina.
rectoscopia	rectoscopy Visualization of the rectum with a scope.
rectosigmoidectomíe	rectosigmoidectomy Surgical resection of the rectum and sigmoid colon.
recuento sanguíneo completo	complete blood count An assay that includes white blood cell, red blood cell, platelet count, hemoglobin, hematocrit and white blood cell differential.
recuento sanguíneo diferencial de glóbulos blancos	differential leukocyte count The percentage of different types of leukocytes.
recuerdo	recollection Memory.
recumbente	recumbent Lying down.
reducción	reduction Return of a dislocated joint or fractured bone to its proper position.
reducción abierta de fracturas	open reduction of fractures

Spanish	English
reducción cerrada de fracturas	closed reduction of fractures
reductor de colesterol	lipid-lowering agent A medication used to treat hyperlipidemia.
reflejo abdominal	abdominal reflex Elicited by stroking the abdomen lightly from mid-axillary line to umbilicus. A normal response is contraction of the umbilicus toward the stimulated side.
reflejo biceps	biceps reflex The biceps brachii tendon is hit with a reflex hammer and results in flexion of the forearm as a normal response. This assesses the C5-C6 region.
reflejo de arcada	gag reflex Contraction of the pharynx muscles when the back of the pharynx is stimulated by touch.
reflejo de prensión	grasp reflex Flexion of the fingers or toes when stimulated.
reflejo de sacudida de la rodilla	knee jerk reflex Contraction of the quadriceps, yielding leg extension when the quadriceps tendon is tapped.
reflejo del cuádriceps	quadriceps jerk (reflex)
reflejo del tríceps	triceps reflex A tendon reflex causing extension of the arm when the triceps tendon is gently tapped.
reflejo espinal	spinal reflex A reflex that has an arc passing through the spine.
reflejo gastrocólico	gastrocolic reflex Peristalsis of the colon produced by food entering the stomach.
reflejo hepatoyugular	hepatojugular reflex
reflejo plantar (reflejo de Babinski)	Babinski's sign A reflex that occurs when the plantar surface of the foot is stimulated. The great toe turns upward- normal in infancy but when it turns upward in an adult it means there is central nervous system injury.
reflejo plantar (reflejo de Babinski)	extensor plantar response Great toe extension indicating a positive Babinski sign.
reflejo tendinoso profundo	deep tendon reflex Reflexes exhibited by the stretching of a tendon.
reflejo tendón	tendon reflex A deep reflex elicited by gently tapping the tendon.
reflexo del tendón de Aquiles	Achilles tendon reflex The normal response to tapping the achilles tendon with a reflex hammer is the plantar flexion of the foot.
registro médico	medical record
registro médico	patient chart
registro operación	operative note A detailed description of a surgical procedure performed on a specific patient.
regurgitación	regurgitation 1. Backflow of blood in the heart. 2. Movement of gastric contents into the mouth.
regurgitación mitral	mitral regurgitation Backflow of blood from the left ventricle to the left atrium because of dysfunctional valve.
reír	laugh, to
relacionado	related to
relaciones sexuales	sexual intercourse
relajante	relaxant Term generally used to refer to a muscle relaxant.
relaxina	relaxin A hormone secreted by the placenta which dilates the cervix.
remisión	remission A decrease in severity or a temporary resolution.
renal	renal Referring to the kidney.
rendimiento cardíaco	cardiac output Amount of blood pumped by the heart in liters per minute.
renina	renin A renal enzyme that facilitates the production of angiotensin.
repetición de sonidos	echoing sounds

Spanish	English
repuesta inmune	immune response The body's reaction to what is perceived as a foreign substance.
resección	resection The removal of tissue.
resfrío	cold Viral upper respiratory tract infection.
resina	resin An organic substance that is insoluble in water. There are many types. Cholestyramine resin is used for hypercholesterolemia.
resistencia	stamina Ability to maintain physical or mental exertion for a long period.
resonancia magnética nuclear	nuclear magnetic resonance (NMR) A type a diagnostic body imaging utilizing electromagnetic radiation in a magnetic field.
respiración	breath
respiración asistido	assisted ventilation The act of helping one breathe through artificial means.
respiración boca a boca	mouth to mouth resuscitation A form of emergency management of respiratory failure.
respiración de Kussmaul	Kussmaul respiration The slow, deep breathing noted in patients with acidosis.
respirador	respirator A device used to artificially ventilate a patient.
respiratorio	respiratory Referring to respiration or the organs of respiration.
resplandor	glare
restitución de la cadera	hip replacement
restricción	confinement
resucitación boca a boca	mouth to mouth A manner of artificial respiration.
resultado clínico	disease outcome The response obtained from treatment.
resultado labatororio	lab result
retener	withhold
reticular	reticular Referring to a matrix of membranous tubules inside the cytoplasm of a eukaryotic cells.
reticulocito	reticulocyte A red blood cell without a nucleus.
reticulocitosis	reticulocytosis An abnormal increase in circulating reticulocytes.
reticuloendotelial	reticulo-endothelial Referring to the system of phagocytes involved in the immune system.
retina	retina The innermost of three layers of the eyeball; it surrounds the vitreous body and is continuous with the optic nerve.
retina desprendida	retinal detachment A tear or hole in the retina caused by vitreous traction.
retinitis	retinitis Inflammation of the retina.
retinoblastoma	retinoblastoma A tumor consisting of retinal germ cells.
retinopatía	retinopathy Any one of a number of retinal inflammatory conditions.
retículo endoplasmático	endoplasmic reticulum A framework of tubules within the cytoplasm of eukaryotic cells.
retorcijones de estómago	stomach cramps
retracción	retraction Being drawn back.
retractor	retractor A device for pulling back tissue during surgery.
retrofaríngo	retropharyngeal Referring to the area posterior to the pharynx.
retroperitoneo	retroperitoneal Situated or referring to the area posterior to the peritoneum.
retrógrado	retrograde Referring to backward movement.
reumatismo	rheumatism Any condition exhibited by inflammation and pain in the joints and muscles.

Spanish	English
reumático	rheumatic Referring to rheumatism.
reventar	burst, to
régimen medicina	dose regimen The amount, frequency and length of treatment of a medication.
riboflavina	riboflavin Also called vitamin B2, this essential vitamin is present in food such as eggs and is synthesized in the small bowel.
ricino	castor bean A bean that can yield the poisonous compound ricin.
rickettsias	rickettsia A disease transmitted by ticks or fleas, caused by a bacterium from the genus Rickettsieae. Rocky Mountain Spotted fever is one of many diseases caused by this bacterium.
rigidez abdominal	wooden belly A rigid abdomen.
rigidez de descerebración	decerebrate rigidity Rigid extension of the arms which is an abnormal posture associated with increased intracranial pressure.
rigidez en navaja	clasp knife reflex The lengthening of the extensor muscles resulting in flexion.
rigidez en rueda dentada	cog wheel As in cogwheel rigidity which is a jerky passive movement after there was increased tone.
rigor mortis	rigor mortis The normal stiffening of the muscles and joints that occurs a few hours after death.
rinitis	rhinitis A viral infection or allergic reaction exhibited by nasal mucosal inflammation.
rinoplastia	rhinoplasty Plastic surgery performed on the nose.
rinorrea	rhinorrhea Abundant nasal mucosal drainage.
rinoscopia	rhinoscopy Examination of the nasal passages.
riñón	kidney One of two glandular organs that form urine.
riñón en herradura	horseshoe kidney Anomalous renal development.
risa canina	risus sardonicus A spasm of the facial muscles causing what appears to be a smile on one's face.
ritma de galope	cantering rhythm Gallop rhythm.
ritmo	rhythm
ritmo circadiano	circadian rhythm Naturally recurring fluctuations in a 24 hour period.
rizotomía	rhizotomy Interruption of the spinal nerve roots within the spinal canal.
rígido	stiff
RNA robosómico	ribosomal RNA Four chains designated by their appropriate coefficients.
roce	rub
roce de fricción	friction rub A noise heard during cardiac auscultation in patients with pericarditis, for example.
rodilla	knee
rodilla de atleta	patellofemoral stress syndrome Overuse syndrome causing anterior knee pain from excessive lateral motion.
rodilla de Brodie	Brodie's knee Also referred to as chronic hypertrophic synovitis of the knee.
rodilla de mucama	housemaid's knee Also referred to as prepatellar bursitis.
rodilla inestable	unstable knee A condition with giving way of the knee due to ligamentous or cartilaginous dysfunction.
rodopsina	rhodopsin A reddish purple light sensitive pigment in the human retina.
roedor	rodent
roentgen	Roentgen One unit of ionizing radiation named after the German physicist Wilhelm Conrad Röntgen.
romboide	rhomboid A back muscle that elevates, retracts and adducts the scapula.
roncha	wheal

Spanish	English
ronco	frog in the throat, to have
ronco	hoarse A rough, harsh sounding voice.
ronquido	rhonchus A coarse, dry sound heard on auscultation of the lungs.
ronquido	snore, to
rosácea	rosacea Erythema of the cheeks and nose caused by chronic vascular and follicular dilation.
rostro, cara	face
rotación	rotation
roto	torn
rotulectomía	patellectomy Surgical excision of the patella.
rótula	kneecap
rótula	patella The bone situated in the anterior portion of the knee.
rubefaciente	rubefacient A substance that reddens the skin.
rubeola	German measles (rubella) A contagious viral infection.
rubéola	rubella
rubio	fair
rueda de andar	treadmill
ruido	bruit An abnormal sound heard through a stethoscope indicating turbulent blood flow.
ruido carotídeo	carotid bruit An abnormal noise heard over the carotid artery that may be a sign of stenosis or aortic valvular disease.
ruidos respiratorios	breath sound The noise heard upon auscultation with a stethoscope.
rupia	rupia A sign of tertiary syphilis in which there are bullae or vesicles formed on the skin that erupt and form crusts.
ruptura	rupture
rusucitación cardiopulmonar	cardiorespiratory assistance Use of artificial means to support respiration and circulation.
sabio	wise
sacral	sacral Referring to the sacrum.
sacralización	sacralization The fusion of the fifth lumbar vertebra to the sacrum.
sacro	sacrum The bone formed by five fused vertebrae that is situated between the two hip bones.
safena	saphena Referring to either of the two superficial saphenous veins.
sal	salt
sala de emergencia	emergency room
sala de hospital	ward
sala de recuperación	recovery room
salida	emergence Coming into prominence.
salida pélvica	inferior pelvis strait The pelvic outlet.
salino	saline A solution of sodium chloride.
saliva	saliva
salivación	salivation The process of secreting saliva.
salpingectomía	salpingectomy Surgical resection of the fallopian tubes.
salpingitis	salpingitis Inflammation of the fallopian tubes.
salpingografía	salpingography Roentgenography of the fallopian tubes after administration of contrast media.
salpingostomía	salpingostomy A surgical procedure involving cutting the fallopian tube.

Spanish	English
salpullido	prickly heat A rash with small vesicles that is pruritic and associated with a warm moist environment.
salud	health
salud de centro	health center
salurético	saluretic An agent that promotes excretion of sodium and chloride in the urine.
sangrado	bleeding
sangrado uterino	uterine bleeding
sangre	blood
sangre oculta	occult blood Presence of blood from an unknown source.
sanguijuela	leech An annelid used in some tropical regions for drawing out blood; they have an anticoagulant effect locally and have been attached to digits of persons with acute peripheral ischemia.
sano	healthy
sano	sound
saponificar	saponify The creation of soap from oil using an alkali.
saprofito	saprophyte Any organism living on dead organic material.
sarampión	measles A childhood viral, infectious disease exhibited by rash and fever.
sarcoide	sarcoid Referring to sarcoidosis.
sarcoidosis	sarcoidosis A chronic disease characterized by lymphadenopathy and widespread granulomas.
sarcolema	sarcolemme The sheath that covers skeletal muscle fibers.
sarcoma	sarcoma A non-epithelial malignant tumor.
sarna	scabies A skin condition exhibited by intense pruritis and a macular rash commonly in the perineal and interdigital spaces.
sartorio	sartorius muscle The thigh muscle that runs from the pelvis to the proximal, medial aspect of the tibia.
saturación	saturation An amount, expressed in a percentage, that expresses the degree something is absorbed versus the maximal absorption possible.
sábana	sheet (bed)
sclera	sclera The white outer covering of the eyeball.
sebáceo	sebaceous Referring to a sebaceous gland or what it secretes.
seborrea	seborrhea Abnormal amount of sebum production.
sección transversal	cross-section
seco	dry
secreción	secretion The discharge of substances from cells or glands.
secretina	secretin A hormone that increases secretion from the pancreas and liver.
secuela	sequela A medical problem related to an initial injury or disease.
secuestro	sequestrum Necrotic bone present in an injured or diseased bone.
secundinas	afterbirth The tissue expelled after the birth of a child that includes the placenta and allied membranes.
sed	thirst
sedante	sedative A medication used to facilitate sleep or calm a person.
sedimento	sludge A viscous fluid.
sedimento urinario	urinary sediments The debris that settles in a urine sample when left undisturbed.
segmentación	cleavage A sharp division or demarcation.
segmento	limb
según	according to

Spanish	English
sellado	seal
semanal	weekly
seminoma	seminoma A malignant tumor of the testis.
senescencia	senescence The normal process of deterioration with age.
senil	senile Generally referring to mental deterioration associated with aging.
senilidad	senility The process of being senile.
seno esfenoidal	sphenoidal sinus Part of the sphenoid bone; it communicates with the most superior aspect of the nasal meatus.
seno paranasales	paranasal sinuses Any of the sinuses (ethmoidal, frontal, maxillary or sphenoidal) that communicate with the nasal cavity.
senos frontales	frontal sinuses
sensación	sensation A perception when one is touched.
sensación de calor o pesadez	sensation of warmth or heaviness
sensibilidad	sensibility Ability to feel or perceive.
sensibilización	sensitization The change in an organ by a hormone so it will respond to another stimulus.
sensibilizar	sensitized Being abnormally sensitive to a substance.
sensible	sensible
sentir	feel, to
sentir mejor	feel better, to
sepsis	sepsis A condition exhibited by overwhelming inflammation due to infection.
septicemia	septicemia A systemic disease in which microorganisms or their toxins are in the blood stream.
serie	serial
serio	severe
seroso	serous Referring to serum or similar to serum.
serotonina	serotonin A neurotransmitter that constricts blood vessels.
serpiginoso	serpiginous A skin lesion having wavy margin.
seudoartrosis	pseudarthrosis Deossification of weight bearing long bones.
seudomnesia	pseudomnesia Sensing the memory of an event that has never happened.
sexo	sex
séptico	septic Referring to a state of sepsis.
sésil	sessile Having a broad base with no stalk.
shock	shock A condition characterized by systemic hypoperfusion.
shock espinal	spinal shock Hypotension related to injury or intervention of the spine.
shunt	shunt An alternate path for blood or fluid.
sialadenitis	sialadenitis Inflammation of a salivary gland.
sialogogo	sialogogue A substance that increase salivary flow.
sialolito	sialolith A calculus in a salivary duct.
sicosis	sycosis A bacterial infection affecting the hair follicles on a person's face.
SIDA	AIDS
siderosis	siderosis Excess iron in the blood or a pulmonary disease from iron inhalation called Pneumoconiosis.
sierra	saw
siesta	nap
sigmoide	sigmoid Referring to the portion of the colon that leads into the rectum.

Spanish	English
sigmoidoscopia	sigmoidoscopy Visualization of the sigmoid colon with a scope.
sigmoidostomía	sigmoidostomy Formation of an opening in the sigmoid colon that communicates with the outside of the body.
signo de Argyll Robertson	Argyll Robertson symptom Presence of small pupils that do not react to light but will constrict when the person focuses on a near object.
signo de la cimitarra	scimitar sign An abnormal radiologic finding associated with anomalous pulmonary venous drainage.
signos vitales	vital signs The designation for blood pressure, pulse, respirations and temperature.
silbar	whistle, to
silbilancia	wheeze
silicosis	silicosis Grinders's disease; fibrotic lung disease caused by inhalation of silica.
silla de ruedas	wheelchair
simbiosis	symbiosis The living together of two organisms.
simetría	symmetry Being equally bilaterally.
simpatectomía	sympathectomy The surgical resection of a sympathetic nerve to reduce undesired effects.
simulación	malingering Feigning illness.
simultáneo	simultaneous
sin hogar	homeless
sin sentido	meaningless
sin tener en cuenta	regardless of
sinapsis	synapse The intersection of two nerve cells.
sinartrosis	synarthrosis Adjacent bones connected by a joint but the joint is fixed.
sincondrosis	synchondrosis A joint with little motion that uses cartilage such as the vertebral bodies.
sinequia	synechia The adhesion of two body parts, such as synechia vulvae in which the labia minora are congenitally adherent.
sinistrocardia	sinistrocardia Location of the heart toward the left (more than normally seen).
sinistrotorsión	sinistrotorsion Distorsion toward the left; in reference to the eye generally.
sinistrómano Zurdo	left handed
sino carvernoso	cavernous sinus Large venous sinus located adjacent to the sphenoid bone and posterior to the petrosal sinuses.
sinoauricular	sinoatrial Referring to the cardiac node of the same name.
sinovectomía	synovectomy Surgical resection of a synovial membrane.
sinovitis	synovitis Inflammation of the synovium.
sinusitis	sinusitis Inflammation of the sinuses.
sinusoide	sinusoid An irregular vessel having almost no adventitia that is found in the liver, heart, parathyroid, spleen and pancreas.
siringomielia	syringomelia A condition exhibited by fluid-filled cavities in the spinal cord.
sistema métrico	metric system
sistema nervioso autonómico (a)	autonomic nervous system Responsible for regulation of cardiac muscle, smooth muscle and glandular activity.
sistema nervioso autonómico (a)	central nervous system (CNS) The brain and spinal cord.
sistema nerviso simpático	sympathetic nervous system The nerves responsible for the flight or fight response.

Spanish	English
sistólico	systolic Referring to systole or that which occurs during systole.
sitio	site
sífilis	syphilis A infectious disease caused by Treponema pallidum that causes a painless penile ulcer in the primary stage but can lead to irreversible brain damage in the untreated tertiary stage.
sífilis congénita	congenital syphilis Passed to the child in utero, the child may have failure to thrive, fever and a flattened bridge of the nose.
síncope	syncope Sudden loss of consciousness.
síncope del seno carotídeo	carotid sinus syncope Dizziness and syncope that results from hyperactivity of the carotid sinus reflex.
síndrome alcohólico fetal	fetal alcohol syndrome A condition caused by acohol use by the mother during pregnancy and exhibited by poor intrauterine growth, decreased muscle tone, delayed development and widened palpebral fissures.
síndrome de Aicardi	Aicardi syndrome A rare genetic anomily in which the corpus collosum is absent or insufficient. It is characterized by seizures, microphthalmos, coloboma and developmental delays.
síndrome de aplastamiento	crush syndrome Rhabdomyolysis occurring as a result of muscle injury from mechanical stress.
síndrome de asa aferente	afferent loop syndrome The obstruction of the duodenum or jejunum after gastrojejunostomy, resulting in duodenal distention.
síndrome de asa ciego	blind loop syndrome A condition in which there is a non-functional section of the bowel that is thought to be responsible for malabsorption and Vitamin B12 deficiency.
síndrome de Barrett	Barretts's esophagus A condition characterized by varying degrees of esophageal injury from gastric acid.
síndrome de Brown Séquard	Brown-Séquard syndrome Unilateral spinal cord lesions, proprioception loss and weakness occur ipsilateral to the lesion, while pain and temperature loss occur contralateral.
síndrome de Cushing	Cushing's syndrome Characterized by trunkal obesity, moon face, acne, abdominal striae, hypertension, decreased carbohydrate tolerance, protein catabolism, psychiatric disturbances, and osteoporosis.
síndrome de dificultad respiratoria	respiratory distress syndrome A disease in infants that is caused by a surfactant deficiency.
síndrome de Down	Down's syndrome A congenital chromosomal defect (trisomy 21) that caused diminished intellectual function, short stature and a broad face.
síndrome de encierro	locked-in syndrome A neurologic condition characterized by a person being conscious of their surroundings but being unable to verbally communicate that understanding.
síndrome de Henri	Henri, syndrome of Congenital anomaly exhibited by different sized external orifices of the nostrils.
síndrome de Hunter	mucopolysaccharidosis type II Also referred to as Hunter syndrome, persons with this inherited condition cannot produce iduronate sulfatase. There are mild to severe forms but all forms have deafness, coarse facial features, hypertrichosis and macrocephaly.
síndrome de Hurler	mucopolysaccharidosis type I Also referred to as Hurler syndrome, persons cannot make lysosomal alpha-L-iduronidase which breaks down glycosaminoglycans.
síndrome de inmunodeficienia adquirida (SIDA)	Acquired Immunodeficiency Syndrome (AIDS) Presence of an AIDS defining illness or having a CD4 of less than 200/mm3.
síndrome de la muerte súbita del lactante	sudden infant death syndrome A leading cause of death of infants from one month to one year; the etiology is unknown.

Spanish	English
síndrome de las piernas inquietas	restless legs Associated with a syndrome exhibited by continuous movement of the legs from uncertain etiology.
síndrome de Marfan	Marfan syndrome A connective tissue disease exhibited by long limbs, joint laxity and cardiovascular defects.
síndrome de Maroteaux-Lamy	mucopolysaccharidosis type VI Also referred to as Maroteaux-Lamy syndrome. It is characterized by hydrocephalus, macroglossia and coarse facial features but normal intelligence.
síndrome de Morquio	mucopolysaccharidosis type IV Also referred to as Morquio syndrome, persons do not produce galactosamine-6-sulfatase or in some cases beta-galactosidase. Symptoms include hypermobile joints, macrocephaly, short stature and wide spaced teeth.
síndrome de respiración de Cheyne -Stokes	Cheyne-Stokes respirations A breathing pattern characterized by alternating apnea with hyperpnea.
síndrome de Rett	Rett syndrome. A rare inherited disorder causing developmental delays and is seen mostly in girls.
síndrome de Sanfilippo	mucopolysaccharidosis type III Also referred to as Sanfilippo syndrome, persons cannot catabolize the heparan sulfate sugar chain. Symptoms include stiff joints, thick eyebrows, coarse facial features and developmental delays.
síndrome de Scheie	mucopolysaccharidosis type Is Also referred to as Scheie syndrome, persons cannot produce lysosomal alpha-L-iduronidase. Symptoms include cloudy cornea, hirsutism, prognathism and stiff joints.
síndrome de Sjogren	Sjogren's syndrome. Characterized by dryness of the mouth and eyes, it is sometimes linked to rheumatoid arthritis.
síndrome de trisomía 21	trisomy 21 A congenital anomaly in which chromosome 21 is effected and results in Down's syndrome.
síndrome de vaciamiento gástrico demasiado rápido	dumping syndrome Characterized by rapid bowel evacuation after eating in patients with prior gastric surgery.
síndrome del intestino irritable	irritable bowel syndrome A condition exhibited by chronic diarrhea or constipation and abdominal pain; it is sometimes associated with a labile emotional state.
síndrome del maullido de gato	cat cry syndrome A hereditary congenital disorder exhibited by microcephaly, hypertelorism, and cognitive deficits.
síndrome del mentón entumecido	numb chin syndrome. Generally associated with metastatic breast or prostate cancer, it is characterized by unilateral sensory loss of the chin and lower lip.
síndrome del robo de la subclavia	subclavian steal syndrome Retrograde vertebral artery flow due to ipsilateral subclavian artery stenosis.
síndrome del tunel del carpio	carpal tunnel syndrome Paresthesia that results from compression of the median nerve.
síndrome premenstrual	premenstrual syndrome A cluster of emotional, behavioral, and physical symptoms that occur in the premenstrual phase of the menstrual cycle and resolve with the onset of menstruation.
síntoma	symptom
síntoma presente	presenting symptom The initial subjective complaint that initiated a visit.
sístole	systole The phase of the cardiac cycle in which the ventricles contract.
sofocación	suffocation
sollozar	sob, to
solpo	murmur An abnormal heart sound heard with a stethoscope.
soltar	blurt out, to
soltero	single (not married)
soltura	looseness

Spanish	English
solución fisiológica	physiological saline 0.9% normal saline.
solvente	solvent Able to dissolve with other chemicals.
somático	somatic Referring to the body.
somnolencia	somnolence Drowsiness.
sonambulismo	somnambulism Sleepwalking.
sonda	probe A device used for exploration.
sonda gastrogavaje	gavage tube A tube used for instillation of liquids into the stomach.
sonroharse	blush, to
soplo cardíaco	heart murmur
sopor	drowsiness
soporífico	soporific Promoting drowsiness or sleep.
soportar, resistir	bear, to To endure or resist.
soporte tobillo	ankle support (device)
sorber	sip, to
sordera	deafness
sordo, sorda	deaf
sordomudo, sordomuda	deaf-mute
sostener	sustain, to
sóleo	soleus muscle Assists with ankle plantar flexion.
spica	spica A figure of eight bandage.
status matrimonial	marital status
status vacuna	vaccine status
subagudo	subacute A stage between acute and chronic.
subaracnoideo	subarachnoid The layer of the brain covering between the arachnoid and pia mater.
subclavio	subclavian Refers to the area under the clavicle; the subclavian vein runs below the clavicle.
subdural	subdural The area between the dura mater and the arachnoid membrane.
suberosis	suberosis A type of hypersensitivity pneumonitis related to inhalation of moldy cork dust.
subfrénico	subphrenic Referring to below the diaphragm.
sublingual	sublingual Situated under the tongue.
submaxilar	submaxillary Situated below the maxilla.
subyacente	underlying
succionar	suck, to As in, to suction fluid.
sucio, sucia	dirty
sucusión	succussion The presence of a splashing sound when a body cavity is moved indicating presence of both air and fluid.
sudamina	sudamina White vesicles noted because of retained sweat in the layers of the epidermis.
sudar	sweat, to
sudor	sweat
sudor excesivo durante el sueño	night sweats
suelto	loose
sueño	dream
sueño	sleep

Spanish	English
suero	serum The fluid that isolates out when blood coagulates.
sufrimiento fetal	fetal distress Term used to describe an abnormal heart rate or rhythm in a fetus indicating the need for urgent childbirth.
sufrir	suffer, to
suicida	suicide
sulfonamidas	sulfonamide A class of drugs derived from sulfanilamide that are antibacterial.
superfetación	superfecundation The fertilization of two different ova by spermatozoa of two different males.
superficie corporal	body surface area Dubois formula is: (weight in kilograms)to the 0.425th power x (height in centimeters) to the 0.725th power x 0.007184.
superior	superior
supinación	supination Turning the sole of the foot or the palm of the hand upward..
supino	supine
supositorio	suppository
supranormal	greater than normal
supraorbitario	supraorbital Situated above the orbit.
suprapúbico	suprapubic Situated above the pubis.
suprarrenal	adrenal Referring to being near the kidney.
supresión	withdrawal
supuración	suppuration Formation of purulent material.
supurar	weep, to
sural	sural Referring to the calf of the leg.
surco	sulcus A groove, like in the brain.
surfactante	surfactant A substance that reduces surface tension in the lungs.
surrar	whisper, to
suspirar	sigh, to
sustancia blanca	white matter The brain tissue consisting of myelin sheaths and nerve fibers.
sustancia gris	gray matter The section of the brain and spinal cord composed of branching dendrites and nerve cell bodies.
sustancia lipotrófico	lipotrophic substance A compound which causes an increase in body fat.
susurro	whisper
sutura	suture
sutura continua	running suture A method of sewing a wound in which there is a knot at each end and continuous otherwise.
sutura coronal	coronal suture The line of intersection of the frontal bone and the two parietal bones.
sutura de colchonero	mattress suture
sutura lambdoidea	lambdoid The suture connecting the parietal bones with the occipital bone.
sutura quirúrgica absorbible	resorbable suture (chromic)
sutura quirúrgica no absorbible	non-resorbable suture (nylon)
sutura sagital	sagittal suture The line where the two parietal bones meet.
tabaquera anatómica	anatomical snuff-box The area on the back of the hand near the base of the thumb that is between the extensor pollicus longus and extensor pollicus brevis.
tabique	septum A wall separating two chambers, the nasal septum for example.
tabique nasal desviado	deviated septum Characterized by deviation of the nasal septum.

273

Spanish	English
tabique rectovesical	rectovesical septum The wall between the rectum and the urinary bladder.
tableta	tablet
tableta de acción sostenida	sustained release tablet Describes a medicine that is slowly dispersed so it has a lasting effect.
tablilla de yeso	plaster cast Use of gypsum impregnated gauze to immobilize fractured extremities.
tacto	touch
taladro	drill
talasemia	thalassemia A hereditary hemolytic anemia first observed in people from the Mediterranean area.
talidomida	thalidomide A drug used originally as a sedative, after it was found to cause congenital anomalies, its use was restricted. Now it is used for a few conditions such as multiple myeloma.
talipes calcáneo	talipes calcaneus A foot deformity exhibited by abnormal dorsiflexion.
talipes equino	talipes equinus A foot deformity exhibited by abnormal plantar flexion.
talipes equinovaro	talipes equinovaro Medical term for what is commonly known as club foot.
tallo encefálico	brain stem An organ that consists of the medulla oblongata, pons and midbrain.
talón	heel
tamaño	size
tampón	tampon Disposible intravaginal product used to collect blood from menstruation.
taponamiento	tamponade 1. Stopping bleeding during surgery with a cotton pledget. 2. When referring to cardiac tamponade, it is the limitation of cardiac contraction because of blood or fluid accumulation in the pericardial sac.
taquicardia	tachycardia Heart rate higher than physiologic normal.
taquicardia ventricular polimorfo	torsade de pointe Ventricular cardiac rhythm disturbance.
taquipnea	tachypnea
tarántula	tarantula
tarde	late
tarea	task
tarsal	tarsal Referring to any bone in the tarsus.
tarsalgia	tarsalgia Pain in any of the tarsal bones.
tarsectomía	tarsectomy Surgical excision of all or part of the tarsus.
tarso	tarsus The group of seven bones of the ankle or foot (three cuneiform bones, talus, calcaneus, navicular, cuboid bones).
tarsorrafia	tarsorrhaphy Suturing the eyelids in order to tighten the palpebral fissure.
tartamudeo	stammering The impulse to repeat the first letter of words and involuntary pauses while speaking.
tartamudez	stuttering Involuntary repetition of the first consonant.
tasa respiratoria	respiratory rate The number of breaths per minute.
tatuaje	tattoo
táctil	tactile Able to be felt.
tálamo	thalamus
teca	theca A tendon or ovarian follicle sheath.
tecoma	thecoma A tumor composed of theca cells.
tectum	tectum A roof-like body.

274

Spanish	English
tejido	tissue
tejido de granulación	granulation tissue
telangiectasia	telangiectasis A condition exhibited by red, dilated capillaries on the skin.
telemetría	telemetry Use of radio signals to transmit patient data. The most common form is for electrocardiography in a patient who is ambulatory.
temblar	shaking
temblor	tremor
temblor de aleteo Asterixis.	asterixis Commonly known as a flapping tremor, it is characterized by involuntary jerking movements of the hands and is seen commonly in hepatic encephalopathy.
temblor intencional	intention tremor The tremulous movement noted when a person is beginning to perform a task but not seen at rest.
temor	fear
temperatura	temperature
tenazas	tongs A medical device used for holding or grasping.
tendencioso	biased Prejudiced.
tendinitis	tendinitis Inflammation of a tendon.
tendinitis de De Quervain	De Quervain tenosynovitis Inflammation of the tendons of the wrist including the abductor pollicis longus and extensor pollicis brevis.
tendones de la corva	hamstrings Tendons of the posterior thigh.
tendón	tendon
tenesmo	tenesmus The attempt to defecate but attempts elicit pain and are ineffective.
tenia	tapeworm A parasitic, intestinal flatworm.
tenoplastia	tenoplasty Surgical repair of a tendon.
tenorrafia	tenorrhaphy The surgical repair with suture of a separated tendon.
tenosinovitis	tenosynovitis Inflammation and swelling of an articulation.
tenotomía	tenotomy Incision of a tendon as is done for strabismus.
tensión	stress
tensión de gases en sangre arterial	arterial blood gas Measurement of the arterial concentration of carbon dioxide and oxygen.
terapeuta habla	speech therapist
terapéutica de choque	electroconvulsive therapy (ECT) The electrical stimulation of the brain to treat mental disorders.
terapia ocupación	occupational therapy Rehabilitation focusing on activities of daily living.
terapia con oxígeno	oxygen therapy Utilization of supplemental oxygen.
terapia fisico	physical therapy Treatment of disease by heat, massage and exercise as opposed to medications.
terapia física	physiotherapy Physical therapy.
teratoma	teratoma A tumor made up of tissue not usually at the location (a mass of hair, teeth and gingival tissue in a leg tumor for instance).
teratógeno	teratogen A substance that induces fetal anomalies.
tercer molar	wisdom tooth Third molar.
terciario	tertiary
terebrante	terebrant Having a piercing quality.
termómetro	thermometer
testículo	testicle One of a pair of organs in the male scrotum that produces sperm.
testosterona	testosterone This steroid hormone produces secondary male sexual characteristics.

Spanish	English
tetania	tetany A condition caused by the hypocalcemic effect of hypoparathyroidism, exhibited by periodic muscle spasms, convulsions, and peri-oral numbness.
tetraciclina	tetracycline An antibiotic used for gram positive and gram negative infections.
tetradáctilo	tetradactylous Referring to a condition of having only four digits on a hand or foot.
tetralogía de Fallot	Fallot, tetrology of Congenital cardiac defects including ventricular septal defect, pulmonic valve stenosis or infundibular stenosis, and dextroposition of the aorta.
técnica del anticuerpo fluorescente	fluorescent antibody test (FTA test)
técnico ortopédico	bonesetter A person who sets bones without being a physician.
tétanos	tetanus A condition caused by Clostridium tetani which produces spasm and rigidity of voluntary muscles.
tiamina	thiamine Also called vitamin B1; a deficiency causes beriberi.
tibia	tibia The larger of two long bones in the lower leg.
tibio	tepid
tic	tic
tic doloroso Neuralgia del trigémino	tic douloureux
tiempo de sangrado	bleeding time The time of bleeding after a controlled standardized puncture of the earlobe.
tienda de oxígeno	oxygen tent A manner of giving supplement oxygen to a neonate.
tijeras	scissors
timectomía	thymectomy Surgical excision of the thymus.
timina	thymine A chemical with a pyrimidine base found in DNA.
timo	thymus A body organ located in the neck and it produces T cells to improve immune function.
timocito	thymocyte A lymphocyte located in the thymus.
timoma	thymoma A tumor composed of thymic tissue and is sometimes associated with myasthenia gravis.
timpano del oído	ear-drum
timpanoplastia	tympanoplasty Restoration of the tympanic membrane's continuity.
timpánico	tympanic Referring to the tympanic membrane or having a resonant quality to percussion.
tinnitus	tinnitus Medical term for ringing in the ears. It is associated with Meniere's syndrome among other conditions.
tintura	tincture 1. A very small amount of something. 2. A medicine dissolved in alcohol.
tiña	ringworm A fungal skin infection exhibited by pruritic well circumscribed patches on the scalp or feet.
tiña	tinea Medical term for ringworm.
tiña de la barba	tinea barbae
tiña de la región genitocrural	tinea cruris
tiña de las uñas	onychomycosis Fungal disease of the toenails or fingernails.
tiña de los pies	tinea pedis
tiña del cuero cabelludo	tinea capitis
tiña del cuerpo	tinea corporis

Spanish	English
tirarse un pedo	fart, to Slang term for releasing flatus.
tiroidectomía	thyroidectomy Surgical resection of all or part of the thyroid.
tiroides	thyroid A gland in the neck that secretes hormones regulating metabolism.
tirosina	tyrosine An amino acid important in the synthesis of hormones.
tirotoxicosis	thyrotoxicosis Abnormal increase in thyroid activity exhibited by thinning hair, hypertension, tachycardia and at times atrial fibrillation.
tirotoxina	thyroxine An iodine containing hormone, referred to T4.
tirón de la ingle	groin pull A muscle strain in the inguinal region.
tirón de la ingle	pull, to
toalla higiénica	feminine pad Gauze specially designed to absorb menstrual flow.
tobillo	ankle
tobillo chichón	ankle swelling
todo	every
todos los días	every day
tomografía axial computarizada	CT scan Computerized axial tomography.
tomografía de los huesos	bone scan Bone imaging using technetium 99m (99mTc) diphosphate.
tomografía por emisión de positrones	PET scan Positron emission tomography.
tonómetro	tonometer A device used to measure ocular pressure in glaucoma.
tonsilectomía	tonsillectomy Excision of the tonsils.
tonsilitis	tonsillitis Inflammation of the tonsils.
tonto	silly
toracentesis	thoracentesis Insertion of a needle into the pleural space to drain and or obtain a specimen for analysis.
toracoplastia	thoracoplasty Surgical removal of ribs.
toracoscopia	thoracoscopy Visualization of the thoracic cavity with a scope.
toracotomía	thoracotomy Surgical incision of the thorax.
torácico	thoracic Referring to the thorax.
tornasol	litmus A dye that turns red with low pH and blue with high pH.
torniquete	tourniquet A device tied tightly around an extremity to diminish blood flow or blood loss.
torpor Embotamiento.	torpor Unresponsiveness to normal stimuli.
torrente sanguíneo	blood stream Common term or the arterial or venous systems.
torsión	torsion Refers to twisting. Testicular torsion is the twisting of the spermatic cord that can lead to ischemia and gangrene of the testicle.
torsión de los testículos	testicular torsion
torso	torso The trunk of the body.
tortícolis	torticollis A condition exhibited by the head being turned to one side continuously.
tos	cough
tos ferina	whooping cough Pertussis
tos seca recurrente	coughing fit
toxemia	toxemia The release of toxic substances into the blood stream from a local infection. Toxemia of pregnancy is a synonym for preeclampsia.
toxicología	toxicology The study of the nature, effects and detection of poisons.
toxina	toxin A poison of plant or animal origin.

Spanish	English
toxoide	toxoid A chemically modified toxin that can be used as a vaccine.
toxoplasmosis	toxoplasmosis A disease caused by an organism from the genus Toxoplasma. One can have simple malaise to central nervous system involvement.
tórax	thorax The part of the body between the neck and abdomen.
tórax en embudo	funnel chest Anterior thorax funnel shaped depression, also called pectus excavatum.
tórax inestable	flail chest The term used when one has multiple rib fractures causing a segment of the chest wall to move incongruently with the rest of the chest wall.
tórax, pecho	chest
tóxico	toxic
tóxico monóxido de carbono	carbon monoxide poisoning This tasteless, odorless gas causes constitutional symptoms but can lead to death upon inhalation.
trabeculectomía	trabeculotomy A surgery for open angle glaucoma.
trabécula	trabecule A connective tissue strand that goes from a capsule to the enclosed organ.
tracción	traction
tracción esquelética	skeletal traction
tracoma	trachoma An infection of the cornea and conjunctiva caused by Chlamydia.
tracto	tract
tracto extrapiramidal	extrapyramidal tract Motor nerves that are not part of the pyramidal tract.
tracto gastrointestina	gastrointestinal tract The alimentary canal from the distal esophagus to the cecum.
traer	bring, to
tragarse	slurring
trago	tragus The fleshy prominence anterior to the opening of the ear.
tranquilizante	tranquilizer A medication used to diminish anxiety.
tranquilo	quiet
transabdomino	transabdominal Through the abdominal wall.
transaminasas	transaminase An enzyme that facilitates the transfer of an amino group to an amino acid.
transdérmico	transdermal Through the skin.
transfusión	transfusion Administration of blood products intravenously.
transpirar	transpire, to To release vapor from the skin or respiratory mucosa.
trapecio	trapezium The lateral bone in the distal row of carpal bones.
trapezius	trapezius muscle The muscle with an origin of occipital bone and seventh cervical vertebra, insertion of clavicle and scapula, and it draws the scapula backward.
trapezoide	trapezoid The bone between the trapezium and capitate bones.
traqueítis	tracheitis Inflammation of the trachea.
traquelorrafia	trachelorrhaphy Surgical repair of a lacerated cervix.
traqueobronquitis	tracheobronchitis Inflammation of the trachea and bronchi.
traqueostomía	tracheostomy Creation of a surgical opening in the trachea so a tube could be placed in the trachea.
traqueotomía	tracheotomy Surgical incision of the trachea.
trasplantar	transplant To move a body part from one location to another.
trasplante	transplantation The grafting of tissues.
trasplante corneal	corneal transplant

Spanish	English
trastorno alimenticio	eating disorder General term for pathologic eating habits.
trastorno de conversión	conversion When referring to a psychiatric condition it is the exhibition of physical symptoms as a manifestation of mental disease.
trastornos afectivo (a)	affective disorders Manic-depressive psychosis.
trastornos cognitivo	cognitive disorders Any disease process that involves altered cognition.
trasudación	transudation The movement of body tissue through a membrane that is usually the result of inflammation.
tratamiento	treatment
tratamiento nebulizador	nebulizer treatment Administration of medication such as albuterol via a fine mist using a nebulizer.
trauma	trauma
traumatismo cervical	whiplash
traumatismo del cráneo	head trauma Any injury to the brain.
traumatismo múltiple	polytrauma A condition exhibited by multiple injuries from blunt or penetrating trauma.
tráquea	trachea The ringed canal between the pharynx and bronchi.
trefina	trephining Cutting away a circular disc of bone or the cornea.
trematodo	trematoda A parasitic fluke such as Schistosoma.
treonina	threonine An amino acid needed for the growth in infants.
triángulo femoral	femoral triangle An area that is bordered by the sartorius muscle, the adductor longus muscle and the inguinal ligament.
tricofitosis	trichophytosis A skin or nail fungal infection caused by Trichophyton.
tricomoniasis vaginitis	trichomoniasis vaginitis
trigeminal	trigeminal Generally refers to the fifth cranial nerve.
tripanosomiasis	trypanosomiasis A disease caused by a protozoa of the genus Trypanosoma that can cause sleeping sickness and Chagas' disease.
triplejía	triplegia Paralysis of three extremities.
triploide	triploid Referring to a cell with three homologous sets of chromosomes.
tripsina	trypsin An enzyme whose precursor is secreted by the pancreas that breaks down proteins in the intestine.
tripsinógeno	trypsinogen The precursor to trypsin that is secreted by the pancreas.
triptófano	tryptophan An amino acid that is a precursor of serotonin. If present in the body in appropriate levels it can prevent pellegra even if niacin levels are low.
triquiasis	trichiasis Inversion of the eyelashes.
triquinosis	trichinosis A disease caused by meat infected by Trichinella spiralis causing fever and gastrointestinal effects.
trismo	trismus Commonly called lockjaw, it is a spasm of the muscles supplied by the trigeminal nerve and is an early symptom of tetanus.
trisomía	trisomy A general category of congenital anomalies in which there is an extra set of chromosomes in the cell nucleus.
tristeza	sadness
trivial	trivial
tríceps	triceps Referring to something having three heads like the triceps muscle.
trídimo	triplets
trígono vesical	trigone of bladder Refers to the area at the base of the bladder between the openings of the ureters and the urethra.
trocar	trocar A device enclosed in a catheter that is used to withdraw fluid from a body cavity.

Spanish	English
trocánter	trochanter Refers to the greater or lesser trochanter; the prominences on the femoral neck.
troclear	trochlear Referring to a trochlea.
trofoblasto	trophoblast A layer of endodermal tissue that helps attach an ovum to the uterine wall.
trombectomía	thrombectomy Excision of a thrombus from a vein or artery.
trombina	thrombin An enzyme that is a catalyst for the conversion of fibrinogen to fibrin in the formation of a clot.
tromboangitis	thromboangiitis Inflammation and thrombosis in a blood vessel.
tromboarteritis	thromboarteritis Thrombosis of an inflammed artery.
trombocitopenia	thrombocytopenia Abnormal decrease in the number of blood platelets.
tromboflebitis	thrombophlebitis Inflammation of a venous wall associated with a thrombus.
trombosis	thrombosis Formation of a clot in a vein or artery.
trombosis del seno cavernoso	cavernous sinus thrombosis A blood clot in the base of the brain.
trombosis venosa profunda (TVP)	deep vein thrombosis (DVT)
trompa de Eustaquio	pharyngotympanic tube Synonym for eustachian tube.
trompas de Falopio	fallopian tubes
tronarse los nudillos	crack one's knuckles
troncal	truncal Referring to the trunk of a body or a nerve.
tróclea	trochlea A pulley-shaped structure such as the groove at the distal humerus.
tubario	tubal Referring to a tube, as in fallopian tube.
tuberculina	tuberculin A solution containing M. tuberculosis or M. bovis that is used to test for tuberculosis by injecting the solution intradermally and looking for a reaction.
tuberculoma	tuberculoma 1. A tuberculous growth in the brain. 2. A mass that is produced from enlargement of a caseous tubercle.
tuberculosis	tuberculosis Any infectious disease caused by Mycobacterium.
tuberculoso	tuberculous Referring to tuberculosis.
tuberosidad	tuberosity A protuberance. For instance the iliac tuberosity is a prominence on the surface of the ilium.
tubérculo	tubercle 1. A granulomatous nodule produced by Mycobacterium tuberculosis. 2. A small prominence on a bone.
tubo balón Inflable esférico utilizado para retenertubos o catéteres.	cuffed tube A cannula that has an balloon on the tip that can be inflated with air or fluid.
tubo de drenaje	drainage tube A cannula used to allow outflow of fluids.
tubo de ensayo	test tube
tubo intravenoso	intravenous tubing
tubo nasogástrico	nasogastric tube A tube that is inserted into the nose with the distal tip in the stomach; it is used for irrigation or drainage of gastric contents.
tuboovárico	tubo-ovarian Referring to the fallopian tube or ovary.
tubular	tubular Referring to a hollow, round-shaped organ.
tularemia	tularemia An infectious disease caused by Francisella tularensis. The symptoms range from mild constitutional complaints to septic shock.
tumefacción	swelling
tumefacción	tumefaction An area of swelling.

280

Spanish	English
tumor	tumor A benign or malignant overgrowth of tissue.
turbinectomía	turbinectomy Surgical excision of a turbinate bone.
turgor	turgor Referring to the elasticity of skin. If one pinches skin and it remains in place the patient is dehydrated.
turno nocturno	night shift
túbulos seminíferos	seminiferous tubules Used for transport of semen.
túnel tarsiano	tarsal tunnel syndrome Characterized by impingement of various nerves of the ankle.
túnica	tunica Generally a covering of a body part or organ. The tunica mucosa nasi is the mucous membrane lining the nasal cavity.
túrgido	turgid Congested and swollen.
ulceroso	ulcerative Referring to ulceration.
ultrasonido	ultrasound A sound or vibration of ultrasonic frequency.
ultrasonido transrectal	transrectal ultrasound
ultrasonido transvaginal	transvaginal ultrasound
ultrasonografía	ultrasonography Visualization of body structures with the echoes of ultrasound pulses.
umbilicado	umbilicated Referring to depressed areas that resemble the umbilicus.
umbilicus	umbilicus The scar that denotes the end of the umbilical cord.
unciforme	unciform Another term for hamate bone in the wrist.
uncinado	uncinate bone Hamate bone.
uncinaria	hookworm A parasitic infection of the family Strongylidae that can cause anemia.
uncinariasis	uncinariasis Hookworm infestation of genus Uncinaria.
undulado	undulant Wave-like appearance.
ungüento	ointment
unicelular	unicellular A term describing organisms like protozoans that only have cell.
unidad motor	motor unit The complex of one motor cell and its attached muscle fibers.
unigrávida	unigravida Term used to describe a woman's first pregnacy.
unilateral	unilateral One side only.
uniovular	uniovolar Referring to one fertilized ovum.
unión estrecha	tight junction An intercellular junction with an impermeable membrane.
uña	nail
unípara	uniparous Refers to a single birth.
uña del pie	toenail
uña en cuchara	spoon nail Also referred to as koilonychia, the nail is concave and is generally associated with anemia.
uña en pico de loro	parrot-beak nail A curved fingernail.
uña encarnada	ingrown nail Also referred to as onychocryptosis.
uraco	urachus A connection between the bladder and the allantois in the fetus.
urato	urate The salt of uric acid.
urea	urea A nitrogenous product of protein metabolism; excreted in urine.
uremia	uremia An excess of urea and creatinine in the blood.
ureteral	ureteral Referring to one of two tubes from the kidneys to the bladder that carry urine.
ureterectomía	ureterectomy Surgical resection of one or both ureters.

Spanish	English
ureteritis	ureteritis Inflammation of the ureter.
ureterocele	ureterocele Protrusion of the distal portion of the ureter into the bladder.
ureterolithotomía	ureterolithotomy Removal of a ureteral stone.
ureterolito	ureterolith Presence of a stone in the ureter.
ureterovaginal	ureterovaginal Referring to the ureter and vagina.
ureterovesical	ureterovesical Referring to the ureter and urinary bladder.
uretra	urethra The canal connecting the urinary bladder with the outside of the body.
uretral	urethral Referring to the urethra.
uretritis	urethritis Inflammation of the urethra.
uretrocele	urethrocele A prolapse of the urethra through the meatus.
uretroplastia	urethroplasty Surgical repair of the urethra.
uretrorrafía	urethrography Imaging of the urethra after instillation of contrast media.
uretroscopia	urethroscope A scope used to visualize the inside of the urethra.
uretrotomía	urethrotomy A surgical opening of the urethra.
uréter	ureter The conduit between each kidney and the urinary bladder.
urgencia	urgency
urinario	urinary Referring to the urine.
urinómetro	urinometer A device for measuring urine specific gravity.
urobilina	urobilin A brownish pigment that is an oxidized form of urobilinogen.
urobilinógeno	urobilinogen A colorless substance produced in the intestines when bilirubin is reduced.
urocromo	urochrome A yellow pigment in the urine that gives urine its color.
urodinamia	urodynamics
urogentital	urogenital Referring to the urinary and genital systems.
urografía	urography Roentgenography of the urinary tract after administration of contrast media.
urolito	urolith Urinary calculi.
urología	urology Surgical specialty involving medical and surgical treatment of the urogenital system.
urticaria	urticaria A diffuse pruritic macular rash, caused by an allergy.
usual,normal	usual
uterino	uterine Referring to the uterus.
uterovesical	uterovesical Referring to the uterus and urinary bladder.
utrículo	utricle A small sac. It can refer to a division of the membranous labyrinth.
uveítis	uveitis Inflammation of the uvea.
uvulectomía	uvulectomy Excision of the uvula.
uvulitis	uvulitis Inflammation of the uvula.
úlcera	ulcer A concave wound caused by a break in the integrity of skin or mucous membrane.
úlcera de decúbito	pressure ulcer Loss in skin integrity due to a portion of the body being in the same position for too long and possibly other factors.
úlcera de herpes simple	cold sore A perioral blister caused by herpes simplex.
úlcera duodenal	duodenal ulcer
úlcera gastroduodenal	gastroduodenal ulcer A lesion in the mucosal lining of the stomach or duodenum.
úlcera por decúbito	decubitus ulcer A wound caused by laying in one position for too long; also referred to as a pressure ulcer.

Spanish	English
úrico	uric Uric acid is a purine-derived product of nitrogen metabolism that can increase the risk of gout and calculi.
útero	uterus The hollow organ in the female pelvis where a fertilized ovum embeds and grows.
útero retroflexionado	retroflexed uterus Bending back of the uterus so that the top portion pushes against the rectum.
úvula	uvula A fleshy pendent at the back of the soft palate.
vaciado; vaciado de yeso	cast; plaster cast
vacío	empty
vacuna	vaccine A solution of attenuated microorganisms given to prevent or treat a disease.
vacunación	vaccination The act of receiving a vaccine.
vacuola	vacuole A cavity that develops in a cell.
vagal	vagal Referring to the vagus nerve.
vagido uterino	vagitus An infant cry that can be further defined as vagitus vaginalis in which the infant cries while its head is in the vaginal canal.
vagina	vagina The canal in a female that extends from the vulva to the cervix.
vaginal	vaginal Referring to the vagina.
vaginismo	vaginismus Involuntary contraction of the vagina muscles that causes a painful spasm.
vagotomía	vagotomy Incision of the vagus nerve.
vaina	sheath A covering.
valgus	valgus Refers to a joint being abnormally angulated away from the midline of the body.
valina	valine An essential amino acid that assists with nitrogen equilibrium.
valva, cúspide	leaflet Cusp.
valvultomía	valvulotomy Surgical incision of a valve.
variable	unsteady
varicela	varicella A virus that causes chickenpox and shingles. Also called herpes zoster.
varicella	chicken pox, varicella
varicocele	varicocele A cluster of varicose veins in the scrotum.
varicoso	varicose Referring to an abnormally distended, irregular vein.
varus	varus Refers to a joint being abnormally angulated toward the midline of the body.
vascular	vascular Referring to a blood vessel.
vasculitis	vasculitis Inflammation of a blood vessel.
vasectomía	vasectomy The surgical separation of each vas deferens with the intent of producing a sterile person.
vasoconstricción	vasoconstriction The process of making the blood vessels smaller which increases blood pressure.
vasodilatación	vasodilatation The process of making the blood vessels larger which decreases blood pressure.
vasoespasmo	vasospasm The abrupt constriction of a blood vessel.
vasomotor	vasomotor Referring to the constriction or dilation of vessels.
vasopresina	vasopressin A hormone secreted by the pituitary that facilitates the retention of sodium and water and also increases blood pressure.

Spanish	English
vasovagal	vasovagal Referring to overstimulation of the vagus nerve, exhibited by hypotension, pallor, nausea and diaphoresis.
válvula aórtica	aortic valve The valve situated between the left ventricle and the aorta.
válvula ileocecal	ileocecal valve The membranous folds between the ileum and cecum.
válvula mitral	mitral valve The valve with two cusps between the left atrium and ventricle.
válvula tricúspide	tricuspid valve The cardiac valve located between the right atrium and right ventricle.
várice	varix A twisted, distended vein, artery or lymph vessel.
vector	vector An organism that transmits disease.
vegetación	vegetation Abnormal growth, such as cardiac valve vegetations as found in endocarditis.
vejiga	bladder
vejiga urinaria	urinary bladder The organ collecting urine from the ureters prior to discharge via the urethra.
vello	hair (of body)
vello púbico	pubic hair
vellosidad	villus A small vascular prominence from a membrane surface.
vellosidad coriónicas	chorionic villus Cord-like projections of a fertilized ovum.
velloso	villous Covered with many villi.
velo	velum A veil-like part.
vena	vein
vena cava	vena cava The large vein that carries deoxygenated blood to the right atrium.
vendaje	bandage
vendaje circular	banding The process of encircling with a thin piece of material.
vendaje elástico	elastic bandage A stretch gauze used for compression of an extremity.
vendaje oclusivo	occlusive dressing A synthetic covering for a wound that has a semipermeable membrane.
vendaje, apósito	dressing The gauze applied to a wound.
veneno	poison
veneno	venom
veno basílica	basilic vein A vein in the hand that joins the brachial veins to form the axillary vein.
venografía	venography Roentgenography of a vein after administration of contrast media.
venoso	venous Referring to the veins.
ventilación	ventilation The movement of air into the lungs; generally meant to suggest by an artificial process.
ventral	ventral Referring to the underside but in humans, a ventral hernia, for example, refers to an abdominal hernia.
ventriculografía	ventriculography Roentgenography of the ventricles after administration of contrast media.
ventriculostomía	ventriculostomy
ventrículo	ventricle 1. One of two chambers of the heart. 2. The four inter-connected cavities in the center of the brain.
venula	venula The vessels that connect the capillary plexuses to veins.
verdad	truth
verminoso	verminous Referring to presence of worms.
verruga	verruca A hyperplastic epidermal lesion, sometimes referred to as plantar wart.
verruga	wart

284

Spanish	English
verruga genital	genital wart
verruga plantar	plantar wart A viral epidermal growth on the bottom of the foot.
verruga venérea Condiloma acuminado.	venereal wart
vesical	vesical Referring to the urinary bladder.
vesicovaginal	vesicovaginal Referring to the urinary bladder and vagina.
vesiculitis	vesiculitis Inflammation of the urinary bladder.
vesícula biliar	gallbladder The organ adjacent to the liver that stores bile and secretes it into the duodenum.
vestibular	vestibular Referring to a vestibule.
vestido de camisa	gown
vestigial	vestigial Rudimentary.
vértebra	vertebra A term for each bone surrounding the spine.
vértice	vertex The crown of the head.
vértice del corazón	apex of heart Normally found 8cm to the left of the midsternal line in the 5th intercostal space.
vértigo	vertigo A sensation of imbalance with many possible causes.
viable	viable Referring to a fetus that can survive childbirth.
vial	vial
vibración	vibration
victima de accidente	casualty
vida media	half-life
VIH virus de inmunodeficiencia humano	HIV Abbreviation for human immunodeficiency virus.
violar	rape Forced sexual relations.
violeta de genciana	gentian violet An antiseptic derived from rosaniline.
virilización	virilization The result of androgen; a process of development of masculine characteristics.
virología	virology The study of viruses.
viruela	smallpox Variola.
viruela bovina	cowpox; vaccinia A viral disease of cows that was used for an original smallpox vaccine.
viruela de los monos	monkeypox A viral disease that is similar to smallpox which occurs primarily in monkeys and rarely in humans.
virulencia	virulence The potential severity of a disease or poison.
viscosímetro	viscometer A device used to measure viscosity.
viscoso	viscous Having a thick, sticky consistency.
visión	vision
visión borroso	blurred vision
visión en túnel	tunnel vision
vista	eyesight
vitelino	vitelline Referring to the yolk of an egg or ovum.
vivisección	vivisection Animal surgery done for purposes of research.
vías urinarias	urinary tract The organs and canals associated with urine secretion including the kidneys, ureters, bladder and urethra.
vísceras	viscera Referring to the organs in the abdominal or thoracic cavity.
vítreo	vitreous Glass appearance; used to describe the vitreous body of the eye.

Spanish	English
vocal	vocal
volumen corriente pulmonar	tidal volume The amount of air inspired with each breath. One can set a ventilator to deliver a preset number of milliliters of oxygenated air with each breath.
volumen de reserva espiratorio	expiratory reserve volume Amount of air left in the lung after a maximal exhalation, in liters.
volumen de reserva inspiratoria	inspiratory reserve volume The amount of air that can be inhaled after a normal inhalation.
volumen espiratorio forzado	forced expiratory volume per second (FEV1) The amount of air exhaled with maximal effort, measured in liters, over one second.
volumen residual	residual volume (RV) The amount of air left in the lung after a maximal exhalation.
volumen sanguíneo	blood volume
volumen sistólico	stroke volume The amount of blood ejected from the ventricle with each contraction.
voluminoso	bulky
voz	voice
vólvulo	volvulus Twisting of the bowel leading to obstruction and sometimes perforation.
vómito	emesis Vomiting.
vómito	vomit, to
vómito en borra de café	coffee-ground emesis
vómito psicógeno	cyclical vomiting Periods of recurrent vomiting with no apparent pathologic cause and the person has a normal state of health between the episodes.
VPH virus del papiloma humano	HPV human papillomavirus
vulva	pudendum The mons, pubis, labia majora, labia minora and the vagina.
vulvectomía	vulvectomy Surgical resection of the vulva.
vulvitis	vulvitis Inflammation of the vulva.
vulvovaginitis	vulvovaginitis Inflammation of the vulva and vagina.
xantina	xanthine A purine derivative that is found in the blood and urine after the metabolism of nucleic acids to uric acid.
xantocromía	xanthochromia A yellow tone to the skin or spinal fluid.
xantoma	xanthoma A lipid deposition on the skin exhibited by an irregular yellow patch.
xeroderma	xerodermia A mild form of ichthyosis.
xeroftalmía	xerophthalmia A manifestation of Vitamin A deficiency exhibited by dryness of the cornea and conjunctiva.
xerosis	xerosis
xerostomía	xerostomia A dry mouth from salivary gland hypofunction.
xerradiografía	xeroradiography A form of radiography using photoelectric cells.
yeso de París	plaster Dehydrated gypsum that has water added to it in order to immobilize fractured extremities.
yeyunectomía	jejunectomy Surgical removal of the jejunum.
yeyunostomía	jejunostomy Surgical creation of an opening in the jejunum.
yodismo	iodism A condition caused by excessive iodine intake resulting in diarrhea , weakness, and convulsions.
yodo	iodine A chemical used as an antiseptic and a deficiency of it can lead to goiter.

Spanish	English
yugular	jugular Referring to the neck, as in jugular vein.
yuxtaarticulación	juxta-articular Positioned near a joint.
zalea	drawsheet The topsheet of a bed.
zancada	stride
zapato	shoe
zeiosis	zeiosis Resembling a bubbling activity.
zonzo	feeble-minded Antiquated term used to describe a person unable to make seemingly simple decisions because of a cognitive impairment.
zoología	zoology The study of animals.
zoonosis	zoonosis An animal-born disease that can be transmitted to humans, such as rabies.
zónula	zonula A small zone or junction.

www.ingramcontent.com/pod-product-compliance
Lightning Source LLC
Chambersburg PA
CBHW071402170526
45165CB00001B/147